Ruth M. Kleinpell, PhD, ACNP-BC, FAAN, FAANP, FCCM, is currently the director of the Center for Clinical Research and Scholarship at Rush University Medical Center and a professor at Rush University College of Nursing in Chicago, Illinois. She maintains active practice as an acute care nurse practitioner and serves as a visiting professor at Vanderbilt University School of Nursing, assisting with clinical scholarship and research initiatives. She received her diploma in nursing from Lutheran Medical Center School of Nursing, Cleveland, Ohio, and her baccalaureate, master's, and doctoral degrees in nursing from the University of Illinois College of Nursing, Chicago, Illinois. She received her acute care nurse practitioner certification at Rush University College of Nursing. Dr. Kleinpell is known for her work on outcome research and has presented and published in the areas of assessing outcomes of advanced practice nursing, outcome research, and other areas of nursing practice. She is a fellow of the American Academy of Nursing, the American Academy of Nurse Practitioners, the Institute of Medicine of Chicago, and the American College of Critical Care Medicine. Her research and contributions have been recognized with a Sigma Theta Tau International Nurse Researcher Hall of Fame Award, an American Association of Critical-Care Nurses Flame of Excellence Award, a National Organization of Nurse Practitioner Faculties Research Award, and a Society of Critical Care Medicine Norma Shoemaker Award for Critical Care Nursing Excellence, among others.

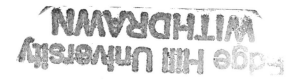

Outcome Assessment in Advanced Practice Nursing

Fourth Edition

Ruth M. Kleinpell, PhD, ACNP-BC, FAAN, FAANP, FCCM

Editor

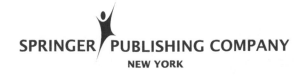

SPRINGER / PUBLISHING COMPANY
NEW YORK

Springer Publishing Company, LLC
11 West 42nd Street
New York, NY 10036
www.springerpub.com

Acquisitions Editor: Joseph Morita
Compositor: Exeter Premedia Services Private Ltd.

ISBN: 978-0-8261-3862-0
e-book ISBN: 978-0-8261-3863-7
Instructor's Manual ISBN: 978-0-8261-3859-0

Instructor's Materials: Qualified instructors may request supplements by e-mailing textbook@springerpub.com

17 18 19 20 / 5 4 3 2 1

The author and the publisher of this Work have made every effort to use sources believed to be reliable to provide information that is accurate and compatible with the standards generally accepted at the time of publication. Because medical science is continually advancing, our knowledge base continues to expand. Therefore, as new information becomes available, changes in procedures become necessary. We recommend that the reader always consult current research and specific institutional policies before performing any clinical procedure. The author and publisher shall not be liable for any special, consequential, or exemplary damages resulting, in whole or in part, from the readers' use of, or reliance on, the information contained in this book. The publisher has no responsibility for the persistence or accuracy of URLs for external or third-party Internet websites referred to in this publication and does not guarantee that any content on such websites is, or will remain, accurate or appropriate.

Library of Congress Cataloging-in-Publication Data

Names: Kleinpell, Ruth M., editor.
Title: Outcome assessment in advanced practice nursing / [edited by] Ruth M.
  Kleinpell.
Description: Fourth edition. | New York, NY: Springer Publishing Company,
  LLC, [2017] | Includes bibliographical references and index.
Identifiers: LCCN 2017007613| ISBN 9780826138620 | ISBN 9780826138590
  (instructor's manual) | ISBN 9780826138637 (e-book)
Subjects: | MESH: Nurse Practitioners—standards | Outcome Assessment (Health
  Care) | Nurse Clinicians—standards
Classification: LCC RT82.8 | NLM WY 128 | DDC 610.7306/92—dc23
LC record available at https://lccn.loc.gov/2017007613

Contact us to receive discount rates on bulk purchases.
We can also customize our books to meet your needs.
For more information please contact: sales@springerpub.com

Printed in the United States of America by McNaughton & Gunn.

Contents

Contributors   *vii*
Foreword   Julie Stanik–Hutt, PhD, CRNP, CCNS, FAANP, FAAN   *xi*
Preface   *xv*

1. Measuring Outcomes in Advanced Practice Nursing: Practice-Specific
    Quality Metrics   *1*
    *April N. Kapu, Corinna Sicoutris, Britney S. Broyhill, Rhonda D'Agostino, and
    Ruth M. Kleinpell*

2. Analyzing Economic Outcomes in Advanced Practice Nursing   *19*
    Kevin D. Frick, Catherine C. Cohen, and Patricia W. Stone

3. Selecting Advanced Practice Nursing Outcome Measures   *45*
    Beth D. Quatrara and Katherine Dale Shaw

4. General Design and Implementation Challenges in Outcome Assessment   *59*
    Ann F. Minnick

5. Locating Instruments and Measures for Advanced Practice Nursing
    Outcome Assessments   *69*
    Marilyn Wolf Schwartz and Roger Green

6. Measuring Outcomes in Cardiovascular Advanced Practice Nursing   *87*
    *Anna Gawlinski, Kathy McCloy, Virginia Erickson, Elizabeth Vandenbogaart, and
    Anna Dermenchyan*

7. Ambulatory Nurse Practitioner Outcomes   *143*
    Mary Jo Goolsby

8. Assessing Outcomes in Clinical Nurse Specialist Practice   *157*
    Judy Elisa Davidson, Melissa A. Morse, Cassia Yi, and Mary C. Hellyar

9. Outcome Measurement in Nurse-Midwifery Practice   *187*
    Julie Marfell

10. Outcome Assessment in Nurse Anesthesia **207**
 Michael J. Kremer and Margaret Faut Callahan

11. Measuring Outcomes of Doctor of Nursing Practice **229**
 Marguerite J. Murphy, Kathy S. Magdic, and Terri L. Allison

12. Resources to Facilitate Advanced Practice Nursing Outcome Research **249**
 *Denise Bryant-Lukosius, Ruth Martin-Misener, Joan Tranmer, Faith Donald,
 Linda Brousseau, and Alba DiCenso*

Index 273

Contributors

Terri L. Allison, DNP, ACNP-BC, FAANP, Director, Doctor of Nursing Practice Program; Associate Professor of Nursing, Vanderbilt University School of Nursing, Nashville, Tennessee

Linda Brousseau, NP, MN, Nurse Practitioner, Halton Clinical Health Services; Doctoral Student and Research Trainee, Canadian Centre for Advanced Practice Nursing Research, McMaster University, Oakville, Ontario, Canada

Britney S. Broyhill, DNP, ACNP-BC, Nurse Practitioner Fellowship Director, Carolinas HealthCare System, Charlotte, North Carolina

Denise Bryant-Lukosius, PhD, RN, Associate Professor, School of Nursing and Department of Oncology; Co-Director, Canadian Centre for Advanced Practice Nursing Research (CCAPNR), McMaster University, Hamilton, Ontario, Canada

Margaret Faut Callahan, PhD, CRNA, FNAP, FAAN, Provost, Health Science Division; Professor, Niehoff School of Nursing, Loyola University Chicago, Chicago, Illinois

Catherine C. Cohen, PhD, RN, Columbia University School of Nursing, New York, New York

Rhonda D'Agostino, MSN, ACNP-BC, CCRN, FCCM, Nurse Practitioner Coordinator, Department of Anesthesiology, Critical Care and Pain, Memorial Sloan Kettering Cancer Center, New York, New York

Judy Elisa Davidson, DNP, RN, FCCM, FAAN, Evidence-Based Practice/Research Nurse Liaison, University of California San Diego Health, San Diego, California

Anna Dermenchyan, BSN, RN, CCRN-K, Senior Clinical Quality Specialist, Department of Medicine, UCLA Health, Los Angeles, California

Alba DiCenso, PhD, RN, Professor Emeritus, School of Nursing and Clinical Epidemiology and Biostatistics, McMaster University, Hamilton, Ontario, Canada

Faith Donald, PhD, NP-PHC, Associate Professor, Daphne Cockwell School of Nursing, Ryerson University, Affiliate Faculty, Canadian Centre for Advanced Practice Nursing Research, Toronto, Ontario, Canada

Virginia Erickson, PhD, RN, Former Coordinator; Staff Nurse Evidence-Based Practice Fellowship, Department of Nursing, Nursing Research and Education, Ronald Reagan UCLA Medical Center, Los Angeles, California

Kevin D. Frick, PhD, Vice Dean for Education, Carey Business School, Johns Hopkins University, Baltimore, Maryland

Anna Gawlinski, PhD, RN, ACNP-BC, CNS-BC, FAAN, Adjunct Professor, UCLA School of Nursing, Los Angeles, California

Mary Jo Goolsby, EdD, MSN, NP-C, FAANP, FAAN, Principal, Institute for NP Excellence, LLC; Associate Professor, Adjunct, College of Nursing, Augusta University, Augusta, Georgia

Roger Green, DNP, FNP, PMHNP, FAANP, Psychiatric and Family Nurse Practitioner, Private Practice, Henderson, Nevada

Mary C. Hellyar, MSN, RN, ACNS-BC, CCRN, Clinical Nurse Specialist, University of California San Diego Health, San Diego, California

April N. Kapu, DNP, APRN, ACNP-BC, FAANP, Associate Chief Nursing Officer, Advanced Practice, Vanderbilt University Medical Center; Associate Professor, Vanderbilt University School of Nursing, Nashville, Tennessee

Ruth M. Kleinpell, PhD, ACNP-BC, FAAN, FAANP, FCCM, Director, Center for Clinical Research and Scholarship, Rush University Medical Center; Professor, Rush University College of Nursing, Chicago, Illinois

Michael J. Kremer, PhD, CRNA, CHSE, FNAP, FAAN, Professor and Director, Nurse Anesthesia Program, Rush University College of Nursing; Co-Director, Rush Center for Clinical Skills and Simulation, Chicago, Illinois

Kathy S. Magdic, DNP, RN, ACNP-BC, FAANP, Assistant Professor and Coordinator, Adult-Gerontology Acute Care Nurse Practitioner Program, University of Pittsburgh, Pittsburgh, Pennsylvania

Julie Marfell, DNP, APRN, FNP-BC, FAANP, Dean of Nursing; Professor, Frontier Nursing University, Hyden, Kentucky

Ruth Martin-Misener, PhD, NP, Professor, School of Nursing, Dalhousie University; Co-Director, Canadian Centre for Advanced Practice Nursing Research, Halifax, Nova Scotia, Canada

Kathy McCloy, RN, MSN, ACNP-BC, Acute Care Nurse Practitioner, Division of Pulmonary and Critical Care Medicine, David Geffen School of Medicine, Los Angeles, California

Ann F. Minnick, PhD, RN, FAAN, Senior Associate Dean for Research; Julia Eleanor Chenault Professor of Nursing, Vanderbilt University School of Nursing, Vanderbilt University, Nashville, Tennessee

Melissa A. Morse, MSN, RN, CNS, CNRN, Clinical Nurse Specialist, Scripps Memorial Hospital, Encinitas, California

Marguerite J. Murphy, DNP, RN, Director, Doctor of Nursing Practice Program–Acute Care, Fuller E. Calloway Endowed Chair, College of Nursing, Augusta University, Augusta, Georgia

Beth D. Quatrara, DNP, RN, CMSRN, ACNS-BC, Advanced Practice Nurse 3–Clinical Nurse Specialist; Director of Nursing Research Program, University of Virginia Health System, Charlottesville, Virginia

Marilyn Wolf Schwartz, MLS, Retired, Library Director, Naval Medical Center, San Diego, California, Redmond, Oregon

Katherine Dale Shaw, DNP, RN, ACNP-BC, Advanced Practice Nurse 3, Neurosurgery, University of Virginia Health System, Charlottesville, Virginia

Corinna Sicoutris, MSN, CRNP, FCCM, FAANP, Director of Advanced Practice, Hospital of the University of Pennsylvania, Philadelphia, Pennsylvania

Patricia W. Stone, PhD, RN, FAAN, Centennial Professor in Health Policy, Columbia University School of Nursing, New York, New York

Joan Tranmer, PhD, RN, Professor and Scientific Director of Nursing and Health Research, School of Nursing, Faculty of Health Sciences, Queen's University, Affiliate Faculty, Canadian Centre for Advanced Practice Nursing Research, Kingston, Ontario, Canada

Elizabeth Vandenbogaart, RN, MSN, CNS, ACNP-BC, Acute Care Nurse Practitioner, Ahmanson—UCLA Cardiomyopathy Center, David Geffen School of Medicine, University of California Los Angeles Medical Center, Los Angeles, California

Cassia Yi, MSN, APRN, CNS, CCRN, Clinical Nurse Specialist, University of California San Diego Health, San Diego, California

Foreword

The ability of advanced practice registered nurses (APRNs) to demonstrate the value we bring to health care systems, and the patients we serve, is more important today than when Dr. Kleinpell published the first edition of this text in 2001. At that time, the text provided APRNs the foundation on which to quantify, document, validate, and evaluate our impact on health care. With this new edition, Dr. Kleinpell and her contributors continue to provide leadership for this important work.

The value of APRN practice is found in our impact on health care quality, especially in "comparative effectiveness data" that documents APRN adherence to best care practices while achieving desired patient health and care system outcomes. Essentially, our value is found in the quality of our care. Today, APRN care processes and health care outcomes form the basis for evaluating provider and practice performance as well as policy initiatives that authorize APRN practice, and also serve an increasing role in reimbursement for services.

Information on care quality is critical to our practice. It is used by a number of groups, including governmental agencies (e.g., health departments, the Patient-Centered Outcomes Research Institute [PCORI]), health care accreditors and organizations (e.g., The Joint Commission, hospitals, group practices), and payers (e.g., Medicare), to determine whether APRN performance meets expectations. It also forms the basis for our individual quality-improvement activities. External audiences, such as individual consumers and businesses, use health care process and outcome data, as well as publicly posted "provider report cards," to make health care choices.

APRNs serve at the front lines of health care and are expected to make even greater contributions in the future to improve our health care system. This is in part because we have developed a reputation for providing accessible, high-quality, cost-effective care. This reputation is based on published data demonstrating excellent APRN care processes and outcomes. As coauthor of the most recently published systematic review of the literature on outcomes of APRN care (Newhouse et al., 2011), I continue to be impressed with the growing number of studies identifying the impact of APRN care. Policy makers use these data to determine APRN practice authority (e.g., scope of practice, practice autonomy). Results from these studies are cited in Federal Trade Commission opinions supporting APRN practice. They have supported recent expansions of APRN practice authority in at least nine states and in the Veterans Administration health care system. Continuing efforts to implement Institute of Medicine APRN practice recommendations, as well as components of the APRN Consensus Model, will require further work to delineate and disseminate data regarding our health care outcomes and processes.

Nongovernmental policy makers (e.g., practice accreditation organizations, credential verification organizations, private payers) use APRN health care outcome and process data to determine who may provide health care services and how we are paid. The Joint Commission requires that data regarding care processes and outcomes be included in credentialing and privileging activities through focused and ongoing professional practice evaluations (Focused Professional Practice Evaluation [FPPE], Ongoing Professional Practice Evaluation [OPPE]). Bipartisan support of the Medicare Access and CHIP (Children's Health Insurance Program) Reauthorization Act of 2015 (MACRA) indicates that implementation of governmental quality and safety programs, as well as value-based payment systems, is likely to continue. By 2019, the existing fee-for-service payment system based on *quantity* of care will be replaced by a merit-based incentive payment system (MIPS) based on *quality* of care in which 50% of provider payment will depend on care quality metrics. To remain competitive, APRNs will need to report care processes and outcomes and participate in quality improvement.

So, what does this mean to APRNs? All APRNs must understand the critical role that data on care processes and outcomes play in evaluating, improving, and changing practice. Armed with this knowledge, individual APRNs must take steps to incorporate assessment of care processes and health care outcomes as a routine component of their day-to-day practice. We need to compare our outcome data to benchmarks and use those data to refine our practice and enhance the profession. APRNs need to be able to discuss outcome data from their practice and how they were achieved. Outcomes, which characterize their patients' health status, are particularly important for nurse-midwives, nurse anesthetists, and nurse practitioners. In addition, for clinical nurse specialists, who spend much of their time behind the scenes ensuring safe and high-quality care delivery, system-related variables are critical to survival in these complex care systems.

How will this book help? This text provides APRN students and educators, practicing APRNs, and the administrators with whom we work up-to-date information on the advanced practice nursing care process as well as patient health- and system-based outcome assessment—the who, what, when, where, how, and why. It includes critical perspectives on not only the health effects of advanced practice nursing but also the economic impact of our practice. Its chapters, which synthesize current data on each APRN role, will guide practice innovations and enhance practice authority. New content regarding identification of metrics, which will help APRNs quantify their impact, is especially relevant. Identified gaps in data will help us prioritize future research and develop new advanced practice nursing care models, which might lead to improvements in health and health care delivery. The authors of this work provide the essential information to accomplish all of these important objectives.

Julie Stanik–Hutt, PhD, CRNP, CCNS, FAANP, FAAN
Professor, The University of Iowa College of Nursing
Iowa City, Iowa

REFERENCE

Newhouse, R. P., Weiner, J. P., Stanik-Hutt, J., White, K. M., Johantgen, M., Steinwachs, D., . . . Bass, E. (2011). Advanced practice outcomes 1990–2008: A systematic review. *Nursing Economics, 29,* 230–250.

Preface

Ongoing changes in health care continue to impact the way care is delivered. As the number of advanced practice registered nurses (APRNs) and their roles expand, the measurement of outcomes is an important parameter by which advanced practice nursing care can be evaluated. Demonstrating outcomes of advanced practice nursing care brings recognition to the multifaceted roles of APRNs and of their impact on outcomes. Since 2001, when the first edition of this book was published, the field of outcome research has further grown and developed. This fourth edition of *Outcome Assessment in Advanced Practice Nursing* has been written to provide APRNs with updated resources and information on measuring outcomes of practice.

The chapters within this book focus on presenting an overview of advanced practice nursing outcomes and discussing outcome measurement in all areas of APRN practice, including clinical nurse specialist, nurse practitioner, certified registered nurse anesthetist, and certified nurse-midwife. Examples of outcome studies are presented from actual research in APRN practice. Additional chapters focus on discussion of outcome assessment in specialty APRN practice, outcomes of advanced practice nursing care that are specifically related to the doctorate of nursing practice (DNP) degree, information on locating instruments and measures for APRN outcome assessment, and information on an international initiative focused on the development of an APRN research data collection toolkit. New to this edition is a focus on practice-specific quality metrics for demonstrating APRN impact and information on a national collaborative launched specifically to showcase outcomes of APRN-led initiatives as part of the Choosing Wisely campaign (www.mc.vanderbilt.edu/aprnchoosingwisely).

The contributors to this fourth edition are recognized expert clinicians, educators, and researchers who collectively offer invaluable insights into the process of conducting outcome assessments in APRN practice. The ever-expanding field of outcome measurement can make conducting an outcome assessment complex. *Outcome Assessment in Advanced Practice Nursing* provides APRNs with up-to-date resources and examples of outcome measures, tools, and methods that can be used in their quest to measure outcomes of care. This fourth edition of the book was written to serve as a resource for assessing outcomes, regardless of the specialty area of practice or clinical setting. Having knowledge of the process of assessing outcomes of practice is important for all APRNs. The true impact of advanced practice nursing care can be established only through continued focus on outcome assessment and evaluation—something that this book encourages readers to actively pursue. **Please note that a supplemental Instructor's Manual for this book, which provides resources for qualified instructors for teaching content related to outcome assessment, is available from Springer Publishing by e-mailing textbook@springerpub.com.**

Ruth M. Kleinpell

CHAPTER 1

Measuring Outcomes in Advanced Practice Nursing: Practice-Specific Quality Metrics

April N. Kapu, Corinna Sicoutris, Britney S. Broyhill, Rhonda D'Agostino, and Ruth M. Kleinpell

Chapter Objectives

1. Discuss the use of practice-specific quality metrics to identify outcomes of advanced practice registered nurse (APRN) care
2. Identify strategies for developing practice-specific quality metrics
3. Highlight examples of using practice-specific quality metrics to demonstrate the effect of APRN care

Chapter Discussion Questions

1. What are two practice-specific quality metrics that can be used to identify outcomes of APRN practice?
2. How can the use of practice-specific quality metrics be used to identify the impact of APRN care?
3. What strategies can be used to measure APRN impact using role-specific metrics? List several examples.

Demonstrating the impact of the APRN role is an essential component of professional practice. The Institute of Medicine (IOM) report on the future of nursing highlighted the importance of promoting the ability of APRNs to practice to the full extent of their education and training and to identify nurses' contributions to delivering high-quality care (IOM, 2010). Demonstrating APRN impact requires an assessment of the structures, processes, and outcomes associated with APRN performance and the care delivery systems in which they practice (Kleinpell & Alexandrov, 2014). An increased focus on assessing the outcomes of APRN practice has resulted from the growing emphasis on outcomes that have become a recognized component of the majority of health care initiatives. The demands for measuring outcomes of care have been emphasized by federal and state regulatory agencies, practice guidelines, employers, and consumer groups. Health care organizations are now actively monitoring outcomes as a means of evaluation as well as requirements for accreditation and certification.

At the same time, a growing number of organizations are utilizing APRNs in a variety of specialty practice roles. Differentiating the impact and value of these roles has become a priority, especially as programs such as the Centers for Medicare & Medicaid Services (CMS) value-based purchasing and Medicare Access and CHIP (Children's Health Insurance Program) Reauthorization Act of 2015 (MACRA) initiatives are being implemented. These programs are aimed at providing quality care while improving value and linking performance to hospital reimbursement structures (CMS, 2016). As outcome evaluation and ongoing performance assessment remain essential components of professional practice, the use of practice-specific quality metrics can be used to demonstrate APRN impact. This chapter discusses strategies for identifying and developing quality metrics to demonstrate impact and value of the APRN role. Institutional exemplars are provided to showcase processes and methods being used to identify APRN outcomes.

CAPTURING APRN IMPACT

A number of single institutional studies and synthesis reviews of APRN outcomes have highlighted the impact of APRN roles (Albers-Heitner et al., 2012; Alexander-Banys, 2014; Hatem, Sandall, Devane, Soltani, & Gates, 2008; Hogan, Seifert, Moore, & Simonson, 2010; Jessee & Rutledge, 2012; Kapu, Kleinpell, & Pilon, 2014; Laurant et al., 2005; Newhouse et al., 2011; Sawatzky et al., 2013). While traditional outcome metrics such as length of stay (LOS) or readmission rates can be used, teasing out the individual impact of the APRN role can be difficult, as often care is provided in team-based and collaborative models of care. Other chapters in this book outline in detail specific studies that have demonstrated APRN outcomes related to the four APRN roles: clinical nurse specialist, certified registered nurse anesthetist, certified nurse-midwife, and nurse practitioner (NP). Collectively these chapters provide a comprehensive review of APRN-role-specific outcomes. Exhibit 1.1 provides several examples of general outcome metrics used to highlight APRN role impact.

When developing processes to measure APRN impact, a number of specific issues need to be considered including the type and number of APRN roles (e.g., do hospital units have 24/7 APRN coverage?), institution-specific practices (type of electronic health record and ability to sort APRN patient panels), and high-value organizational quality goals that can be targeted (e.g., has a clinic had an increase in wait time, or

EXHIBIT 1.1 Examples of Outcome Metrics for APRNs

Blood glucose control
Symptom management
Patient lengths of stay
Costs of care
Smoking cessation
Adverse events (e.g., accidental extubation)
Patient and family knowledge
Patient self-efficacy
Urinary incontinence rates
Lipid management
Blood pressure control
Fall rates
Staff nurse knowledge
Staff nurse retention rates
Nosocomial infection rates
Readmission rates
Nutritional intake
Skin breakdown rates
Restraint use
Hand hygiene compliance
Patient and family satisfaction rates
Nurse satisfaction rates
Caregiver knowledge, satisfaction
Rates of adherence to best practices

APRNs, advanced practice registered nurses.

has a hospital unit had a recent increase in sentinel events?). Garnering administrative support for building system support for data abstraction and ongoing reporting of APRN outcome data is essential. Exhibit 1.2 outlines several considerations for identifying APRN metrics.

Strategies that can be used to measure APRN impact include establishing role-specific metrics, planning for outcome evaluation when any new role is established, and building in outcome assessment as a part of the Ongoing Professional Practice Evaluation (OPPE) processes of an institution. Nationally, a number of organizations are assimilating increasing numbers of APRNs. Focusing on capturing the impact of APRNs becomes

EXHIBIT 1.2 **Considerations for Identifying APRN Outcome Metrics**

What are outcomes valued by the organization/institution?
What are outcomes valued by the practice?
Has there been an APRN-led initiative that could result in comparison of outcomes?
Is there an opportunity to implement an APRN-led project that could result in comparison of outcomes?
Has there been a new practice guideline implemented by the APRN team that could result in comparison of outcomes?
Is there an opportunity to implement a new practice guideline that could result in comparison of outcomes?
What electronic data capture or records are available?
How can data reports be generated and provided to the APRN team?
Consider identifying metrics as positions are developed/formed
Aim to capture metrics that reflect APRN role activities
Garner information systems support for data abstraction and ongoing reporting

APRN, advanced practice registered nurse.

an essential component of demonstrating return on investment and impact of the role. Several institutional exemplars are included to highlight the process of identifying practice-specific quality metrics to quantify APRN role impact.

DEVELOPING QUALITY METRICS: INSTITUTIONAL EXEMPLAR, VANDERBILT UNIVERSITY MEDICAL CENTER

Vanderbilt University Medical Center (VUMC) is a comprehensive cancer, transplant, burn, and children's center and level 1 trauma center, with over 1,100 patient care beds. There are 850 APRNs and physician assistants (PAs) throughout the inpatient and outpatient environment, spanning the adult and pediatric population. With increasing demand for outcomes demonstrating quality of care, VUMC has developed several dashboards to align with and demonstrate effort toward strategic goals. Some of these goals include decreasing nosocomial infections, decreasing wait times for new appointments, decreasing patient harm index, decreasing mortality rates, improving Hospital Consumer Assessment of Healthcare Providers and Systems (HCAHPS) scores, reducing unexpected hospital readmissions, improving patient experience, and facilitating ideal LOS. These metrics are reflective of a team approach with administrators, physicians, APRNs, nurses, and many others directly or indirectly involved in patient care. There are a few metrics that are tracked specifically to APRNs, such as process performance indicators and resource utilization. An example of a performance indicator is that of ordering blood transfusions, using an APRN-specific dashboard (Exhibit 1.3). This dashboard indicates the APRN's name, area of practice, number of blood transfusions ordered per month, and number of transfusions ordered within the organizational blood transfusion protocol.

EXHIBIT 1.3 NP/PA Blood Transfusion Dashboard: Total Number of Blood Transfusions per Month and Percentage Within Transfusion Protocol

Name	Jan	Feb	Mar	Apr	May	June	July	Aug
NP 1	67%	17%	0%	67%	0%	67%	38%	56%
	3	6	1	3	2	6	8	9
NP 2	17%	100%	50%		0%		75%	100%
	6	1	4		1		4	1
NP 3	60%	67%	100%	100%	100%	100%	100%	100%
	5	3	4	1	4	2	1	5
PA 1		0%	50%	13%	29%	25%	50%	50%
		1	2	8	7	4	2	4
PA 2	50%	0%			0%	75%	33%	100%
	2	1			2	4	2	4
NP 4	67%	100%	100%	100%	80%	100%	100%	100%
	3	4	5	3	5	4	6	5

NP, nurse practitioner; PA, physician assistant.

Quality metrics that are impacted by APRNs are discussed and included in the OPPE process. The OPPE process is implemented through the use of a secure, online data collection tool, providing opportunity for peer, physician leader, and APRN leader competency feedback (Figure 1.1). The competencies included are specific to the role, organization, and practice site. Role-specific competencies may include: professionalism, interpersonal communication, leadership, medical/clinical knowledge, and other competencies specific to advanced practice. Organizational competencies may include: chart review of documentation, controlled substance ordering practices, team effort toward organizational goals, and other indicators of measurable goals. Practice-specific competencies might include: knowledge and application of practice-specific protocols, procedural competencies, quality of provider-to-provider communication, peer feedback, and documentation quality.

Outcome measures of success are reviewed not only during OPPE; these measures are followed closely to demonstrate downstream return on investment in APRN practice. Often new practices are implemented on a pilot basis to compare specific APRN-associated metrics before and after adding APRNs to the practice. Given that the success of the team is reflective of quality and sustainability, APRNs are actively involved in the process of identifying the metrics for achievement of outcomes and regular review of outcomes to determine whether improvement measures are necessary. Overall, outcome measurement has been instrumental in the success of the VUMC advanced practice program, allowing for growth and continued demonstration of organizational value.

Competency ratings

	Poor	Needs improvement	Proficient, meets expectations	Advanced, experienced	Expert, consultant	
Professionalism · must provide value	○	○	○	○	○	reset
Patient Care · must provide value	○	○	○	○	○	reset
Medical/Clinical Knowledge · must provide value	○	○	○	○	○	reset
Interpersonal Communication · must provide value	○	○	○	○	○	reset
Systems-based Practice · must provide value	○	○	○	○	○	reset
Practice-based Learning and Improvement · must provide value	○	○	○	○	○	reset
Quality · must provide value	○	○	○	○	○	reset
Leadership · must provide value	○	○	○	○	○	reset

Practice Management

History & Physical (EMR)	O	REQ
Daily Progress Note (EMR)	O	REQ
Death Report & Summary (EMR)	O	REQ
Team Summary / Handover (EMR)	O	REQ
IMPAX Training	O	REQ
Star Panel Training	O	REQ
WIZ/HEO Training	O	REQ
Rx Star/Discharge Wizard	O	REQ

Procedures

Chest tube removal	P	REQ
Tracheostomy downsize/exchange	P	REQ
Tracheostomy decannulation	P	REQ
Enteral feeding tube placement	P	REQ
Complex wound management	P	REQ
Percutaneous drain removal	P	REQ

Clinical Practice

Anemia	P	REQ
Bronchial hygiene	P	REQ
Cervical spine immobilization	P	REQ
Chest wall injury management	P	REQ
Deep vein treatment; Pulmonary er	P	REQ
Fever	P	REQ
Fluid/electrolyte replacement	P	REQ
Glycemic control	P	REQ
Open fracture management	P	REQ
Splenic vaccinations	P	REQ

This practitioner meets expectations required for the following quality indicators:

☑ Inpatient NP/PA Bundle (O/E LOS, Blood transfusion rates, DC before noon, CAUTI, CLABSI, Hand Hygiene) ☑ CVICU
SCIP Measures (BG control, DC periop abx, BB for CABG)

Please review the attached core competencies for practice (click on unit tab) and indicate bel... ...are all met or whether they are some competencies that can be improved.

Attachment: [icon] VUH NP PA Core Competencies for Practice.xlsx (0.03 MB)

Please comment on practitioner's accomplishments, strengths and opportunities for improvement.

FIGURE 1.1 Online data collection tool for APRN OPPE.

APRN, advanced practice registered nurse; BB CABG, beta blockers after coronary artery bypass graft surgery; BG, blood glucose; CAUTI, catheter-associated urinary tract infection; CLABSI, central-line-associated bloodstream infection; DC, discharge; EMR, electronic medical record; NP, nurse practitioner; O/E LOS, observed/expected length of stay; OPPE, Ongoing Professional Practice Evaluation; PA, physician assistant; SCIP, surgical care improvement project; VUH, Vanderbilt University Hospital; WIZ/HEO, order entry system at Vanderbilt.

Source: Vanderbilt University Medical Center.

DEVELOPING QUALITY METRICS: INSTITUTIONAL EXEMPLAR, HOSPITAL OF THE UNIVERSITY OF PENNSYLVANIA

At the Hospital of the University of Pennsylvania (Penn), there has been a long history of measuring the contributions of APRNs. The organization is a large urban academic medical center and regional referral center with a large and growing advanced practice provider (APP) workforce. APPs have been a part of the history at Penn since 1978, and there are well over 1,000 APPs across the health system. Since that time, APPs have been successfully integrated into virtually every clinical service within the hospital and ambulatory settings and are contributing positively to patient care in meaningful and substantive ways.

Historically, much of the early work to assess APP impact had been done in the surgical critical care unit where APPs were integrated into the intensivist-led interprofessional teams since 2002. At that time, a database was developed and designed with use of a Microsoft Access database management system that allowed the tracking of demographic variables including patient identification number, date of birth, and age. Additionally, admission and discharge dates to the intensive care unit (ICU) were documented, along with treatment-specific variables such as ventilator days, ICU diagnosis, complications such as venous thromboembolism (VTE), sepsis, hospital-acquired infections, and gastrointestinal bleed (GIB) to name a few. The database was used to track utilization of resources (labs, x-rays) and compliance with evidence-based clinical practice guidelines (CPGs). Through some of this early work around the integration of APPs in ICUs, differences were observed in compliance with evidence-based CPGs in a surgical ICU population (Gracias et al., 2008), complications and LOS in a trauma patient population (Scaff et al., 2004), nursing satisfaction (Haut et al., 2006), readmission mortality (Martin et al., 2015), and resource utilization (Haut et al., 2004). With data generated from the database and the strong support of clinical and executive leadership at the organization, measurement and reporting could be done to demonstrate the impact and outcomes of team-based care in the surgical ICU.

More recently, the APPs at Penn are focusing on provider-specific metrics to illustrate impact and articulate contribution to patients and our health care organization. This has been more challenging than evaluating team-based outcomes, since there is no clear way to establish attribution between a patient and an APP at the organization. Patients are admitted under an attending physician and the discharging physician on record is used to attribute an admission to a physician. It was not clear, however, if the discharging APP was the appropriate model to use for attribution. In partnership with quality leaders and data analysts at the organization, the advanced practice committee tested several hypotheses including discharging provider, types of orders, number of orders, admitting APP to understand and validate a patient, and APP attribution. Based on the work done by this team, it was found that in a team-based model, when an individual APP wrote more than 25% of the orders for a patient, the attribution of that patient could be made for that individual APP. In the end, the goal of this project was to develop quality metric reports (e.g., provider-specific report cards) similar to those issued to attending physicians with a focus on OPPE quality metrics such as general indicators (LOS, mortality, readmissions), safety indicators (unexpected deaths, central-line-associated bloodstream infection [CLABSI]), and perfect care measures (deep vein thrombosis [DVT] prophylaxis; Table 1.1).

APPs are able to generate value in all settings of care. At the organization, the future of measuring the quality impact of APPs will be focused around this value proposition,

TABLE 1.1   Example of a Provider-Specific Report Card to Showcase APP Outcomes

Discharges Between May 1, 2015 and May 1, 2016							
Service Group	Measure Group		Comparison Service	APP #1	APP #2	APP #3	APP #4
Trauma	Discharges	# Discharges	2,203	637	293	946	327
		LOS	6.4 days	6.1	5.7	7.3	5.9
	Mortality	Expected mortality (%)	0.5	50	60	40	50
		Inpatient mortality (%)	0.5	60	40	50	50
		O/E	1.1	1	1	1.1	1.1
	Readmissions (%)	30-day all-cause	7.8	6.4	9	7.4	8.7
		7-day unplanned	6.6	5.6	5.9	6.7	8
	Perfect care (%)	VTE prophylaxis	96.7	100	100	90	97
		SCIP	100	100	100	100	100
	Indicators	Postop VTE	4	2	0	1	1
		CLABSI	1	0	1	0	0
			Attending physicians included in comparison:				
			MD #1				
			MD #2				
			MD #3				

APP, advanced practice provider; CLABSI, central-line-associated bloodstream infection; LOS, length of stay; MD, medical doctor; O/E, observed/expected; SCIP, surgical care improvement project; VTE, venous thromboembolism.

and aligning the work with organizational goals. Certainly, that includes team-based metrics such as mortality, LOS, hospital complications, and reduction in unnecessary variations of care. However, it also includes things such as access to care, care coordination across settings and time, throughput and efficiency, maximizing revenue, and managing total cost of care. Based on the institutional experience of introducing APPs onto care teams, outcomes and efficiencies are better. An ongoing focus is needed on developing and testing models of care to create the workforce of the future; one that meets the needs of the profession, patients, and organizations. This focus is needed to ensure the continued ability to identify the impact of APRN care on access, availability, cost, outcomes, and quality.

DEVELOPING QUALITY METRICS: INSTITUTIONAL EXEMPLAR, CAROLINAS HEALTHCARE SYSTEM

Carolinas HealthCare System (CHS) is a large health care system that serves patients on a complete care continuum. With more than 40 hospitals and 900 care locations, the opportunities for APRNs and PAs (APPs) are tremendous. Nearly 1,700 APPs are an integral part of the health care delivery system of CHS across seven care divisions and service lines.

Given the size of CHS and the diversity of services delivered by APPs, creating a process for measuring value and quality is a complex process. In 2016, the Medical Group Division created an APP committee to help steer APP practice with developing a system to evaluate value created by APPs as one of its initial projects. It was decided that a formal APP dashboard would be created at first to assess the current state of APPs to begin evaluating their contribution to the organization.

A subcommittee was created that involved APPs, information technology, physicians, quality personnel, and the chief nursing informatics officer. It was decided to focus on the following seven categories: demographics, education, research, productivity, quality, engagement, and patient satisfaction. While this information was reported previously in multiple databases, the goal was to create a single dashboard that could show these metrics for the overall APP workforce, but also be subdivided by care division and service line.

Demographics is the first area of metrics to be added to the dashboard. It is to include routine demographic data such as age, sex, years of experience as an APP, years of service to CHS, and ethnic background. An additional data point will include type of board certification of each provider. Demographic data is critical for evaluating diversity and succession planning needs as the APP workforce grows.

Education of the APP (master's degree, doctorate of nursing practice [DNP], or PhD) serves as the second group of metrics to be evaluated. As the nursing workforce seeks to double its number of doctorally prepared nurses, the organization wants to track this as well. Additionally, the dashboard will measure the number of APP student preceptor hours and potentially the number of lectures provided to enhance medical education by the APPs.

Research is the third element added to the APP dashboard. A metric to assess the number of research studies in which an APP serves as either a principal investigator or coinvestigator will be evaluated. National, state, and local conference presentations as well as publications will also be tracked.

Productivity is the fourth element to be considered in the APP dashboard, and perhaps is the most difficult given the variety of practice locations of the CHS APPs. The committee assessed that there would have to be separate productivity assessments for the ambulatory and inpatient care teams. In the ambulatory setting, productivity can be tracked somewhat easily given that many APPs are responsible for their own patient panels.

In the inpatient setting, however, it is much more difficult to assess, given that most of the care is carried out in teams leading to shared billing, which is many times attributed to a physician partner rather than the APP. The committee looked to the electronic medical record (EMR) to assess productivity within the inpatient setting. If an APP is the primary author of a history and physical, progress note, discharge summary, or procedure note, then an internal attribution of productivity is based on these types of notation in the EMR. The procedure note assessment is also very helpful in terms of reappointment for medical staff privileges.

Quality assessment also was a metric that diverged based on care setting. In the ambulatory setting, quality metrics were assigned to the individual APP by care division and service line and are the same metrics measured for physician colleagues. In the inpatient setting, quality metrics are to be assessed in the initial phase similar to how metrics are being assessed for physician providers; for example, to include LOS, discharge order by 10 a.m., and adherence to the diabetes mellitus order set.

Engagement is the fifth metric included in the APP dashboard, including the engagement scores of the APPs overall, and the engagement scores of each of the care divisions and service lines. This in combination with turnover rates of each of the individual areas of practice will help the APP committee target areas of concern for APPs to prevent unnecessary turnover. In addition to APP engagement, the committee evaluates physician satisfaction scores of those who work with APPs versus those who do not have APP teammates.

Patient satisfaction is the last metric to be added to the dashboard. Individual patient satisfaction scores are to be attributed to the APP in the ambulatory setting, but again are difficult to assess in the inpatient setting given the team-based approach. The patient satisfaction scores is a new section to be added to the inpatient surveys to include whether an APP was involved in a patient's care. While patient satisfaction will not be directly attributed to an individual APP, at a minimum, feedback related to satisfaction with the APP team will be acquired.

By creating a comprehensive dashboard that spans the entire care continuum in which APPs provide care, the organization can assess its advanced practice workforce in detail. The value of APPs to the organization is much broader than revenue and this dashboard works to show all aspects of their contribution. Finally, the dashboard serves as a data pool to aid in strategic planning and workforce development of this vital component of the overall provider workforce.

DEVELOPING QUALITY METRICS: INSTITUTIONAL EXEMPLAR, MEMORIAL SLOAN KETTERING CANCER CENTER

Memorial Sloan Kettering Cancer Center (MSKCC) is a 471-bed oncologic specialty hospital with more than 450 APPs. The critical care APPs, which consist of 41.7 full-time equivalents (FTEs), staff a 20-bed mixed medical–surgical ICU, a 35-bed postanesthesia care unit (PACU), and lead the hospital's rapid response and daytime code team. In total, there are 30 NPs and six PAs, in addition to five NP specialists—who manage education, scheduling, and practice—and one program manager, who manages the hospital-wide sepsis program. The critical care APP program is managed by an NP coordinator.

In the critical care unit at MSKCC, separating APP quality has been, like in many other institutions, historically challenging to measure. The APPs work in conjunction with ICU intensivists; however, their role as rapid response team (RRT) leaders is mainly autonomous and necessitated the exploration of novel quality metrics.

In 2014, the critical care APP group analyzed hospital-wide RRT data, focusing on RRT multiples. These multiples, defined by subsequent call(s) within 24 hours of one another, were further broken down into those where the latter RRT call resulted in an ICU admission and classified as "24hr_admit" (see Figure 1.2).

The data, tracked by the provider, resulted as a percentage: the number of multiple calls divided by total calls within a month. Subsequently, the 24hr_admit multiples were reviewed during monthly staff meetings as case presentations followed by open-ended discussion and assessment regarding appropriateness of care (24hr_admit_reviewed; see Figure 1.3).

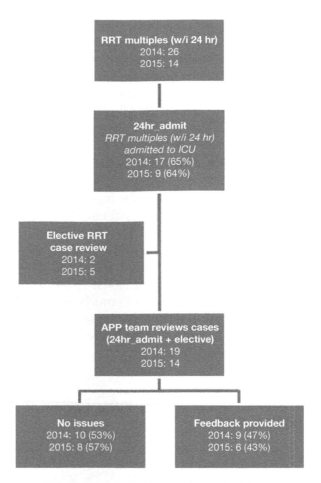

FIGURE 1.2 APP RRT metric methodology.

APP, advanced practice provider; ICU, intensive care unit; RRT, rapid response team; w/i, within.

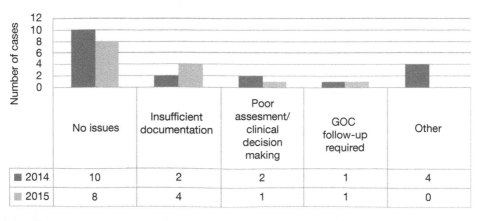

FIGURE 1.3 Individual case review feedback. This figure illustrates monthly staff-meeting case-review recommendations. The most common issues identified were insufficient documentation and poor clinical assessment, both of which decreased by 50% the subsequent year. In 2014, 47% of the cases had quality of care issues requiring feedback compared to 43% in 2015.

GOC, goals of care.

TABLE 1.2 APP RRT Metric Before (24hr_admit) and After Reviewed (24hr_admit_reviewed)

APP	2014		2015	
	24hr_admit (%)	24hr_admit_reviewed (%)	24hr_admit (%)	24hr_admit_reviewed (%)
1	2.6	0	0	0
2	0	0	0	0
3	0	0	0	0
4	0	0	0	0
5	0	0	0	0
6	0	0	5.7	4.7
7	3.2	3.2	5	0
8	0	0	0	0
9	3.8	0	0	0
10	0.8	0	0	0
11	2.9	2.9	3.4	1.7
12	2.9	0	3.3	0
13	0	0	0	0
14	0	0	0	0
15	2.6	0	0	0
16	0	0	0	0
17	4.4	2.2	4.3	4.3
18	1.9	0	0	0

Note: In 2014, 44% of the APPs had cases that were flagged for review compared to 2015, which had only 28%. After the review process took place, only 17% of APPs in 2014 and 2015 had cases with quality of care issues.
APP, advanced practice provider; RRT, rapid response team.

Data were further processed by removing the number of cases where appropriate care was rendered. All feedback was provided to the clinicians regardless of their presence during staff-meeting review. Cases were also reviewed that were internally flagged, either because of unexpected outcomes or internal staff suggestions. The process of case review was found to be extremely valuable to the staff. In total, 19 cases were reviewed in 2014 and 14 cases in 2015 (see Table 1.2).

LESSONS LEARNED

In the first 2 years of tracking and reviewing APP-specific quality metrics, there was a noted increase in elective case review. This was thought to occur because the team anecdotally found the review process to be both educational and appealing, consequently gaining confidence in case presentation and discussion.

It was also recognized that the RRT flagged cases (24hr_admit) decreased from 19 to 14, which may have happened as a result of the process; however, the actual process of review is crucial to the development and quality of care rendered. Therefore, it has been proposed to increase the RRT ICU admit window to 36 hours instead of 24 hours to capture more reviews.

It is important to understand that the initial phase of APP metric utilization should not focus on improving quality of care, although initially a small decrease in quality of care issues was seen (5%; 47%–43%), but rather creating a seamless process. A structured APP metric/improvement method will steer improved APP quality patient care.

In addition, it was helpful to provide a review template, since many of the APPs are new to providing an objective quality analysis. By implementing a template and providing a quick orientation, review presentations have improved and become more efficient in achieving unbiased scholarly discussion.

PRACTICE-SPECIFIC QUALITY METRICS

As described in the exemplars, measuring outcomes of APRN practice involves identifying and choosing metrics to be monitored, along with forming a process to track and monitor the metrics. Identifying practice-specific metrics is a strategy that can be used to define impact of the APRN role. Exhibit 1.4 outlines examples of metrics comparing traditional, quality and safety, and role-specific metrics.

Choosing Wisely®

An emerging opportunity to showcase the impact of the APRN role is through implementing the Choosing Wisely recommendations. The American Board of Internal

EXHIBIT 1.4   Examples of Metrics Used to Highlight Impact of APRN Role

Traditional Metrics:
Length of stay
Readmission rates
Quality/Safety Metrics:
Catheter-associated urinary tract infection rates
Pressure ulcer incidence
Postsurgical glycemic control
Patient satisfaction rates
Role-Specific Metrics:
APRN-led CHF clinic: rates of patient follow-up; ED and hospital readmission rates
APRN 24/7 ICU service: blood transfusion rates; chest-x-ray use; daily lab use; unit discharges by noon
APRN unit-specific staff nurse engagement scores
Patient-reported symptoms with APRN cardiac surgery follow-up

APRN, advanced practice registered nurse; CHF, congestive heart failure; ED, emergency department; ICU, intensive care unit.

Medicine Foundation established the Choosing Wisely campaign in 2012 to promote the use of judicious testing, as well as decrease unnecessary treatment measures such as avoiding antibiotic overuse (www.choosingwisely.org/about-us). The Choosing Wisely campaign identifies tests, procedures, and treatments commonly used but whose necessity should be questioned. More than 70 specialty organizations have identified recommendations to improve decision making and promote appropriate patient-centered care. Each society has developed a list of five to 10 tests, treatments, or services that are commonly overused (Cassel & Guest, 2012). Choosing Wisely initiatives have included best practice campaigns, quality improvement projects, and formal research studies within the United States and globally.

An APRN-led initiative was launched in 2015 at VUMC working in conjunction with an interdisciplinary Choosing Wisely committee. A multidisciplinary daily lab reduction initiative that was completed at the institution served as a guide for implementing the APRN Choosing Wisely project (Iams et al., 2016). For a 12-month period, lab and chest-x-ray use were tracked in six ICUs and in several specialty units to assess the impact of APRN-led unit-based projects. Data were tracked on lab and x-ray use and reviewed at monthly taskforce meetings. An interdisciplinary committee including medical, nursing, quality, lab services, and data analyst support reviewed key metrics on a monthly basis in order to refine data collection and review ongoing project results. Overall, the APRN-led initiative resulted in increased clinician awareness and better ordering practices with a decrease in unnecessary testing and care measures (Kleinpell et al., in press).

As a result of the initiative's success, the Vanderbilt Advanced Practice Nursing Collaborative was launched to enable APRN teams at other institutions to implement a Choosing Wisely initiative, track outcomes, and disseminate results. Participating teams will identify up to three lab or diagnostic test measures to target reduction in unnecessary ordering, or another Choosing Wisely recommendation. An online registration process, Research Electronic Data Capture (REDCap), is used for teams to register to participate and to gain access to the collaborative materials (www.mc.vanderbilt.edu/aprnchoosingwisely). These materials include sample flyers, sample slide deck, examples of data tracking and displays, and lessons learned by Vanderbilt APRN teams. For more information, visit the collaborative website (www.mc.vanderbilt.edu/aprnchoosingwisely).

SUMMARY

Health care restructuring continues to change the way in which care is delivered, and as APRNs' roles expand, the measurement of outcomes is an important parameter by which APRN care can be evaluated. Moreover, as APRNs are involved in providing care to a variety of patient groups and in various settings, they are often the most familiar with the clinical problems that need to be studied and are therefore the ideal practitioners to participate in the development of outcome-based initiatives (Resnick, 2006). Knowledge of the process of outcome measurement and of available resources is essential for all APRNs regardless of practice specialty or setting. The use of practice-specific quality metrics and initiatives such as implementation of the Choosing Wisely recommendations can be used to define impact of the APRN role. The additional chapters in this book outline further examples of practice-based outcome assessments related to APRN practice, including indicators monitored and how outcome assessments were conducted, as well as sources for identifying outcome-related tools.

Answers to Chapter Discussion Questions

1. Several practice-specific quality metrics can be used to identify outcomes of APRN practice. Examples include the incidence of catheter-associated urinary tract infections after an APRN-led initiative to reduce use of unnecessary catheter use, clinic wait time after initiative of an APRN urgent care clinic, or daily lab use after implementation of a Choosing Wisely initiative to reduce the use of unnecessary lab testing in hospitalized patients.

2. Practice-specific quality metrics can be used to identify the impact of APRN care by monitoring changes in metrics after implementation of an APRN-led initiative. Dashboard can be used to measure practice-specific quality metrics such as wait times for new appointments, HCAHPS scores, unexpected hospital readmissions, pressure ulcer incidence, discharges by 11 a.m., or adherence to a diabetes mellitus order set, for example. Practice-specific metrics can be used to define impact of the APRN role through identifying outcome metrics that are directly impacted by the APRN role.

3. Strategies that can be used to measure APRN impact include establishing role-specific metrics, planning for outcome evaluation when any new role is established, and building in outcomes as a part of the OPPE processes of an institution's overall strategic plan to identify impact of the APRN role.

░ REFERENCES

Albers-Heitner, C. P., Joore, M. A., Winkens, R. A., Lagro-Janssen, A. L. M., Severns, J. L., & Berghmans, L. C. (2012). Cost-effectiveness of involving nurse specialists for adult patients with urinary incontinence in primary care compared with care-as-usual: An economic evaluation alongside a pragmatic randomized controlled trial. *Neurology and Urodynamics, 31,* 526–534. doi:10.1002/nau.21204

Alexander-Banys, B. (2014). Acute care nurse practitioner managed home monitoring program for patients with complex congenital heart disease: A case study. *Journal of Pediatric Health Care, 28,* 97–100.

Cassel, C. A., & Guest, J. A. (2012). Choosing Wisely: Helping physicians and patients make smart decisions about their care. *The Journal of the American Medical Association, 307,* 1801–1802. doi:10.1001/jama.2012.476

Centers for Medicare & Medicaid Services. (2016). MACRA: Delivery system reform, Medicare payment reform. Retrieved from https://www.cms.gov/Medicare/Quality-Initiatives-Patient-Assessment-Instruments/Value-Based-Programs/MACRA-MIPS-and-APMs/MACRA-MIPS-and-APMs.html

Gracias, V. H., Sicoutris, C. P., Stawicki, S. P., Meredith, D. M., Horan, A. D., Gupta, R., . . . Schwab, C. W. (2008). Critical care nurse practitioners improve compliance with clinical practice guidelines in "semiclosed" surgical intensive care unit. *Journal of Nursing Care Quality, 23*(4), 338–344.

Hatem, M., Sandall, J., Devane, D., Soltani, H., & Gates, S. (2008). Midwife-led versus other models of care for childbearing women. *Cochrane Database of Systematic Reviews, 2008*(4). doi:10.1002/14651858 .CD004667.pub2

Haut, E. R., Gracias, V. H., Sicoutris, C. P., Meredith, D. M., Reilly, P. M., Auerbach, S., . . . Schwab, C. W. (2004, September). *Decreased laboratory utilization in an "intensivist managed" surgical intensive care unit.* Maui, HI: The American Association for the Surgery of Trauma.

Haut, E. R., Sicoutris, C. P., Meredith, D. M., Sonnad, S. S., Reilly, P. M., Schwab, C. W., . . . Gracias, V. H. (2006). Improved nurse job satisfaction and job retention with a transition from a "mandatory consultation" model to a "semiclosed" surgical intensive care unit: A 1-year prospective evaluation." *Critical Care Medicine, 34*(2), 387–395.

Hogan, P., Seifert, R., Moore, C., & Simonson, B. (2010). Cost-effectiveness analysis of anesthesia providers. *Nursing Economics, 28,* 159–169.

Iams, W., Heck, J., Kapp, M., Leverenz, D., Vella, M., Szentirmai, E., . . . Kripalani, S. (2016). A multidisciplinary house staff-led initiative to safely reduce daily lab testing. *Academic Medicine, 91,* 813–820.

Institute of Medicine. (2010). *The future of nursing: Leading change, advancing health.* Washington, DC: National Academies Press.

Jessee, B. T., & Rutledge, C. M. (2012). Effectiveness of nurse practitioner coordinated team group visits for type 2 diabetes in medically underserved Appalachia. *Journal of the American Academy of Nurse Practitioners, 24,* 735–743. doi:10.1111/j.1745-7599.2012.00764.x

Kapu, A. N., Kleinpell, R., & Pilon, B. (2014). Quality and financial impact of adding nurse practitioners to inpatient care teams. *Journal of Nursing Administration, 44,* 87–96.

Kleinpell, R. M., & Alexandrov, A. W. (2014). Integrative review of outcomes and performance improvement research on advanced practice nursing. In A. B. Hamric, C. M. Hanson, M. F. Tracy, & E. T. O'Grady (Eds.), *Advanced practice nursing: An integrative approach* (pp. 607–636). St. Louis, MO: Elsevier Saunders.

Kleinpell, R. M., Kapu, A., Witherspoon, B., Oliver, L., Gibson, J., Vance, H., . . . Iams W. (in press). Showcasing Outcomes of APRN Practice with the Choosing Wisely® Campaign. *American Nurse.*

Laurant, M., Reeves, D., Hermens, R., Braspenning, J., Grol, R., & Sibbald, B. (2005). Substitution of doctors by nurses in primary care. *Cochrane Database of Systematic Reviews, 2005*(2). doi:10.1002/14651858.CD001271.pub2

Martin, N. D., Pisa, M. A., Collins, T. A., Robertson, M. P., Sicoutris, C. P., Bushan, N., . . . Kohl, B. (2015). Advanced practitioner-driven critical care outreach to reduce ICU readmission mortality. *International Journal of Academic Medicine, 1,* 3–8.

Newhouse, R. P., Weiner, J. P., Stanik-Hutt, J., White, K. M., Johantgen, M., Steinwachs, D., . . . Weiner, J. P. (2011). Advanced practice outcomes 1990–2008: A systematic review. *Nursing Economics, 29,* 230–250.

Resnick, B. (2006). Outcomes research: You do have the time! *Journal of the American Academy of Nurse Practitioners, 18*(11), 505–509.

Sawatzky, J., Christie, S., & Singhal, R. K. (2013). Exploring outcomes of a nurse practitioner-managed cardiac surgery follow-up intervention: A randomized trial. *Journal of Advanced Nursing, 69,* 2076–2087.

Scaff, D. W., Gracias, V. H., Sicoutris, C. P., McMaster, J., Puri, N. K., Sonnad, S., . . . Schwab, C. W. (2004). Reducing ICU complications in trauma patients: The effect of two different clinical delivery systems. *Critical Care Medicine, 32*(12), A37.

CHAPTER 2

Analyzing Economic Outcomes in Advanced Practice Nursing

Kevin D. Frick, Catherine C. Cohen, and Patricia W. Stone

Chapter Objectives

1. Present an overview of five different types of economic evaluations that an advanced practice registered nurse (APRN) may encounter
2. Contrast economic evaluation methodology with that of comparative-effectiveness studies and business case studies
3. Outline appropriate outcome measures for each type of analysis
4. Summarize and critique published examples of each type of economic evaluation
5. Discuss methodological issues of importance to economic evaluations

Chapter Discussion Questions

1. How does comparative-effectiveness research compare with cost-effectiveness research and business case studies?
2. In what scenario would a cost–utility methodology be appropriate? Provide an example.
3. If studying three interventions with no single standard outcome measure (or validated means of clinical outcome aggregation), which methodology may be most appropriate?
4. What is a key assumption required for a successful cost–benefit analysis (CBA)? How are the outcomes of CBAs presented?
5. Use a "two-step" approach to determine cost of a new antibiotic formulation that requires 4 minutes of reconstitution preparation by the RN immediately prior to intravenous infusion.

Cost-effectiveness of health care practice is an increasingly important topic in the delivery of care and consequently in nursing research. The growing proportion of older adults in the U.S. population, various improvements in health care technology, direct-to-consumer advertising for a long list of pharmaceuticals, increasing costs of doing business in other sectors besides health care, and international competitive pressures on wages and benefits have drawn greater attention to the costs of health care over time. U.S. health care spending in 2014 grew 5.3%, which was faster than the rate of inflation and accounted for 17.5% of gross domestic product (Centers for Medicare & Medicaid Services, 2016; Chernew, 2015). Concerns over unsustainable increases in health care spending led to passage of the Affordable Care Act (U.S. national health reform), which within the first 2 years of implementation (2013–2015), contributed to a decline in the number of uninsured Americans at 12.8 million (Rovner, 2016). While U.S. legislation prohibits use of cost thresholds in health care policy decisions, the proportion of the gross domestic product being spent on health care forces policy makers to at least consider the costs as well as the effectiveness of new treatments, devices, or interventions (Neumann, Cohen, & Weinstein, 2014). Health policy makers increasingly request analyses, including projected economic outcomes prior to the approval of funding for or reimbursement of these new activities.

At the same time that the focus on cost has increased, other factors have also raised the importance of studying and contemplating the cost-effectiveness of health care in the United States. These include (a) the scientific recommendations related to the conduct of cost-effectiveness analyses that have been issued in the United States, (b) a format for formulary submissions offered by the Academy of Managed Care Pharmacy, (c) recognition by parties in the United States of other recommendations around the globe, (d) conferences related to cost-effectiveness sponsored by the National Institute of Nursing Research, and (e) authorization of a new organization, the Patient-Centered Outcomes Research Institute (PCORI), by the U.S. Congress in 2010 that emphasizes use of comparative-effectiveness methodology to improve the quality of evidence available to inform health care decision making (PCORI, 2014).

Therefore, in the current economic and health care environment, APRNs need to be knowledgeable about the interpretation of cost, and effectiveness data in particular, when they are combined in a cost-effectiveness study. The increased demand for economic information has resulted in a number of economic evaluations in the literature specific to nursing and a plethora of cost-effectiveness studies (e.g., Bryant-Lukosius et al., 2015; Cohen, Choi, & Stone, 2016; Martin-Misener et al., 2015; Twigg, Myers, Duffield, Giles, & Evans, 2015). Not only are APRNs and other clinicians now expected to review publications containing economic outcomes related to their services, but they must also participate in these analyses and interpret others for appropriateness of implementing findings into practice.

To accomplish these goals, APRNs must understand how to distinguish comparative-effectiveness research from cost-effectiveness analysis (CEA) research and business case analyses. *Comparative-effectiveness research* has been defined as the conduct and synthesis of research comparing the benefits and harms of different interventions and strategies to prevent, diagnose, treat, and monitor health conditions in "real-world" settings; its purpose is to improve health outcomes by developing and disseminating evidence-based information about the everyday effectiveness of interventions (Federal Coordinating

Council for Comparative Effectiveness Research, 2009; Iglehart, 2009; Volpp & Das, 2009). This is in contrast to efficacy research, such as a randomized controlled trial, where the question is typically whether the treatment can work under a controlled environment. Because comparative-effectiveness research is aimed to inform actual patient situations, it is very much patient-centered and thus is also called *patient-centered outcome research*. This methodology not only highlights the everyday needs of the patients, but it may also incorporate many different types of patient outcomes. Cost-effectiveness research is one type of patient-centered outcome research that focuses on economic outcomes of two or more comparable health care interventions and is well suited to be conducted along-side a comprehensive comparative-effectiveness assessment (Garber, 2011; Jacobson, 2007; Stone, 2001a, 2001b). In contrast to both of these, a *business case analysis* is generally from the more narrow perspective of a single organization that may choose to implement an intervention or not. This focuses on the costs and revenue generated for a single organization (and describes data on any health outcomes that are relevant to the organization) and uses an organization's view of the future to compare costs and revenue now with costs and revenue later to calculate return on investment and make an inference about whether to implement.

A number of different methods are employed to address economic outcomes of health care to inform policy or recommendations for adoption. The purposes of this chapter are (a) to present an overview of five different types of economic evaluations an APRN may encounter, (b) discuss appropriate outcome measures for each type of analysis, (c) present and critique published examples of each type of economic evaluation, and (d) discuss methodological issues of importance to economic evaluations.

TYPES OF ECONOMIC EVALUATIONS

Five different methods of economic evaluations are commonly used in assessing the economic impact of new health care interventions and technology. Table 2.1 presents a brief overview of these methods (Drummond, Sculpher, Claxton, Stoddart, & Torrance, 2015). In all of these economic outcome evaluations, alternative strategies are compared and the incremental cost of the competing strategies is computed according to the following formula:

$$\text{Incremental costs} = C1 - C2$$

where C1 represents the cost of the new intervention and C2 represents the cost of the comparator (e.g., the next-best strategy). There is more variation between methods regarding how effectiveness is measured, although the focus remains on incremental changes in effectiveness (e.g., comparing the outcome of one intervention with that of another).

Cost-Minimization Analysis

In a true cost-minimization analysis (CMA), only the costs are evaluated and the alternatives are assumed or have been found to offer equivalent outcomes. Many of these studies begin as cost-effectiveness studies, in which the investigators expected one intervention to be both more effective and more expensive. As a result, in most published

TABLE 2.1 Types of Economic Evaluations

Type of Study	Definition	Effect Measurement
CMA	An analysis that computes the incremental costs of alternatives that achieve the same outcome	Assumed or shown to be the same
CCA	An analysis in which incremental costs and multiple effects are computed, without any attempt to aggregate them	Natural occurring units*
CEA	An analysis in which incremental costs and one type of effects are presented in a ratio	Natural occurring units*
CUA	A special type of CEA, in which quality of life is considered and a metric is used that combines quality and quantity of life	Quality-adjusted life years
CBA	An analysis in which incremental costs and effects are computed, and all benefits and costs are measured in a single currency such as 2016 U.S. dollars	Monetary

*Examples of natural occurring units are life years gained, disability days saved, or cases avoided.
CBA, cost–benefit analysis; CCA, cost–consequence analysis; CEA, cost-effectiveness analysis; CMA, cost-minimization analysis; CUA, cost–utility analysis.

economic evaluations labeled as CMAs, clinical outcomes of the strategies being compared are measured (e.g., Beaver et al., 2009; Schuurman et al., 2009). For example, after establishing similar efficacy of traditional hospital visits and nursing telephone consultations following breast cancer in a randomized control trial, Beaver et al. (2009) then used data from the trial to conduct a CMA. They determined that, from the perspective of the United Kingdom (UK) National Health Service, the telephone consultation arm had higher costs. In the Schuurman et al. (2009) study, comparison of costs for technological versus human approaches to preventing pressure ulcers was performed in conjunction with a prospective cohort study regarding incidence and risk factors for the clinical outcome. While incidence was similar between the two approaches, the technological approach was cost-saving.

Cost-Consequence Analysis

A cost–consequence analysis (CCA) is a study in which the costs and the consequences of two or more alternatives are measured, but costs and consequences are listed separately. This methodology is often chosen when there is no obvious summary measure for the outcomes applicable to the interventions being studied. In a CCA, the analyst expects the decision makers to form their own opinions about the relative importance of the findings. To facilitate decision making, the analysts provide an array of consequences applicable to each strategy. Two studies serve as examples of this methodology being used in the nursing literature. Schoonhoven et al. (2015) compared the consequences of using bed baths or traditional soap and water baths for nursing home residents in a cluster randomized trial that assessed resident skin integrity, resident behavioral problems, costs, and resident and nurse satisfaction. Campbell et al. (2014) determined the costs and consequences of increasing primary care access (operationalized as the number of patient contacts) comparing usual care to (a) general practitioner telephone consultation or (b) nurse telephone consultation.

Cost-Effectiveness Analysis

CEA also measures incremental costs. In CEA, incremental consequences are measured in a single common natural unit, such as life years gained or cases avoided. In addition, costs and effects are summarized in an incremental cost-effectiveness ratio (ICER), which is calculated using the following formula:

$$\text{Cost-effectiveness ratio} = (C1 - C2)/(E1 - E2)$$

where $C1$ represents the cost of the new intervention, $C2$ represents the cost of the comparator, $E1$ represents the effect of the new intervention, and $E2$ represents the effect of the comparator. For CEA, analysts often attach the resource utilization data-collection process to a randomized trial, usually powered on something other than the cost-effectiveness result (e.g., Joen [2015] examined nurse work environment and outcomes in older adults), or employ a decision-analytical approach and model the problem through the use of a decision tree (e.g., Kang, Mandsager, Biddle, & Weber [2012] examined different methods of monitoring for methicillin-resistant *Staphylococcus aureus* in academic hospitals; Fatoye & Haigh [2016] compared ankle brace use vs. taping on patients returning to work after an acute ankle sprain).

The decision is between choosing alternative 1 or alternative 2. Both alternatives have associated probabilities of positive (good) and negative (bad) outcomes. In addition, there are the associated costs of each strategy. The use of decision analysis and decision trees is a defined mathematical modeling technique. "A sample decision tree is diagrammed in Figure 2.1." It is suggested that anyone interested in using this technique seek training opportunities. There are a number of highly readable texts available to the APRN wishing to understand this approach better (Drummond et al., 2015; Haddix, Teutsch, & Corso, 2002; Petitti, 2000).

A number of examples of CEA can be found in the recent nursing literature (Hunter, 2015; Jeon et al., 2015; Kang et al., 2012). Jeon et al. (2015) provide an excellent example of deriving a CEA from a cluster randomized controlled trial. The study sought to improve care of older adults through a year-long intervention among nurse managers to improve management skills to improve work environment, measured by the Work Environment Scale-R (WES-R) score and the Multifactor Leadership Questionnaire (MLQ)–Rater form. The cost of the intervention was monitored as a secondary outcome, the results of which were expressed as a mean ICER. The intervention resulted in a one-point increased mean score in transformational leadership per $1,584 AUD (Australian dollars) spent and a

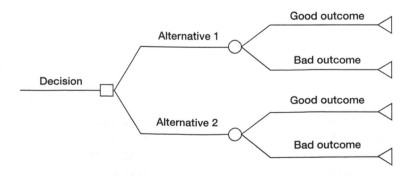

FIGURE 2.1 Example of a decision tree.

one-point increased mean score in overall leadership per $1,343 AUD spent. Although these are acceptable health outcomes, use of the WES-R score and MLQ–Rater form only facilitate comparison with other studies that also focus on interventions for work environment. In contrast, Hunter (2015) used a Markov model (i.e., simulating what happens to a cohort of individuals over multiple periods through time) to estimate the cost-effectiveness of three alternatives to promote antibiotic stewardship for respiratory illness in primary care: standard practice, c-reactive protein point of care testing, and this testing with added communication training. For each option, the author calculated the probability of antibiotic prescribing and the number of respiratory illnesses.

Cost–Utility Analysis

Cost–utility analysis (CUA) considers the effectiveness of the interventions on both the quantity and the quality of life in a single measure, the quality-adjusted life year (QALY). The QALY is a measure of the quantity of life gained weighted by the quality of that life. Quality of life is measured by a utility, which is a measure of preference for a given health state rated on a scale of 0 (death) to 1 (perfect health). Because dollars spent to gain a QALY are not disease specific, the measure is useful for informing health policy decisions and is recommended for such use by the U.S. Public Health Service's Panel on Cost-Effectiveness in Health and Medicine (Neumann, Sanders, Russell, Siegel, & Ganiats, 2016). The QALY is a common outcome unit at this point in time, as it has been recommended by a number of organizations around the world and facilitates comparisons among different studies.

However, variance in the interpretation of what QALYs are actually measuring ("Determinants of health economic decisions in actual practice: The role of behavioral economics," 2006) and estimates for the value of a QALY have ranged from $20,000 to $200,000 (Neumann et al., 2014). In fact, a 2016 meeting of the International Society of Pharmacoeconomics and Outcomes Research (ISPOR) devoted a session to whether more evidence is needed for cost-effectiveness thresholds and if so, how to generate this evidence (ISPOR, 2016). While lack of universal agreement as to what society should be willing to pay to gain a QALY persists, and despite specific U.S. legislation against use of a cost-per-QALY threshold, the figure of $50,000/QALY threshold is still often cited in the United States (Neumann et al., 2014).

Numerous examples exist in the nursing literature of cost–utility analyses. For example, Blakely et al. (2015) examined the cost–utility of a hospital-based nurse cancer care coordinator (vs. having no dedicated coordination service) for stage III colon cancer patients. They determined that the cost per QALY of this program was $15,600 USD, with increased coverage of chemotherapy and reduced time to treatment. In another CUA, Marsden et al. (2015) evaluated different repositioning strategies for the prevention of pressure ulcers from the perspective of the UK National Health Service and determined that while repositioning every 2 to 4 hours is slightly more effective, it is not more cost-effective than repositioning every 4 hours.

Cost–Benefit Analysis

CBA is a form of economic evaluation in which consequences are summarized in monetary units. In CBA, a single monetary figure representing benefits minus costs is calculated. As long as the decision maker agrees with the methods used to place a dollar value on outcomes, this provides the decision maker with a direct indication of whether the value of the benefits is greater than the cost. Wang et al. (2014) used a CBA to help policy makers evaluate the value of the Massachusetts Essential School Health Services program, which employs and maintains an onsite, full-time, baccalaureate-prepared RN in every public school. By including costs of nurse staffing and medical supplies, and the savings (benefits) from reducing medical procedures and protecting teacher and parent productivity, the authors determined that the program yielded a net benefit of $98.1 million during the 2009–2010 school year ($2.20 gained for every $1 invested). Another study used CBA to determine if a safe patient-handling program in an outpatient rehabilitation center would prevent work-related injuries during patient transfers among nurses and other therapy staff. Implementing the program gained $3.71 in benefit for every dollar invested in the program, although the injury reduction rates were not sustained (Theis & Finkelstein, 2014).

COMMON ISSUES IN ALL ECONOMIC EVALUATIONS

The basic steps in conducting economic evaluations are illustrated in Figure 2.2. In addition, because this is essentially a new language to many APRNs, Table 2.2 defines some of the concepts and common terminology used in these analyses.

Selecting the Type of Economic Evaluation

The first step is to select the appropriate type of analysis to conduct. Considerations should include (a) the goal of the analysis (e.g., whether to compare only interventions affecting a single disease with a well-defined most important symptom or to compare interventions for different diseases or interventions for a condition with a complex set of symptoms), (b) whether the effectiveness of the interventions is equivalent (and, if so, this suggests a CMA), (c) the effectiveness measures available (e.g., can QALYs be generated), (d) the potential impact of the interventions on either quality or quantity of life (if both, then a CUA is most appropriate), (e) the availability of data, (f) the expertise available, and (g) ethical issues.

Framing the Analysis

Once the economic method has been selected, the researcher frames the analysis. This includes selecting the appropriate comparator(s) to analyze. For example, when testing the cost-effectiveness of a new educational program, the researcher might consider implementation in a hospital setting, initiation in an outpatient clinic, and a lack of teaching altogether as comparators given that outcomes may be different among them. At the least, the comparison of new interventions should be to the current practice, or status quo. Benchmarking to an established standard of care emphasizes the fact that analyses do not compare an intervention with "doing nothing." In addition, often more than one comparator is appropriate to include in the analysis. This is especially true when multiple alternatives have been found to offer similar clinical outcomes or if there are potentially multiple levels of intensity of the interventions (e.g., increasing home health visits from twice a week to daily).

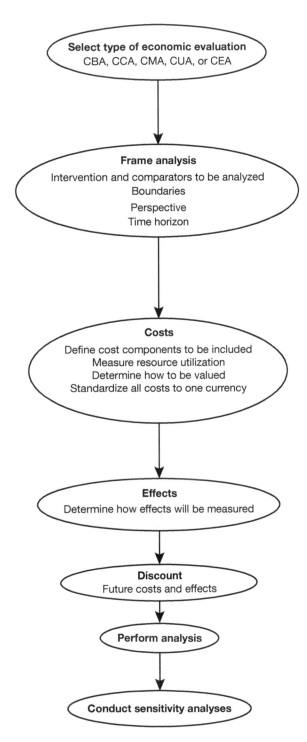

FIGURE 2.2 Basic steps in economic evaluations.

CBA, cost–benefit analysis; CCA, cost–consequence analysis; CEA, cost-effectiveness analysis; CMA, cost-minimization analysis; CUA, cost–utility analysis.

TABLE 2.2   Common Terminology in Economic Evaluations

Term	Definition
Boundaries of the study	The scope of the study
Comparator(s)	The alternative(s) to which the new intervention is compared
CPI	A measure of average change in price over time. This is used to adjust costs that are estimated in different past years to the present
Discounting	The process of converting future costs and effects to the present value
Incremental cost-effectiveness ratio	The ratio of the difference of the costs of two alternatives to the difference in effectiveness between the same two alternatives. Used in cost-effectiveness and cost–utility analyses
Perspective	The viewpoint from which the analysis is conducted
Sensitivity analysis	Calculations in which an input to the calculation (either measured or assumed) is varied and indicates the degree of influence it has on the analysis. Often used when a parameter is uncertain
Time horizon	The period of time for which the costs and effects are measured

CPI, consumer price index.

Boundaries (i.e., the scope) of the study delimit the costs and effects that are included in the analysis. Many interventions have spillover effects that must be considered. The question becomes how far to follow such effects to adequately assess the economic impact of the intervention. For example, if the aim of an educational program for mothers of infants admitted to a neonatal intensive care unit is to decrease the mothers' levels of anxiety and improve the physiologic outcomes of the infants, then it logically follows that the boundaries would include both the mothers and the infants. This intervention may affect the overall parenting skills of the mother, however, and may have additional positive effects on other children in the family. In theory, all these effects are relevant, but in framing the study it is important to draw practical and feasible limits around the analysis.

In all types of economic evaluations, the perspective or viewpoint taken in the analysis also drives the set of costs and benefits included. Studies may be motivated by policy decisions relevant to specific institutions or individuals. In this case, the perspective of primary interest may be that of a managed care organization, hospital, employer, state health department, or another party. An economic evaluation conducted from the perspective of the hospital (e.g., providing a result most relevant to a hospital decision maker) should not consider costs (or savings) associated with family caregiving in the home. If the goal of the analysis is to affect broad resource allocation and health policy issues, however, then the societal perspective is appropriate and recommended (Neumann et al., 2016). This perspective incorporates all costs and all health effects regardless of who incurs them. This is advantageous because, if a systematic analysis is performed to compare the results of multiple studies and all have used the societal perspective, it makes comparison easier. Gathering data for the societal perspective also allows any other perspective to be calculated as a subset of the societal perspective. Indeed, the Second Panel on Cost-Effectiveness in Health and Medicine recommend that two reference cases should be reported: one from the health care perspective and one from the societal perspective (Neumann et al., 2016).

The time horizon refers to the period of time for which the costs and benefits are measured in the analysis. The time horizon may vary from less than 1 year to the patient's entire life span. The appropriate time horizon to consider will depend on the probable length of effect of the interventions being compared. Once the framing of the analysis is complete, the analyst is ready to estimate costs. The distinction between the time of the intervention and the time horizon for the analysis must be kept in mind. An intervention that lasts less than 1 year (e.g., nurses providing counseling to adolescents on high-risk behaviors) may have effects that last a lifetime.

Costs

Terminology pertaining to costs of resources has traditionally been divided into "direct" and "indirect" costs (Gold et al., 1996), with other labels like "friction costs" sometimes being applied to the cost of hiring a new employee and sometimes being applied to an entire method of valuing productivity (Brouwer & Koopmanschap, 2005; Gold et al., 1996). However, because economists and accountants do not use the same definitions and sometimes even economists have not been able to agree on a universal set of definitions, the terminology has become complicated. In health economics, direct costs have been defined as changes in resource use directly attributable to the provision of care, whereas indirect costs have referred to costs associated with the loss of productivity from morbidity and/or mortality (Liljas, 1998). Accountants, on the other hand, refer to direct costs as variable costs (e.g., supplies) and indirect costs as fixed costs (e.g., rent; Young, 2012). In light of these past inconsistencies in defining and measuring costs, the APRN conducting an economic evaluation should be sure to clarify and clearly communicate how the cost terms are defined. The trend in the CEA literature is to avoid the term "indirect." Given this trend and the potential for confusion, we urge APRNs to likewise avoid using this term.

Economists and analysts often use a "two-step" approach to determine the costs attributable to an intervention. The first step in the estimation is determining the amount of resources attributable or consumed. Once the attributable resources have been determined, the "money" valuation or costs of the resources may be estimated. Using a two-step approach increases the clarity and transparency of the analysis and allows readers of the analysis to understand how the costs of attributable resources may be similar or different in their own setting.

The resources and associated costs can be categorized as in Exhibit 2.1, which is an adaptation of a grouping that appeared earlier in the literature (Luce, Manning, Siegel, & Lipscomb, 1996). In CEA, financial health care costs are directly related to the intervention itself and associated costs or savings of future health care, which the intervention may impact. For example, financial health care costs associated with a hepatitis B virus (HBV) immunization program should include the costs of obtaining and administering the immunization. In addition, they should include "downstream" costs (as well as savings), such as hospitalizations, outpatient visits, and other treatment costs associated with the diagnosis of HBV itself. Financial costs associated with other related diseases, such as cirrhosis or cancer, should also be included. Similarly, the value of the time a patient spends either seeking care or participating in an intervention constitutes a real use of resources for the individual and society. Thus, relevant patient time costs may include both the time involved in receiving the treatment and the time spent waiting to receive care.

EXHIBIT 2.1   Cost Components to Consider for Inclusion

Direct health care costs*
Intervention
Hospitalization
Outpatient visits
Long-term care
Other health care
Direct non-health care
Transportation
Family/caregiver time
Social services
Productivity costs*
Other

*Not recommended for inclusion in cost–utility analyses by the Second Panel on Cost-Effectiveness in Health and Medicine.
Source: Neumann et al. (2016).

Consumption of resources other than those associated with the provision of health care also should be considered in economic evaluations conducted from the societal perspective. Examples of financial non-health care costs may include child care costs for a parent attending a smoking cessation program, increase in a family's food expenditure as a result of a dietary prescription, the cost of transportation to and from a clinic, and the like.

Historically, patient time and other non–health care resources have not been consistently included in analyses (Jacobs & Fassbender, 1998; Stone, Chapman, Sandberg, Liljas, & Neumann, 2000). Nonetheless, if an analysis is conducted from the societal perspective, inclusion of such factors is recommended (Neumann et al., 2016). In addition, because health care is becoming more community based, nursing interventions may directly influence these costs. For example, a home visit by an APRN case manager may not only increase the ability of the APRN to conduct a holistic assessment, but may also save resources related to patient time, transportation, and family caregiving. Bhandari (2011) included patient transportation costs of an iron supplementation therapy in a cost-minimization study and found that new iron preparations reduced these costs compared to standard of care.

Productivity costs are the costs associated with morbidity or mortality. Morbidity costs are those associated with lost or impaired ability to work or to engage in leisure activities (e.g., loss of income due to time for recuperation or convalescence after coronary bypass surgery). Mortality costs are related to loss of life and are usually measured according to what the individual would have been capable of earning. Two issues are important to note concerning productivity costs.

First, the U.S. Public Health Service's Panel on Cost-Effectiveness in Health and Medicine recommended that productivity costs be excluded from CUAs (Gold et al., 1996). The authors expressed concern that including both productivity costs and QALYs would represent a double counting because people may be considering productivity and earning potential when responding to trade-offs involving health and quality of life. Thus, when QALYs are used, productivity is already included in the denominator of the cost-effectiveness ratio.

Second, the assumption that productivity costs should be excluded from CUAs is controversial and has been debated by experts in the field (Krol, Brouwer, & Rutten, 2013). In light of this controversy, some analysts have presented results both with and without the inclusion of productivity costs (Krahn, Guasparini, Sherman, & Detsky, 1998; Moradi-Lakeh, Shakerian, & Esteghamati, 2012). APRNs conducting CUAs may also wish to present results both with and without the inclusion of productivity costs as well as continue to monitor recommendations made in the United States and elsewhere.

Some interventions (e.g., a successful smoking cessation program) extend life. Costs related to resource consumption in "added life years" are recommended for inclusion in economic evaluations. Added life-year costs are related to the consumption of health care resources (financial health care costs) and other types of consumption (all other cost categories). Because not all analyses increase life expectancy (e.g., use of cochlear implants or an educational intervention program aimed at decreasing parental anxiety), resource consumption in added life years is not always applicable. Sometimes, living longer and healthier can cost less annually but sum to more over a lifetime (van Baal et al., 2008). Generally, only the added health care costs and not added general consumption are included in the analysis.

Finally, income transfers, such as Social Security payments, are redistributions of money and are therefore not real costs to society. Consequently, although these "transfer costs" may be tracked and may be important for analyses from the government's perspective, they should not be included with other societal costs. What should be included in a societal cost analysis are the costs of administering an income transfer program.

When trying to determine which costs to include, the process should begin with an outline of the categories of costs included, using the list in Exhibit 2.1. Once this is complete, a researcher should consider the cost "ingredients" that the intervention impacts under each category (Drummond et al., 2015). After the ingredients are identified, discussions about which costs are most relevant and which are important to measure can take place. Moreover, the perspective of the analysis will drive the decisions about which cost component to include. The treatment of the cost component (e.g., productivity costs captured in quality of life adjustments) is determined by the specific economic-analytical method chosen.

Once the consumption of resources has been estimated, the resource must be assigned a dollar value. Economists use the term "opportunity costs," which reflects the value of the next-best alternative use of the resources. Determining the actual opportunity cost of a resource is difficult. Following are some general guidelines for assigning a dollar value to a resource.

In many markets, market prices (or charges) equate to opportunity costs. This does not apply in health care as often as in other fields. This incongruence is particularly notable for charges associated with hospitalizations. Although health care institutions bill for standard amounts, some payers are able to successfully negotiate lower charges for care. However, payers who are willing to pay higher levels of reimbursement or unable to negotiate lower levels of reimbursement will ultimately pay more for the same care. The practice of obtaining higher payments from some patrons is termed "cost shifting."

Therefore, for these institutional categories, an adjustment to prices is necessary to accurately represent exchange of funds, the cost. In fact, many customers, such as large insurance organizations, pay only a fraction of these charges. Large payers negotiate payment rates for services rendered based on the cost of the service and allowed profit margins (or excess revenues for not-for-profit institutions). Payers with the least market power (e.g., uninsured individuals) are the only ones who are likely to pay anything near the actual cost. If a hospital were just to break even based on the negotiated rates, then it is clear that the actual amount charged does not represent anything close to the actual cost.

Instead of using charges, a common source of valuation for hospital costs is the hospital's own cost-accounting system. For researchers internal to the institution, these will often be easy to access. These cost-accounting systems are developed by finance departments to help administrative decision making and are based on past accounting studies and algorithms. Although the market price of medical care often does not represent actual costs, the market prices of the goods in the cost-accounting system are expected to represent the relevant costs of inputs to care. If a cost-accounting system is available, the APRN can usually determine the specific monetary health care cost components, such as variable costs (e.g., staffing and supplies) and fixed overhead costs (e.g., rent and percentage of administration costs).

Another alternative is to use hospital cost-to-charge ratios, which are calculated by dividing the total costs in a cost center by the total charges for the same resource. Cost-to-charge ratios are recognized as a gross adjustment to charges. This type of adjustment is better than using charges alone, but is not preferable to cost-accounting systems when they are available. Published sources also are often used as the source of valuation of the resource (Stone et al., 2000). Governmental fee schedules are also often used to represent costs of particular procedures (Armstrong, Malone, & Erder, 2008).

When cost estimates come from various sources, it is important to standardize all costs to the same currency and year. For example, non-U.S. currency figures may be converted into U.S. dollars using the appropriate foreign exchange factor for that time period (Board of Governors of the Federal Reserve System, www.federalreserve.gov/releases/g5a/current/default.htm). A recent review article in the nursing literature demonstrates the concept of applying exchange rates to cost estimates to compare across geographic regions (Cohen et al., 2016). The concept of purchasing-power parity, which not only accounts for the exchange rate but also attempts to yield the capacity to purchase the same quantity of goods, is also commonly used (Penz et al., 2014). In addition, because $1 in 1988 does not have the same purchasing power as $1 in the year 2008, the costs from different years must be adjusted into a standard year format by the use of the consumer price index (CPI), for which U.S. data are available from the Bureau of Labor Statistics (BLS) website (www.bls.gov), and a single year-to-year calculation can be done using the inflation calculator provided at that website (data.bls.gov/cgi-bin/cpicalc.pl). This inflation calculator is based on general market goods inflation. An example of such adjustment is a recent review examining costs of infection prevention activities in long-term care facilities in which the authors converted reported costs into 2013 U.S. dollars so that costs from different studies could be compared more effectively (Cohen et al., 2016). The BLS also calculates a medical inflation rate (www.bls.gov/cpi/cpifact4.htm). Because the costs of health care are rising more rapidly than costs in most other markets, analysts often use the medical inflation rate to inflate costs that pertain only to health care resources. Finally, there is discussion as to whether to use the CPI or the producer price index for inflation adjustment in general. Again, this largely depends on perspective. True opportunity costs are likely to be reflected in the producer price index. However, if the perspective is a payer perspective, then the CPI is likely to be more appropriate.

Discounting

Once all costs and benefits have been calculated, future costs and benefits are discounted to present value. Discounting reflects the principle that suggests people place greater value on something they have today than on something they will have in the future. Interest rates are an example of this principle. Future costs and benefits are discounted to present value using the following formula:

$$F/(1 + r)^n$$

where F is the future value (usually measured in dollars at today's value), r is the discount rate, and n is the number of years in the future (Stone, 1998). Currently, in the United States, experts recommend using the same discount rate to discount both costs and effects (Neumann et al., 2016). However, because prevention interventions are aimed at improving future health, by discounting future benefits, the intervention may not seem as beneficial. Therefore, some analysts are uncomfortable discounting future health benefits and only discount costs (Stone et al., 2000). Thus, to increase the comparability of analyses, APRNs in the United States should discount both costs and effects at 3% and, if desired, the results without discounting may also be presented. Moreover, the discount rate for a business case analysis is likely to be higher and represent the expected return on alternative uses of resources.

Analysis

In conducting economic evaluations, data gathered may include resource utilization, value of resources, effectiveness of treatment, and preferences regarding health outcomes. Based on the data gathered, the "base-case" analysis is computed. A best practice when presenting results is to include a table listing all parameters, the value assigned to each parameter, and the source of the value.

Sensitivity Analysis

Many of the data points gathered include some assumptions or uncertainty in the inputs. For clarification, the analysis based only on the best point estimates is referred to as the "base case," regardless of whether the recommendations of the panel are followed. Thus, any CEA includes a base case, but not all base-case analyses are reference-case analyses.

The assumptions that are made in the base case should be clearly stated before the results are presented to increase the transparency of the analysis. In addition, sensitivity analyses should be conducted to explore the implications of alternative assumptions. Sensitivity analysis is an important element of a sound economic evaluation (Drummond et al., 2015; Gold et al., 1996).

Sensitivity analyses are calculations in which a parameter is varied. These analyses indicate the degree of influence the particular value has on the analysis. The range used for a parameter should be specified along with the point estimate in Table 2.2.

A *univariate* sensitivity analysis examines the degree to which changing a single assumption changes the outcome of the entire analysis. By varying the value of the variable over a reasonable set of parameters, the investigator is able to determine how that variable may impact the results under different assumptions. The impact on the results has multiple interpretations. One is how the magnitude of the cost-effectiveness ratio changes; in other words, whether the ratio changes from spending $10,000/QALY gained to $30,000/QALY gained. However, a second level of interpretation is whether the decision to implement or not implement a new intervention changes. If a decision maker believes that any program costing less than $50,000 is a candidate for implementation, then the change from $10,000/QALY to $30,000/QALY will not change the decision about whether to consider a new intervention for implementation. Ryan, Revill, Devane, and Normand (2013) used a series of univariate sensitivity analyses to explore the extent of cost minimization between midwife-led maternity care and midwife care for only low-risk cases across the UK. Taking parameter estimates from three different clinical studies, the authors generated and evaluated eight different possible scenarios and determined that the cost difference between the alternatives ranged from −£253.38 to £108.12 per case.

Although univariate sensitivity analyses are insightful, looking at one source of uncertainty by itself is usually inadequate. The alternative is multivariate sensitivity analysis. A *multivariate* sensitivity analysis examines multiple sources of uncertainty at one time and may generate a more accurate understanding of the uncertainty of the cost-effectiveness results. This can be done by changing all parameters to their most or least favorable levels—but still working with predetermined levels of the values for each variable. A second approach makes use of the fact that variables can sometimes be expected to change together; in such cases, the analyst might explore how the cost-effectiveness ratio changes as the two variables are varied over their ranges. Finally, an analyst can conduct what is referred to as a *probabilistic* sensitivity analysis.

In this case, the analyst must define distributions from which the values for parameters may be drawn. A random draw is then taken from each distribution and the results of the analysis are calculated. The results of the first analysis are recorded and the process is repeated—at least thousands and sometimes tens of thousands of times. The analyst must then describe the range of results by describing the distribution of ratios. Fatoye and Haigh (2016) use this technique to describe the distribution of cost-effectiveness results in a study to compare the use of semirigid ankle brace versus taping to prevent recurrent acute ankle sprains. In this study, the estimated mean costs were assumed to have normative distributions, thereby identifying a range of possible cost values to be included in the Monte Carlo simulation model. The authors found that although taping was less expensive, the ICER for the brace versus taping was £263/QALY (well below the recommended ICER). However, due to skewed willingness to pay, there was a 46% probability of cost-effectiveness. A decision maker faced with this information would have to determine whether being 46% certain of a favorable economic result is sufficient to move forward with a policy change.

SUMMARY

The checklist in Exhibit 2.2 may be useful when communicating the results of an economic evaluation. This checklist draws on criteria for high-quality cost-effectiveness studies and draws on a number of sets of criteria that have been specified in related literature (Drummond et al., 2015; Eldessouki, 2012; Gold et al., 1996).

A second checklist for economic evaluations is the Consolidated Health Economic Evaluation Reporting Standards (CHEERS). This checklist, shown in Exhibit 2.3, may be particularly useful when reading and evaluating reported economic analyses, as well as designing and publishing these analyses (Husereau et al., 2013).

With the continuing development of new treatments, technologies, and models of care delivery, health-economic evaluations have become increasingly important. The demand for economic outcome research is growing, as is the number of published analyses. In this chapter, we have introduced various methods used in economic evaluation and have described the concepts and terminology used in these analyses.

EXHIBIT 2.2   **CEA Checklist for Journal Report**

1. **Framework**
   - Background of the problem
   - General framing and design of the problem
   - Target population for the intervention
   - Other program descriptors
   - Description of comparator programs
   - Boundaries of the analysis
   - Time horizon
   - Statement of the perspective of the analysis

2. **Data and methods**
   - Description of event pathway
   - Identification of outcomes of interest in the analysis
   - Description of model used
   - Modeling assumptions
   - Diagram of event pathway/model
   - Software used
   - Complete information about the sources of effectiveness data, cost data, and preference weights
   - Methods for obtaining estimates of effectiveness, costs, and preferences
   - Critique of data quality
   - Statement of year costs
   - Statement of method used to adjust costs for inflation
   - Statement of type of currency
   - Sources and methods for obtaining expert judgment
   - Statement of discount rates

(continued)

EXHIBIT 2.2 CEA Checklist for Journal Report (*continued*)

3. Results
▪ Results of model validation
▪ Reference case results (discounted and undiscounted): total costs and effectiveness, incremental costs and effectiveness, and incremental cost-effectiveness ratios
▪ Results of sensitivity analyses
▪ Other estimates of uncertainty, if available
▪ Graphical representation of cost-effectiveness results
▪ Aggregate cost and effectiveness information
▪ Disaggregated results, as relevant
▪ Secondary analyses using 5% discount rate
▪ Other secondary analyses, as relevant
4. Discussion
▪ Summary of reference case results
▪ Summary of sensitivity analysis assumptions having important ethical implications
▪ Limitations of the study
▪ Relevance of the study results for specific policy questions or decisions
▪ Results of related CEAs
▪ Distributive implications of the intervention
5. Technical report available upon request

CEA, cost-effectiveness analysis.
Source: Adapted from Gold et al. (1996).

EXHIBIT 2.3 CHEERS Checklist for Journal Report

Section/Topic	#	Recommendation	Reported on page no./line no.
Title			
Title	1	Identify the study as an economic evaluation, or use more specific terms such as "cost-effectiveness" and describe the interventions compared	
Abstract			
Structured summary	2	Provide a structured summary of objectives, perspective, setting, methods (including study design and inputs) results (including base-case and uncertainty analyses), and conclusions	
Introduction			
Background and objectives	3	Provide an explicit statement of the broader context for the study. Present the study question and its relevance for health policy or practice decisions	

(*continued*)

EXHIBIT 2.3 CHEERS Checklist for Journal Report (*continued*)

Section/Topic	#	Recommendation	Reported on page no./line no.
Methods			
Target population and subgroups	4	Describe characteristics of the base-case population and subgroups	
Setting and location	5	State relevant aspects of the system(s) in which the decision(s) need(s) to be made	
Study perspective	6	Describe the perspective of the study and relate this to the costs being evaluated	
Comparators	7	Describe the interventions or strategies being compared and state why they were chosen	
Time horizon	8	State the time horizon(s) over which costs and consequences are being evaluated and say why appropriate	
Discount rate	9	Report the choice of discount rate(s) used for costs and outcomes and say why appropriate	
Choice of health outcomes	10	Describe what outcomes were used as the measure(s) of benefit in the evaluation and their relevance for the type of analysis performed	
Measurement of effectiveness	11a	Single study-based estimates: Describe fully the design features of the single effectiveness study and why the single study was a sufficient source of clinical effectiveness data	
	11b	Synthesis-based estimates: Describe fully the methods used for identification of included studies and synthesis of clinical effectiveness data	
Measurement/valuation of preference based outcomes	12	If applicable, describe the population and methods used to elicit preferences for outcomes	
Estimating resources and costs	13a	Single study-based economic evaluation: Describe approaches used to estimate resource use associated with the alternative interventions. Describe primary or secondary research methods for valuing each resource item in terms of its unit cost. Describe any adjustments made to approximate to opportunity costs.	
	13b	Model-based economic evaluation: Describe approaches and data sources used to estimate resource use associated with model health states. Describe primary or secondary research methods for valuing each resource item in terms of its unit cost. Describe any adjustments made to approximate to opportunity costs.	
Currency, price, date, and conversion	14	Report the dates of the estimated resource quantities and unit costs. Describe methods for adjusting estimated unit costs to the year of reported costs if necessary. Describe methods for converting costs into a common currency base and the exchange rate.	
Choice of model	15	Describe and give reasons for the specific type of decision-analytical model used. Providing a figure to show model structure is strongly recommended	

(*continued*)

EXHIBIT 2.3   CHEERS Checklist for Journal Report (*continued*)

Section/Topic	#	Recommendation	Reported on page no./line no.
Assumptions	16	Describe all structural or other assumptions underpinning the decision analytical model	
Analytical methods	17	Describe all analytical methods supporting the evaluation. This could include methods for dealing with skewed, missing, or censored data; extrapolation methods; methods for pooling data; approaches to validate or make adjustments (e.g., half-cycle corrections) to a model; and methods for handling population heterogeneity and uncertainty.	
Results			
Study parameters	18	Report the values, ranges, references, and, if used, probability distributions for all parameters. Report reasons or sources for distributions used to represent uncertainty where appropriate. Providing a table to show the input values is strongly recommended	
Incremental costs and outcomes	19	For each intervention, report mean values for the main categories of estimated costs and outcomes of interest, as well as mean differences between the comparator groups. If applicable, report incremental cost effectiveness ratios	
Characterizing uncertainty	20a	Single study-based economic evaluation: Describe the effects of sampling uncertainty for the estimated incremental cost and incremental effectiveness parameters, together with the impact of methodological assumptions (e.g., discount rate, study perspective)	
	20b	Model-based economic evaluation: Describe the effects on the results of uncertainty for all input parameters, and uncertainty related to the structure of the model and assumptions	
Characterizing heterogeneity	21	If applicable, report differences in costs, outcomes, or cost-effectiveness that can be explained by variations between subgroups of patients with different baseline characteristics or other observed variability in effects that are not reducible by more information	
Discussion			
Study findings, limitations, generalizability, and current knowledge	22	Summarize key study findings and describe how they support the conclusions reached. Discuss limitations and the generalizability of the findings and how the findings fit with current knowledge	
Other			
Sources of funding	23	Describe how the study was funded and the role of the funder in the identification, design, conduct, and reporting of the analysis. Describe other non-monetary sources of support	
Conflicts of interest	24	Describe any potential for conflict of interest of study contributors in accordance with journal policy. In the absence of a journal policy, we recommend authors comply with International Committee of Medical Journal Editors recommendations	

CHEERS, Consolidated Health Economic Evaluation Reporting Standards.
Source: Adapted from Husereau et al. (2013).

The quality of studies has been variable and not necessarily improving. As more studies are conducted and submitted for peer-reviewed publication, editors are not always able to find reviewers with the appropriate expertise; hence, studies that are poorly conducted in general or for which specific elements are poor can make their way into print. APRNs who plan to read these analyses need to understand methodology enough to recognize what makes a good study and what makes a study that is barely acceptable or even fails the test of acceptability.

APRNs interested in exploring this type of outcome evaluation are encouraged to seek additional training in these methods.

If APRNs participate in and conduct economic evaluations concerning the care they provide, the cost-effectiveness of APRN care may be demonstrated. When the analysis uses a standard methodology and the assumptions are transparent, the results are more easily interpreted. If the outcome measure is a standard ratio, such as dollars per QALY gained, the results may furnish a strong argument to health policy decision makers concerning the funding and continued recognition of APRNs as cost-effective health care providers.

Answers to Chapter Discussion Questions

1. Both comparative effectiveness and cost-effectiveness are forms of research that determine relative effectiveness of an intervention, diagnostic procedure, or preventive strategy in a real-world environment. Cost-effectiveness methodology contrasts two or more interventions by including economic outcome(s). Comparative-effectiveness methodology compares a potentially broader range of benefits and harms in the everyday environment, but does not necessarily include economic outcomes or analysis. A business case analysis focuses on monetary outcomes for a single organization using the organization's own comparison of current and future costs and revenue. Relevant health care results are described but not included directly in a calculation.

2. CUA presents outcomes in terms of cost per QALY gained. Therefore, scenarios in which quality of life, mortality, as well as cost are of interest would be appropriate. For example, Biesheuvel-Leliefeld et al. (2012) designed a cost–utility study to test the quality of life improvement of a nursing-led intervention for recurrent major depressive disorder, and reported in cost per QALY gained.

3. Cost–consequence methodology is intended for subjects with multiple relevant outcome measures, often when these outcomes cannot be summarized into a single measure. Cost and consequences are listed from each intervention of interest in the results and analysis.

4. CBA requires that the benefits of the tested interventions be monetized. Therefore, a researcher must assume a particular monetary value that accurately represents derived benefit or QALY gained, which may be controversial. The outcome measure for CBA is a dollar amount that is the sum of all costs minus the benefits. In this way, the costs and benefits are compared in the same units, which is particularly helpful if potential benefits include nonclinical parameters (Riegelman, 2012).

5. The first step is to identify all the factors that will influence the total cost of the therapy. These may include the price of the antibiotic itself, the nurse's time for preparation, the patient's time in the clinical setting, and any physical materials for preparation (e.g., needle, syringe, tubing) depending on the study perspective. Benefits may include shortened time in the hospital, reduced complications, and fewer rehospitalizations. The second step would be assigning a dollar value to each cost and benefit, as exemplified in the methods of Weiss, Yakusheva, and Bobay (2011).

WEB LINKS

- CEA Registry website: A database of medical publications containing CEA that have been audited by the Center for the Evaluation of Value and Risk in Health (CEVR), part of the Institute for Clinical Research and Health Policy Studies at Tufts Medical Center. All papers included are original analyses, written in English, and use QALY outcome measure(s). The website also includes a dictionary of relevant economic terms among other resources.
  healtheconomics.tuftsmedicalcenter.org/cear4/Home.aspx
- Board of Governors of the Federal Reserve System: On this website, the Federal Reserve offers exchange rates between the U.S. dollar and foreign currencies annually, monthly, and daily, recorded as far back as 1971. These data are useful if research analyses require converting values to or from U.S. currency for the sake of comparison between or aggregation of costs in a common monetary unit.
  www.federalreserve.gov/releases/g5a/current/default.htm
- BLS: The BLS website (www.bls.gov) lists CPI, which allows comparison for the real value of money between time periods. The CPI calculator can determine conversion of the U.S. dollar's value between any years ranging from 1913 to present.
  data.bls.gov/cgi-bin/cpicalc.pl
- Federal Reserve Bank of St. Louis Economic Data (FRED): This website offers extensive economic indicator data useful for economic analyses. For example, these data include the U.S. inflation rate by day, month, or year.
  research.stlouisfed.org
- Health Economics Resource Center (HERC): HERC is a resource for cost-effectiveness research that includes help identifying costs, definitions of economic concepts, and a bibliography of over 300 cost-effectiveness studies. This U.S. Department of Veterans Affairs website also contains actual Veterans Affairs health-economic data with registration.
  www.herc.research.va.gov/include/page.asp?id=cost-effectiveness-analysis
  www.herc.research.va.gov/include/page.asp?id=budget-impact-analysis

REFERENCES

Armstrong, E. P., Malone, D. C., & Erder, M. H. (2008). A Markov cost-utility analysis of escitalopram and duloxetine for the treatment of major depressive disorder. *Current Medical Research and Opinion*, 24(4), 1115–1121. doi:10.1185/030079908X273309

Beaver, K., Hollingworth, W., McDonald, R., Dunn, G., Tysver-Robinson, D., Thomson, L., . . . Luker, K. (2009). Economic evaluation of a randomized clinical trial of hospital *versus* telephone follow-up after treatment for breast cancer. *British Journal of Surgery, 96*(12), 1406–1415. doi:10.1002/bjs.6753

Bhandari, S. (2011). Update of a comparative analysis of cost minimization following the introduction of newly available intravenous iron therapies in hospital practice. *Therapeutics and Clinical Risk Management, 7,* 501–509. doi:10.2147/TCRM.S25882

Biesheuvel-Leliefeld, K. E., Kersten, S. M., van der Horst, H. E., van Schaik, A., Bockting, C. L., Bosmans, J. E., . . . van Marwijk, H. W. (2012). Cost-effectiveness of nurse-led self-help for recurrent depression in the primary care setting: Design of a pragmatic randomised controlled trial. *BMC Psychiatry, 12,* 59. doi:10.1186/1471-244X-12-59

Blakely, T., Collinson, L., Kvizhinadze, G., Nair, N., Foster, R., Dennett, E., & Sarfati, D. (2015). Cancer care coordinators in stage III colon cancer: A cost-utility analysis. *BMC Health Services Research, 15,* 306. doi:10.1186/s12913-015-0970-5

Brouwer, W. B., & Koopmanschap, M. A. (2005). The friction-cost method: Replacement for nothing and leisure for free? *Pharmacoeconomics, 23*(2), 105–111.

Bryant-Lukosius, D., Carter, N., Reid, K., Donald, F., Martin-Misener, R., Kilpatrick, K., . . . DiCenso, A. (2015). The clinical effectiveness and cost-effectiveness of clinical nurse specialist-led hospital to home transitional care: A systematic review. *Journal of Evaluation in Clinical Practice, 21*(5), 763–781. doi:10.1111/jep.12401

Campbell, J. L., Fletcher, E., Britten, N., Green, C., Holt, T. A., Lattimer, V., . . . Taylor, R. S. (2014). Telephone triage for management of same-day consultation requests in general practice (the ESTEEM trial): A cluster-randomised controlled trial and cost-consequence analysis. *The Lancet, 384*(9957), 1859–1868. doi:10.1016/S0140-6736(14)61058-8

Centers for Medicare & Medicaid Services. (2016, August 10). NHE fact sheet. *National Health Expenditure Data.* Retrieved from https://www.cms.gov/research-statistics-data-and-systems/statistics-trends-and-reports/nationalhealthexpenddata/nhe-fact-sheet.html

Chernew, M. (2015). Interpreting new data on health care spending growth. *Health Affairs Blog.* Retrieved from http://healthaffairs.org/blog/2015/12/02/interpreting-new-data-on-health-care-spending-growth

Cohen, C. C., Choi, Y. J., & Stone, P. W. (2016). Costs of infection prevention practices in long-term care settings: A systematic review. *Nursing Economic, 34*(1), 16–24.

Determinants of health economic decisions in actual practice: The role of behavioral economics. (2006). Summary of the presentation given by Professor Daniel Kahneman at the ISPOR 10th Annual International Meeting First Plenary Session, May 16, 2005, Washington, DC, USA. *Value Health, 9*(2), 65–67. doi:10.1111/j.1524-4733.2006.00084.x

Drummond, M. F., Sculpher, M. J., Claxton, K., Stoddart, G. L., & Torrance, G. W. (2015). *Methods for the economic evaluation of health care programmes* (4th ed.). Oxford, UK: Oxford University Press.

Eldessouki, R., & Smith, M. D. (2012). Health care system information sharing: A step toward better health globally. *Value Health Regional, 1,* 118–120.

Fatoye, F., & Haigh, C. (2016). The cost-effectiveness of semi-rigid ankle brace to facilitate return to work following first-time acute ankle sprains. *Journal of Clinical Nursing, 25*(9–10), 1435–1443. doi:10.1111/jocn.13255

Federal Coordinating Council for Comparative Effectiveness Research. (2009). *Report to the President and the Congress*. Washington, DC: U.S. Department of Health and Human Services.

Garber, A. M. (2011). How the Patient-Centered Outcomes Research Institute can best influence real-world health care decision making. *Health Affairs, 30*(12), 2243–2251. doi:10.1377/hlthaff.2010.0255

Gold, M. R., Siegel, J. E., Russell, L. B., & Weinstein, M. C. (1996). *Cost effectiveness in health and medicine*. New York, NY: Oxford University Press.

Haddix, A. C., Teutsch, S. M., & Corso, P. S. (2002). *Prevention effectiveness: A guide to decision analysis and economic evaluation* (2nd ed.). New York, NY: Oxford University Press.

Hunter, R. (2015). Cost-effectiveness of point-of-care C-reactive protein tests for respiratory tract infection in primary care in England. *Advances in Therapy, 32*(1), 69–85. doi:10.1007/s12325-015-0180-x

Husereau, D., Drummond, M., Petrou, S., Carswell, C., Moher, D., Greenberg, D., . . . Loder, E. (2013). Consolidated Health Economic Evaluation Reporting Standards (CHEERS) statement. *The European Journal of Health Economics, 14*(3), 367–372. doi:10.1007/s10198-013-0471-6

Iglehart, J. K. (2009). Prioritizing comparative-effectiveness research—IOM recommendations. *The New England Journal of Medicine, 361*(4), 325–328. doi:10.1056/NEJMp0904133

International Society for Pharmacoeconomics and Outcomes Research. (2016). ISPOR 21st Annual International Meeting: Released Presentations. Retrieved from http://www.ispor.org/Event/ReleasedPresentations/2016Washington

Jacobs, P., & Fassbender, K. (1998). The measurement of indirect costs in the health economics evaluation literature: A review. *International Journal of Technology Assessment in Health Care, 14*(4), 799–808.

Jacobson, G. A. (2007). *CRS report for Congress: Comparative clinical effectiveness and cost-effectiveness research: Background, history and overview*. (Vol. RL34208). Washington, DC: Congressional Research Service.

Jeon, Y. H., Simpson, J. M., Li, Z., Cunich, M. M., Thomas, T. H., Chenoweth, L., & Kendig, H. L. (2015). Cluster randomized controlled trial of an aged care specific leadership and management program to improve work environment, staff turnover, and care quality. *Journal of the American Medical Directors Association, 16*(7), 629.e19–629.e28. doi:10.1016/j.jamda.2015.04.005

Kang, J., Mandsager, P., Biddle, A. K., & Weber, D. J. (2012). Cost-effectiveness analysis of active surveillance screening for methicillin-resistant *Staphylococcus aureus* in an academic hospital setting. *Infection Control & Hospital Epidemiology, 33*(5), 477–486. doi:10.1086/665315

Krahn, M., Guasparini, R., Sherman, M., & Detsky, A. S. (1998). Costs and cost-effectiveness of a universal, school-based hepatitis B vaccination program. *American Journal of Public Health, 88*(11), 1638–1644.

Krol, M., Brouwer, W., & Rutten, F. (2013). Productivity costs in economic evaluations: Past, present, future. *PharmacoEconomics, 31*(7), 537–549. doi:10.1007/s40273-013-0056-3

Liljas, B. (1998). How to calculate indirect costs in economic evaluations. *PharmacoEconomics, 13*(1, Pt. 1), 1–7.

Luce, B. R., Manning, W. G., Siegel, J. E., & Lipscomb, J. (1996). Estimating costs in cost-effectiveness analysis. In J. E. S. M. Gold, L. Russell, & M. Weinstein (Ed.), *Cost-effectiveness in health and medicine* (pp. 176–213). New York, NY: Oxford University Press.

Marsden, G., Jones, K., Neilson, J., Avital, L., Collier, M., & Stansby, G. (2015). A cost-effectiveness analysis of two different repositioning strategies for the prevention of pressure ulcers. *Journal of Advanced Nursing, 71*(12), 2879–2885. doi:10.1111/jan.12753

Martin-Misener, R., Harbman, P., Donald, F., Reid, K., Kilpatrick, K., Carter, N., . . . DiCenso, A. (2015). Cost-effectiveness of nurse practitioners in primary and specialised ambulatory care: Systematic review. *BMJ Open, 5*(6), e007167. doi:10.1136/bmjopen-2014-007167

Moradi-Lakeh, M., Shakerian, S., & Esteghamati, A. (2012). Immunization against Haemophilus Influenzae Type b in Iran; Cost-utility and cost-benefit analyses. *International Journal of Preventive Medicine, 3*(5), 332–340.

Neumann, P. J., Cohen, J. T., & Weinstein, M. C. (2014). Updating cost-effectiveness—the curious resilience of the $50,000-per-QALY threshold. *The New Englad Journal of Medicine, 371*(9), 796–797. doi:10.1056/NEJMp1405158

Neumann, P. J., Sanders, G. D., Russell, L. B., Siegel, J. E., & Ganiats, T. G. (Eds.). (2016). Cost-effectiveness in health and medicine (2nd ed.). New York, NY: Oxford University Press.

Patient-Centered Outcomes Research Institute. (2014, October 6). About us. Retrieved from http://www.pcori.org/about-us

Penz, E. D., Mishra, E. K., Davies, H. E., Manns, B. J., Miller, R. F., & Rahman, N. M. (2014). Comparing cost of indwelling pleural catheter vs talc pleurodesis for malignant pleural effusion. *Chest, 146*(4), 991–1000. doi:10.1378/chest.13-2481

Petitti, D. B. (2000). *Meta-analysis, decision analysis, and cost-effectiveness analysis: Methods for quantitative synthesis in medicine* (2nd ed.). New York, NY: Oxford University Press.

Riegelman, R. K. (2012). *Studying a study and testing a test* (6th ed.). Philadelphia, PA: Lippincott Williams & Wilkins.

Rovner, J. (2016, September 13). A record percentage of Americans now have health insurance. *Time.* Retrieved from http://time.com/money/4490196/health-insurance-coverage-census-2015

Ryan, P., Revill, P., Devane, D., & Normand, C. (2013). An assessment of the cost-effectiveness of midwife-led care in the United Kingdom. *Midwifery, 29*(4), 368–376. doi:10.1016/j.midw .2012.02.005

Schoonhoven, L., van Gaal, B. G., Teerenstra, S., Adang, E., van der Vleuten, C., & van Achterberg, T. (2015). Cost-consequence analysis of "washing without water" for nursing home residents: A cluster randomized trial. *International Journal of Nursing Studies, 52*(1), 112–120. doi:10.1016/j .ijnurstu.2014.08.001

Schuurman, J. P., Schoonhoven, L., Defloor, T., van Engelshoven, I., van Ramshorst, B., & Buskens, E. (2009). Economic evaluation of pressure ulcer care: A cost minimization analysis of preventive strategies. *Nursing Economic, 27*(6), 390–400, 415.

Stone, P. W. (1998). Methods for conducting and reporting cost-effectiveness analysis in nursing. *Image—the Journal of Nursing Scholarship, 30*(3), 229–234.

Stone, P. W. (2001a). Dollars and sense: A primer for the novice in economic analyses (Part I). *Applied Nursing Research, 14*(1), 54–55. doi:10.1053/apnr.2001.21025

Stone, P. W. (2001b). Dollars and sense: A primer for the novice in economic analyses (Part II). *Applied Nursing Research, 14*(2), 110–112. doi:10.1053/apnr.2001.22379

Stone, P. W., Chapman, R. H., Sandberg, E. A., Liljas, B., & Neumann, P. J. (2000). Measuring costs in cost-utility analyses: Variations in the literature. *International Journal of Technology Assessment in Health Care, 16*(1), 111–124.

Theis, J. L., & Finkelstein, M. J. (2014). Long-term effects of safe patient handling program on staff injuries. *Rehabilitation Nursing, 39*(1), 26–35. doi:10.1002/rnj.108

Twigg, D. E., Myers, H., Duffield, C., Giles, M., & Evans, G. (2015). Is there an economic case for investing in nursing care–what does the literature tell us? *Journal of Advanced Nursing, 71*(5), 975–990. doi:10.1111/jan.12577

van Baal, P. H., Polder, J. J., de Wit, G. A., Hoogenveen, R. T., Feenstra, T. L., Boshuizen, H. C., . . . Brouwer, W. B. (2008). Lifetime medical costs of obesity: Prevention no cure for increasing health expenditure. *PLOS Medicine, 5*(2), e29. doi:10.1371/journal.pmed.0050029

Volpp, K. G., & Das, A. (2009). Comparative effectiveness–thinking beyond medication A versus medication B. *The New England Journal of Medicine, 361*(4), 331–333. doi:10.1056/NEJMp0903496

Wang, L. Y., Vernon-Smiley, M., Gapinski, M. A., Desisto, M., Maughan, E., & Sheetz, A. (2014). Cost-benefit study of school nursing services. *JAMA Pediatrics, 168*(7), 642–648. doi:10.1001/jamapediatrics.2013.5441

Weiss, M. E., Yakusheva, O., & Bobay, K. L. (2011). Quality and cost analysis of nurse staffing, discharge preparation, and postdischarge utilization. *Health Services Research, 46*(5), 1473–1494. doi:10.1111/j.1475-6773.2011.01267.x

Young, D. W. (2012). *Management control in nonprofit organizations* (9th ed.). Cambridge, MA: Crimson Press.

CHAPTER 3

Selecting Advanced Practice Nursing Outcome Measures

Beth D. Quatrara and Katherine Dale Shaw

Chapter Objectives

1. Discuss reasons why measuring outcomes of advanced practice registered nurses (APRNs) is essential to the role of the APRN
2. Identify at least three outcome measure categories that can be influenced by an APRN
3. Discuss the benefits and pitfalls of using benchmark/aggregate data to measure APRN outcomes
4. Describe methods to measure and monitor APRN outcome data

Chapter Discussion Questions

1. Why is establishing a clear goal and defined outcome an important step early in the assessment process?
2. Why are some data points considered less desirable APRN outcome measures than others?
3. Why is a trending data over time a valuable strategy for recording APRN outcomes?
4. What are the key elements of APRN outcome measures?

Changes in the health care landscape are emphasizing the need for providers to demonstrate outcomes. Government regulatory agencies, insurance companies, and institutional administrators expect high-quality patient care outcomes at the individual and aggregate levels in order to improve overall health and reduce fiscal waste. Standard process outcomes such as productivity and adherence are no longer as valued as the results of the care provided or the services rendered. Data pointing to the volume of patients seen or compliance with an established guideline is often considered inadequate if it fails to further demonstrate a resulting improvement in patient care.

As health care providers, APRNs are increasingly being asked to demonstrate the effectiveness of their roles. In some cases, the inability of an APRN to do so results in the dissolution of the role. APRNs must be thoughtful in demonstrating their effectiveness and "value-added" benefit to the institutions and communities in which they practice.

Well-controlled studies on APRN outcomes continue to be relatively scant (Bryant-Lukosius et al., 2015; Donald et al., 2015; Newhouse et al., 2011; Stanik-Hutt et al., 2013). However, some do exist and suggest that APRNs "provide safe, effective, quality care to a number of specific populations in a variety of settings" (Newhouse et al., 2011; Stanik-Hutt, 2013). The studies on APRN outcomes are extremely helpful as guides to APRN practice. While more studies are needed on APRN roles in specific settings, clinicians in practice must continue to demonstrate the effectiveness of their roles in less labor-intensive ways than performing research studies on a day-to-day basis. To that end, the purpose of this chapter is to describe a number of different methods and outcome measures that might be used to evaluate an APRN's contributions to quality patient care. Examples of actual APRN outcome projects will illustrate the methods and demonstrate the importance of determining appropriate outcome data for measurement.

SELECTING APRN ROLE-SENSITIVE OUTCOME MEASURES

A common approach used to determine APRN outcomes is to attempt to link aggregate data such as length of stay (LOS) and cost per case to APRN practice. While these types of measurements are important and helpful in some cases, they are generally not sensitive enough to clearly demonstrate the APRN's unique contribution. Rarely does aggregate data show the causal effect of an individual on a patient population; there are simply too many intervening variables that may have contributed to the effect (this is discussed in depth later in the chapter). Thus, it is important to consider other, more sensitive indicators. There is also a practical reason for carefully selecting outcome variables; APRNs are busy and data collection takes time. The data that the APRN collects should be easy to obtain and should be specific to the APRN's role. With the proliferation of electronic health records (EHRs) and other electronic systems and databases, data collection should be simplified through the generation of reports. However, the data collected should be limited to carefully selected role-sensitive indicators and the tendency to pull a plethora of semirelated data elements avoided. Reviewing unnecessary and tangentially related data distracts from the true outcome measure and wastes valuable APRN time. If hand-collected data are required they should be minimized to essential elements only. If the data-collection burden is too great, it is unlikely that the required metrics will be routinely collected. Unfortunately, many APRNs are averse to collecting data and having to demonstrate the value of their efforts. In addition, the APRNs may feel that data collection distracts them from their primary roles as clinical experts. But, if the outcome measures are carefully selected, the data will not only help to clarify the APRN's value to the health care system, but may also be used to focus the role accordingly.

When an APRN is hired, the administrator and physician (if applicable) to whom the APRN will report will generally have a specific role or function in mind (clinical nurse specialist [CNS], nurse practitioner [NP], certified registered nurse anesthetist [CRNA], or certified nurse-midwife [CNM]). Following role negotiation, the APRN should begin establishing targeted outcome measures that are mutually agreed upon by the APRN and the individual who hired the APRN. Setting the outcome measures early in the role negotiation process (or prior to starting any new project) allows the APRN to identify currently available data sources and define the specific metrics within a defined time frame, which will be attributable to his or her efforts. Examples of role-specific outcome measures follow and an example of an APRN outcome planning, tracking, and reporting worksheet is found in Exhibit 3.1.

ACUTE CARE NURSE PRACTITIONER FOR A MEDICAL ACUTE CARE UNIT

If the role is that of acute care nurse practitioner (ACNP) for a medical acute care floor, the collaborating physician and institutional leadership may be interested in the number of ACNP-managed patients requiring 30-day readmissions within a selected time interval. These data are relatively easy to collect and can be obtained from institutional EHRs or clinical data repositories. The ACNP will need to maintain a secure database of his or her discharged patients in order to query the system on a regular basis (e.g., every 2 months, quarterly, yearly). It may be desirable to compare these to other health care provider data as well, while being mindful that readmissions to outside facilities may not be easy to determine and are important for the accuracy of the report. The ACNP may consider further focusing his or her efforts on strategies to reduce 30-day readmissions within a specific high-risk population. For example, chronic obstructive pulmonary disease patients may be a complex population that warrants the attention of the ACNP. Further analyzing the 30-day readmission rates for this provider within the subcategory of a patient population could produce valuable insights into the care of these patients.

ACUTE OR CRITICAL CARE CLINICAL NURSE SPECIALIST

The role of CNS generally encompasses all the domains of advanced practice (e.g., clinical management, education, research, consultation, and change agency). However, it may be that outcome measures may focus on only one or two measures of role effectiveness and that these may change over time. For example, the administrator and CNS may agree that one key objective for the year is to improve medication safety (i.e., medication errors). The CNS in this example might partner with the quality assurance (QA) department to track unit medication errors following the implementation of a CNS educational and evidence-based practice change initiative. A trended line chart might be used to graphically demonstrate the change in percentage of medication errors per time interval. In this case, the APRN does not actually need to collect data but instead partners with the QA department to ensure that the intervention date (i.e., training of staff and evidence-based change) is marked accurately on the chart. Very few examples like this one would be needed to demonstrate the APRN's

EXHIBIT 3.1   **APRN Outcome Planning, Tracking, and Reporting Worksheet**

APRN Name _____

Date _____

Manager _____ Administrator _____

Area of Outcome Focus: Brief title summarizing the activities described below.

Problem Statement: Briefly describe needed practice change and rationale.

Specific Goals: The APRN and administrator meet to mutually agree on the goals for each evaluation time period.

Process/Methods/Interventions: Describe intended approach and evolution of plans, if any.

Describe the data-collection method:

- Existing data source _____
- Data prospectively collected _____

IRB Approval Number: _____ (if needed for your initiative)

Describe Measurable Goals	Source for Measurement	Timeline
1. (add rows as needed)		Progress by: Completion by:

Progress Reports: As appropriate, APRN should log and date periodic notes for each goal.

Measurement and Reporting of Outcomes: Brief summary of findings and lessons learned. Graphical representation of the outcome variable of interest pre- and postintervention/initiative is encouraged.

Outcomes Apply to:

- Metrics important to the institution (e.g., LOS, UTI). Describe: _____
- Implement and sustain an evidence-based unit or institutional practice change. Describe: _____
- Improve metrics over time in a patient population. Describe: _____
- Improve satisfaction, knowledge, adherence to guidelines, and development of others. Describe: _____
- Other. Describe: _____

Staff Assisting With Outcome Activities: Give names and credentials.

References: Evidence-based literature/guideline that supports the change.

APRN, advanced practice registered nurse; IRB, institutional review board; LOS, length of stay; UTI, urinary tract infection.
Source: Adapted for use with permission of University of Virginia Professional Nursing Staff Organization, University of Virginia, Charlottesville, VA (copyright 2011).

worth to the institution. More importantly, the APRN can use the data to readjust or change the intervention if necessary. See Figure 3.1 for an example of a trended line chart.

The CNS may also monitor the effect of a change initiative on practice and patient outcomes. Perhaps the initiative is one designed to incorporate prone positioning into the care management protocol for patients with acute respiratory distress syndrome (ARDS). A prospective audit by the CNS following implementation of the educational and competency-based initiative would be relatively easy to accomplish while the CNS is on the unit. Elements to track would be protocol adherence (i.e., was it implemented), accuracy (i.e., was it done correctly), and the patient outcome (i.e., what was the patient's response: PaO_2 following prone positioning, physiologic tolerance). Little data collection

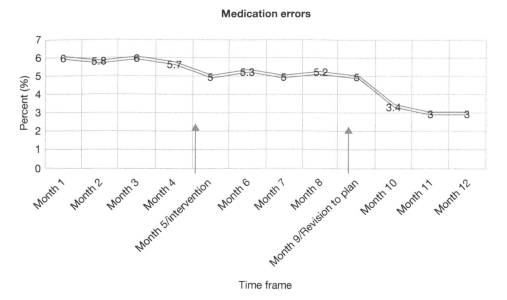

FIGURE 3.1 Trended line chart.

Note: Baseline data demonstrated a higher than desired percentage of medication error. The goal of the medication error initiative was to reduce the percentage of errors below 5. The initial intervention at month 5 demonstrated a reduction but did not achieve the goal. The subsequent revision to the plan at month 9 succeeded in achieving the goal. The trended line chart allowed the clinical nurse specialist to follow progress over time, intervene as appropriate, and demonstrate sustained improvement.

would be necessary since the patient population is discrete and maneuver is generally used infrequently. The reason such an initiative is a reasonable one to use as a CNS outcome is because the procedure is potentially risky and is almost entirely nurse managed. The CNS's effectiveness in safely implementing such a protocol is essential as it speaks to integration of all the CNS role components and demonstrates effective leadership and follow-through. In addition, the CNS can use the data to quickly adapt and adjust the protocol as needed. This "real-time" monitoring with short cycles of intervention, evaluation, and correction ensures quality.

Some specific categories of outcome measures and the associated issues with each are discussed in the text that follows.

CATEGORIES OF APRN OUTCOME DATA

A variety of indicators may be used to demonstrate the effectiveness of an APRN. The strengths and weaknesses of the indicators are described in examples that follow.

Satisfaction (Patient, Family, Caregivers, and Physician)

Satisfaction is a variable that speaks directly to the institution's "market share" of customers. If customer satisfaction is not good, the customer will not return. In addition, the customer's negative advertisement of the hospital will have far-reaching implications for the institution. As noted in the business industry, 95% of customers will share a bad experience while 87% will share a good experience (Dimensional Research, 2013). Furthermore, 54% will share the bad experience with more than five people while 33% will share a good experience with more than five people (Dimensional Research, 2013). Few hospitals exist today that are arrogant enough to ignore satisfaction as an outcome measure. However, as we know, satisfaction is not always synonymous with quality. Regardless, it is an important variable to monitor, particularly for hospitals that participate in the Centers for Medicare and Medicaid's Hospital Consumer Assessment of Healthcare Providers and Systems (HCAHPS) surveys. These publicly reported ratings of patient perceptions of care are measures with significant impact on financial outcomes.

Most institutions routinely measure patient satisfaction in a global manner. Like other aggregate data, it is hard to specifically attribute the outcomes to APRN practice. For example, in many cases, the satisfaction instrument will not distinguish the APRN from the bedside nurse or the physician. Further complicating the matter, many institutions collect data related only to the service line (i.e., medicine or surgery). Thus, for satisfaction to be linked to APRN practice, a separate survey may be necessary. However, even this may be a stumbling block. In some institutions, patient satisfaction surveys are closely controlled and may be distributed only via the institutional mechanism in place. There are good reasons for this; the institution does not want the patients and families "bothered" with numerous forms and questionnaires. Further, more specific and detailed questions are difficult to design, take the patient additional time to complete, and often require interpretation. If satisfaction is a desired APRN outcome measure, it is necessary to determine whether the existing institutional survey is sensitive enough. If not, the APRN may need to design his or her own survey, if permissible within the institutional structure.

If an institutional survey is used to measure APRN satisfaction outcomes, it is best to directly target a specific question(s). This is exemplified by an ACNP who wanted to improve patients' pain management satisfaction scores. She identified the following survey questions as targeted outcome measures for unit: "how well was pain controlled" and "nurses kept me informed." She designed a project to address these specific satisfaction measures by providing education about medication availability, timing, and by involving patients in their own pharmacologic pain management regimen. This nursing intervention provided patients with the information they needed to improve their pain management and empowered them to control the discomfort. The intervention was successful. Using the institutional survey data, the ACNP was able to demonstrate a sustained improvement in satisfaction scores, a valuable institutional outcome (Figure 3.2).

However, there are times when a broad institutional survey cannot address the unique attributes of a particular customer service initiative. Although difficult as described, it may be possible to use a separate survey to determine customer satisfaction with a specific intervention without overtaxing the survey process or overburdening patients and families. A key to success lies with introducing a well-timed, brief, and focused survey. For example, an operating room (OR) clinical research team implemented a new perioperative communication plan to evaluate the effect on family member anxiety and satisfaction. The communication plan included regularly scheduled OR nurse updates to a designated family member from the perioperative team on his or her loved one's status throughout the surgery. With minimal intrusion, family members who were receiving

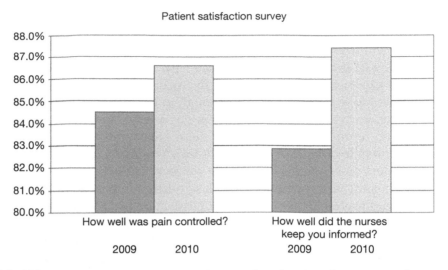

FIGURE 3.2 APRN-directed pain management intervention: Results of patient satisfaction survey.
APRN, advanced practice registered nurse.

the status updates responded to a short questionnaire about the experience. The survey participation rate was high. The satisfaction data directly demonstrated customer satisfaction with the new communication plan (Figure 3.3). Such interventions can directly contribute to an increased overall customer service rating but the outcome cannot be attributed to the APRN-led project without specific data.

Surveys of staff and physician satisfaction may also be an effective and useful measure of APRN practice. The satisfaction of caregivers is important because their dissatisfaction can affect recruitment, retention, quality of care, and other financial outcomes. According to the 2016 National Health Care Retention Survey, institutional costs

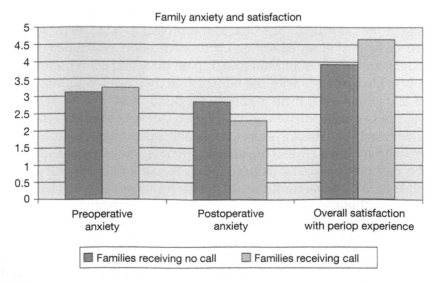

FIGURE 3.3 Survey results comparing preoperative and postoperative satisfaction of patients' families related to communication intervention.

of nursing turnover are cited to be $37,700 to $58,400 (United States) per nurse (NSI Nursing Staffing Solutions, 2016). Additionally, frequent turnover makes the assurance of quality care difficult. It is costly (in time and money) to provide enough training to ensure the basic competency of "safe" care delivery following orientation. In this time of a "nursing shortage," retention is essential, and nurses' satisfaction with their work environment, professional development opportunities, and ability to "make a contribution in a collaborative manner" are important variables to consider. The APRN may well have an important part to play in satisfaction as it relates to one or more of these variables. Satisfaction surveys related to these and other specific aspects of APRN practice may be useful and relatively easy to accomplish via mechanisms such as the unit or service line intranet.

Physician satisfaction is another variable that may be measured. The physician generates revenue and the APRNs with whom they work contribute to the efficiency and effectiveness of the physicians' practice. In these cases, physician satisfaction with the collaborative relationship and the results of the same are important to follow.

Additional considerations for the APRN with regard to the development and use of satisfaction surveys include decisions related to whether or not the project must be reviewed and approved by the facility's institutional review board (IRB) before implementation. If the information received from the survey is de-identified, it is likely that the project will receive an "exempt status" approval from the IRB. However, in some institutions, a satisfaction survey must seek approval via the QA department or sometimes a nursing research department. It is the responsibility of the APRN to proceed via appropriate channels. A second and important consideration when designing satisfaction surveys is that of the validity and reliability of the instrument. If it is not a tested instrument, the survey may provide inaccurate and erroneous answers. To avoid this potential stumbling block, use of an existing tested instrument is preferable.

Clinical Outcome Measures

APRN-sensitive clinical outcomes may be difficult to identify because many factors may potentially affect them. It is important to remember that clinical outcome measures need not be inclusive of everything the APRN practice may affect, but rather those that are the most easily and clearly attributed to the APRN practice. For example, consider the NP charged with managing the care of a neurosurgical patient population. Because, in this case, the NP's role is focused on managing the medical aspects of care of the patients, selected aspects of care may yield sensitive indicators of effectiveness. Examples include such indicators as urinary tract infection (because the NP is responsible for ordering catheter removal), decubitus ulcer formation (secondary to initiation of mobilization), and selected discharge outcomes.

A common error made by APRNs who manage large groups of patients is to collect a large data set in the hope that it will show something. This approach, "fishing in the data," is unnecessary and a poor use of the APRN's time. A rule of thumb, as with any research study, is that the question should be clear and the variables of interest, measurable. For example, perhaps the APRN's role is focused on improving the outcomes of patients who require prolonged mechanical ventilation. It is important that the APRN have benchmark data available on ventilator duration so that a comparison may be made. LOS, though sometimes related to ventilator duration, may not be directly affected by the APRN since the clinician's role may not extend to the unit to which the patient is transferred following successful weaning. In contrast, duration of ventilation may be attributable if the APRN is the one charged with ensuring proper application of, and adherence to, a weaning protocol. In this example, the data are relatively easy to collect because they are congruent with the role of the APRN and can be easily collected in the course of a practice day.

Another outcome directly attributable to an APRN may be defined through attention to the details of medication reconciliation. The 2016 National Patient Safety Goals for Hospitals includes this requirement:

> Record and pass along correct information about a patient's medicines. Find out what medicines the patient is taking. Compare those medicines to new medicines given to the patient. Make sure the patient knows which medicines to take when they [sic] are at home. Tell the patient it is important to bring their [sic] up-to-date list of medicines every time they [sic] visit a doctor. (The Joint Commission, 2016)

For one inpatient ACNP who works in an academic medical center, managing medication orders placed by different care providers is a daily activity. As the ACNP accurately verifies or properly adjusts medications to meet the needs of an individual patient, she records these data points and demonstrates her unique contribution to patient safety. By presenting her daily work in terms of her effort to meet regulatory requirements and enhance patient safety, she is actively showcasing her influence on institutional outcomes. As with any selected outcome measure, it is essential that monitoring be done long enough that the effect can be evaluated accurately. As noted earlier, clinical outcomes should be those that are directly attributable to the APRN intervention.

Efficiency (Time-Saving) Outcomes

Time and efficiency are appropriate outcome measures for APRNs and can be measured in a number of different ways. Again, the appropriateness of the measures is dependent on the specific role of the APRN. For example, if the role of the APRN is to enhance the efficiency of care for patients with sepsis, the APRN will want to evaluate the timing of the steps of the sepsis protocol as it is operationalized. Representative categories such as time until identification, time until fluids started, time until blood culture sent, and time until antibiotic administered might be selected. These details can be monitored in time segments. Once summarized, the time elements may represent opportunities for system efficiencies that ultimately influence patient outcomes. Using the timed steps, the APRN can direct interventions to target specific segments of the sepsis protocol that require modification.

In another example, an ACNP was hired to manage congestive heart failure (CHF) patients in the cardiology clinic. Prior to the ACNP's practice in the clinic, clinic patients would learn of test results upon returning to the clinic or would call the secretary or doctor to learn the results. The ACNP quickly identified that this practice was not optimal and assumed responsibility for this component of the practice, as well as management of the patients during clinic visits. Her collaborative practice allowed for an increase in the total volume of patients cared for in the clinic. Patient and family satisfaction has increased and the collaborating physician has noted that his efficiency has been enhanced. Increased physician efficiency and patient satisfaction in combination with a decreased readmission rate and increased patient volumes since the NP began her practice is convincing evidence that she is effective in her role.

Other time-related measures may demonstrate the APRN's effectiveness as well. An example might be an initiative that emerges because emergency department patients are not being seen in a timely manner and satisfaction has suffered. APRNs are frequently charged with system initiatives like this one but often do not measure the effects of the initiatives. In this case it would be appropriate to measure satisfaction and waiting times resulting from the initiative. Though in any system initiative there are numerous people who also play a role in making the approach successful, the APRN heading the project could use the results as an indication of his or her effectiveness.

Time is money, and the translation of time to money (i.e., cost savings) is relatively easy to do. This type of measure is underused by APRNs who frequently play a very important role in improving the quality and efficiency of care initiatives.

Financial Outcomes

While virtually any outcome measure can be translated into financial outcomes, some financial data are especially of interest to institutions. Financial outcomes can be presented in terms of dollars saved. Although aggregate data are difficult to relate to an individual intervention, there are times when these measures are appropriate for the situation. For example, when an acute care CNS introduced a guideline to manage patients with pancreatitis, improving LOS while simultaneously reducing readmission rates was a natural outcome to track. Once adherence was determined through chart audits, the CNS was able to use an institutional database to measure the influence of the guideline. The CNS was able to demonstrate an association between the decreased LOS and readmission rate with guideline use because she also had a strong understanding of additional variables that might contribute to these data. Although other factors were at play during the time of the guideline introduction, the guideline was the most influential change and had the largest influence on the 19.1- to 14.7-day decrease in LOS. A 4.4-day LOS change can readily be converted into institutional dollars saved.

Similarly, infection reductions can demonstrate cost savings and the benefit of the APRN role contribution to enhanced patient outcomes. When a team of APRNs introduced chlorhexidine bathing to all patients at risk for a catheter-associated urinary tract infection or central-line-associated bloodstream, they noted a significant reduction in both types of infections. Using a return on investment calculation, they translated the reduced infection rates into both lives saved and dollars retained.

Financial outcomes such as those noted previously are a clear opportunity for APRNs to designate their contributions to the fiscal health of the institution and the well-being of their patients. However, the APRN needs to establish a collaborative relationship with the quality department, supply chain, and finance team to obtain and interpret the data. Pulling upon the skills of these essential team members will help the APRN to share clean and valid results.

Aggregate Data and/or Hospital Benchmark Data

As noted earlier, aggregate data are defined as data collected and reported by organizations and/or departments (i.e., QA, clinical data repositories, or EHRs) as a sum or total over a given time period (i.e., monthly or quarterly). The data are helpful and attractive to organizations because they can be translated into financial savings (or in most cases estimates of financial savings). Despite the common use of such outcome data, it is rarely possible to attribute such data to any one source unless the outcome element is carefully selected as in the examples provided previously. For example, when a team led by an APRN wanted to develop an intervention to improve outcomes for newborns in the community, the use of aggregate data helped to establish a baseline and demonstrate a need for services. The aggregate data was further drilled down to understand the nuances of the conditions afflicting the newborns so that interventions specifically directed at the source could be established. Continuing to follow the aggregate data over time allowed the team to test the effectiveness of the initial rollout of the community-based newborn program. Paying close attention to the conditions that were cited as the rationale for the strategic interventions, the APRN can trend the results of the program with a moderate degree of certainty that the initiation of the newborn program is the primary factor at play. However, the APRN also needs to acknowledge the limitations of the aggregate set. Additional community influences should be referenced and listed as potential confounding factors. Openly expressing the limitations of any outcome report maintains the credibility of the APRN and opens the door for future improvement opportunities along a similar path.

Aggregate data are sometimes referred to as *hospital benchmark data* and are often used to compare institutional outcomes to those of other similar type facilities (academic medical centers, community hospitals, etc.). Given the volume of data available in institutional data banks, it is easy to understand why administrators and clinicians alike attempt to assign causality to this type of aggregate outcome data. The assumption that the data represent the effect of specific interventions or care is often unwarranted. This is especially a problem when an attempt is made to infer the reasons for the outcomes and impose solutions. Those upon whom the solutions are to be imposed comment that the data are not representative of their patients, that they are "sicker" or "different," and that the data are not sensitive enough to stratify appropriately. In fact, the approach often engenders irritation, frustration, and lack of buy-in for the initiative. For example, say the APRN has been charged with a hospital-wide initiative on wound care. The APRN learns that pressure ulcer rates can be retrieved from the institutional data banks by service center. Unfortunately, when the APRN tries to separate the data by specific units, she or he learns that the data are not available in that form. In fact, the data do not distinguish which patients had preexisting ulcers (and where they originated) or where the majority of the care was delivered when the ulcer developed since the "service line" designation is by discharge unit, not the unit in which the pressure ulcer developed. Thus, the data may be helpful in looking at overall hospital trends but will be less useful if a targeted intervention is to be developed. In this case, unless the APRN can drill down by examining the site of origin or use prospectively collected data to find the answers, the intervention might be applied to all the units though it may be warranted only in one.

The use of aggregate data may be helpful in following trends but may require an in-depth understanding of the variable of interest to ensure accurate interpretation. An example is the use of LOS data. Take, for example, LOS data related to patients with tracheostomies. If one institution is able to transfer patients to discharge facilities with the tracheostomies in place (and requiring mechanical ventilation), the data on LOS may be inaccurately compared to an institution where similar transfer facilities do not exist. If this fact is not understood, erroneous comparisons between the two hospitals may be made. Instead, a more sensitive indicator of quality for these patients may be weaning, reintubation rates, and ventilator duration. Institutional aggregate data are useful in some cases; however, a thorough understanding of the data is necessary if the outcomes are to be attributable to APRN practice.

SUMMARY

The current health care climate calls for attention to outcome measures. APRNs are essential to the quality system initiatives that occur in hospitals. Their work directly influences patient care outcomes, consumer satisfaction, system efficiencies, and cost savings, but too often it is not recognized because it is "invisible." Using carefully selected data to demonstrate the APRN's effect on some of these system initiatives is possible and important if APRNs are to demonstrate their "value-added" contributions. Though system outcomes may be hard to ascribe to any one individual, the contributions of APRNs are more likely to be acknowledged if data are available.

This chapter provides some examples of outcome measures that may be selected and used to accurately demonstrate the impact of APRN practice. It is essential that APRNs recognize that the measures should be selected carefully and be clearly linked to the APRN role. Aggregate data are perhaps the least sensitive in being able to demonstrate the effectiveness of individuals but may be used to demonstrate trends in system approaches led by the APRN. While financial data are an appropriate indicator of APRN "value-added" contributions in some cases, they may be less so in others, especially if the role is not specifically linked to direct patient management. APRNs are essential to the provision of cost-conscious, quality patient care. Not only are they responsible for a wide variety of evidence-based practice changes and system initiatives, they are also responsible for the direct provision of evidence-based care. APRN practice outcomes can and should be monitored to more strongly demonstrate the APRN's positive contributions to health care.

Answers to Chapter Discussion Questions

1. Establishing a clear goal and defined outcome early in the assessment process creates role clarification and professional accountability with administration and the APRN. Clarity in goal direction allows for discussions about available data sources and realities of measurements. Defining outcome expectations also provides the APRN with

focus. It deters the APRN from seeking multiple data points that are not relevant to the designated project or administrative agendas.

2. Aggregate data are often relatively easy to obtain but are rarely associated with the specific APRN intervention under examination. Aggregate data are influenced by multiple factors. It is very difficult to relate these large and variable groupings to individual interventions because the effect of the intervention cannot be appreciated on such a hefty scale. An APRN who is striving to demonstrate the value of his or her practice by using aggregate data is often not fully demonstrating his or her contributions. Smaller, more specific outcome measures are better able to capture an APRN's influence.

3. Patterns of normal variation exist in every practice setting. Trended data allow for leniency with normal variations. Using established goals and previous trends, normal variation is apparent and true changes in outcomes are evident. If the APRN does not trend data over time, she or he will be reacting to normal variation and constantly adjusting the intervention to meet an artificial outcome measure. Real and sustainable outcomes are best measured over time.

4. APRNs need to identify outcome measures that are specific to their daily practice. The outcome measures must also be important to the institution in terms of patient care, satisfaction, efficiency, or dollars saved. It is important that outcome measures be derived from data that is easy to collect and the data should account for a period of time so that the outcomes may be translated into sustained improvement as a direct result of APRN practice. The outcome measures may be unique to the APRN, his or her role and practice setting, but the key elements should be included.

REFERENCES

Bryant-Lukosius, D., Carter, N., Reid, K., Donald, F., Martin-Misener, R., Kilpatrick, K., . . . DiCenso, A. (2015). The clinical effectiveness and cost-effectiveness of clinical nurse specialist-led hospital to home transitional care: A systematic review. *Journal of Evaluation in Clinical Practice*, 21(5), 763–781.

Dimensional Research. (2013). Customer service and business results: A survey of customer services from mid-size companies. Retrieved from http://cdn.zendesk.com/resources/whitepapers/Zendesk_WP_Customer_Service_and_Business_Results.pdf

Donald, F., Kilpatrick, K., Reid, K., Carter, N., Bryant-Lukosius, D., Martin-Misener, R., . . . DiCenso, A. (2015). Hospital to community transitional care by nurse practitioners: A systematic review of cost-effectiveness. *International Journal of Nursing Studies*, 52(1), 436–451.

Newhouse, R. P., Stanik-Hutt, J., White, K. M., Johantgen, M., Bass, E., Zangaro, G., . . . Weiner, J. P. (2011). Advanced practice nurse outcomes 1990–2008: A systematic review. *Nursing Economics*, 29, 230–250.

NSI Nursing Staffing Solutions. (2016). *2016 National Healthcare Retention & RN Staffing Report*. Retrieved from http://www.nsinursingsolutions.com

Stanik-Hutt, J., Newhouse, R. P., White, K. M., Johantgen, M., Bass, E. B., Zangaro, G., . . . Weiner, J. P. (2013). The quality and effectiveness of care provided by nurse practitioners. *The Journal for Nurse Practitioners, 9*(8), 492–500.

The Joint Commission. (2016). Hospital: 2016 national patient safety goals. Retrieved from http:// www.jointcommission.org/assets/1/6/2016_NPSG_HAP_ER.pdf

CHAPTER 4

General Design and Implementation Challenges in Outcome Assessment

Ann F. Minnick

Chapter Objectives

1. Ensure that the outcome assessment (OA) design can meet the project's purpose
2. Select outcomes
3. Maximize the ability to link cause and effect
4. Select a design that is amenable to resolving analytic quandaries

Chapter Discussion Questions

1. What five steps would you take to ensure saliency of the outcome?
2. What three steps will help achieve the necessary qualities of reality and "common currency" for your project?
3. What seven challenges establish cause and effect in nonexperimental designs?
4. Considering your outcome of interest, what analytic issues do you anticipate?
5. What four implementation challenges exist within OA projects? Suggest a solution for each challenge.

The conduct of OA studies is expensive, especially in terms of human resources that might be applied to any number of other important activities. The results of OA projects are needed to determine public policies and institutional efforts. Both of these uses of OA results make it imperative that the studies be designed to avoid common design flaws and make parsimonious use of resources during their execution. Simply put, you need to avoid wasting your time and someone else's money while producing valuable information.

This chapter is based on the assumption that few practitioners want to simply describe a single outcome but rather are trying to devise assessments that will help them improve care in multiple ways. This chapter discusses solutions to the four most common design problems and four implementation challenges to achieving this goal. Recognition of these basic problems and challenges will lead to the discovery of other issues that can be threats to the execution of OA studies. Although the list of potential solutions presented in this chapter is not exhaustive, it is designed to arm the person embarking on such projects with a basic set of effective responses.

SOLVING DESIGN CHALLENGES

Four common design problems in OA are (a) ensuring that the design can meet the project's purpose, (b) selecting outcomes, (c) maximizing the ability to link cause and effect, and (d) selecting a design that is amenable to resolving analytic quandaries.

Linking Purpose and Design

Challenges

The first and perhaps most important step is to determine what question(s) the OA project seeks to answer. Many novices have found themselves implementing a design only to discover that they never determined the specific questions they sought to answer. This occurs most often when clinicians note that some naturally occurring event, such as a change in practice at one site, will result in what seems like experimental and control groups. They then begin to track outcomes, but, because specific questions were never posed, find that they neglected to collect data on some important variable or that the pre- or postintervention design they used cannot really capture the additional ongoing practice changes at the sites.

A second problem in linking purpose and design is the failure to plan a project that could have answered, with only a few design changes, many more questions that are of interest to the larger world of institutional and public policy making. Many practitioners can verbally explain the larger issues for which OAs are needed, but they design studies that do not help inform the important debates over outcomes and how best to improve them. At a minimum, any OA usually needs to include some exploration of patients' physical and psychosocial outcomes as well as some elements of service costs and impact on the provider.

Solutions

Persons planning to embark on OAs can take the following steps to avoid these two problems:

1. Write the *questions* your OA project seeks to answer. Next, answer the question: How will answering each of these questions lead to actions that will improve outcomes for patients, the practice and/or institution, and the public?

2. For each project question, identify who cares about the answer and the level at which each person/agent functions in terms of making decisions that might influence changes your project might suggest. For example, is it a professional advanced practice registered nurse (APRN) group, the practice manager for your group, or a state agency? Could it be all of them if the design were changed? You will need resources for your study, even if your plans encompass only an assessment of outcomes within your own practice. These people/agencies could be sources of support. The first rule of sales (and gaining support for any type of project) is to meet the customer's needs. Be sure your project does so.

3. If in step 2 you could not identify more than one audience of interest, reconsider the questions. OA projects are too expensive to be one-trick ponies. If you identify someone who has resources but who you believe will not be supportive, consider how at least one question of interest to him or her can be included and be answered as *part* of the assessment. In providing an answer for what the individual or institution may think is the most important aspect of an OA, you will have the opportunity to bring these other questions (and findings) to his or her attention.

4. Verify through literature review and consultation with persons at each of the specified levels that these are the most important questions. "Important" means those questions that arise because there are great gaps in understanding and for which solutions are most urgently needed.

5. Seek consultation to ensure that it is possible to design an assessment that produces data that can answer the questions.

Selecting Outcomes

Challenges

When the preceding five steps are taken, it becomes easier to address the problem of defining outcomes. Each outcome must have three attributes to make a project worth the investment: *salience, objectivity,* and *common currency.*

Salience is the quality of being related to the phenomenon of interest. By performing the five steps already mentioned, salience can be achieved.

Objectivity is the ability of an outcome to be measured without bias. For an outcome to be said to be based in reality, it must be one that has the quality of being true to life. One example of a bias problem that is a lack of objectivity is illustrated by a seemingly simple outcome: rehospitalization within 60 days after treatment. In one study, we had to grapple with the bias inherent in defining rehospitalization as having occurred only if it happened at the single hospital where most APRNs had privileges. There was the chance that some patients were being rehospitalized at several other hospitals at which a few of the APRNs also had privileges.

Another example of this problem involves physical restraint use as an outcome. Once the physical restraint is defined, it should be fairly easy to determine if someone is restrained. The issue arises in counting restrained persons. If patients are transported to a unit in restraints, should they be counted against the receiving unit in a project seeking to assess the outcomes of a restraint-reduction program? If not, how long should the unit be given to implement restraint alternatives before patients are counted as restrained?

Should there be another outcome such as "duration of restraint use for patients admitted in restraint?" How much detail is necessary?

Reality can be defined as the extent to which the outcome definition has some fidelity to nature, that is, is true to life. Depression, quality of life, and spiritual health are examples of outcomes for which there are readily acknowledged problems in capturing the reality of the situation. Other outcomes, although seemingly immune to this problem because they are behaviorally based, are just as vulnerable. Consider the outcome "ambulation sufficient to accomplish five activities of daily living." If the outcome is operationalized as the ability to do this in a setting assumed to be a one-story home, but many patients live in multistory dwellings, there is little that is true to life about the study because many people need to be able to not only just ambulate but also climb stairs. Resources to consult in the definition and measurement of common outcomes are listed at the end of this chapter. The books listed highlight the advantages, disadvantages, and design issues associated with each approach.

A final problem revolves around what outcome researchers often assume is "common currency" in defining outcomes. For example, if death is an outcome and the performance of numerous hospitals is being measured in the OA, the death rates will be very different in the hospital that includes its hospice unit in the report versus those that do not have such a unit. A hospital may include deaths in the emergency department and another may not. If a hospital is the public receiving facility for the pronouncement of death in police and fire cases, should these deaths be included in the operationalization of the definition of death? Responsible persons at each hospital often believe everyone at other hospitals uses the same definitions for outcomes when in fact there is no common currency.

Solutions

Solutions lie in rigorous definitions:

1. Each time an outcome is mentioned in the project's questions, underline it. Within the context of each question, define the outcome in terms that can be objectively applied within the context of the study. It is important that you do this with each question independently. You may find that the outcome you are referring to as "mobility" in question 1 may be very different by question 4.

2. Discuss your definitions at sites where you plan to conduct the assessment to determine if data are currently amassed using your definition. Ask the responsible parties to describe any special situations they may have that could influence their outcomes, even when their definition is the one you propose. Be prepared to give examples of situations. Remember, most people do not believe their situation is the exception.

3. Simultaneous with step 2, complete a review to determine what definitions were used in the most important outcome studies published to date. Although you may choose to define an outcome in a new way and may, in reality, be developing a new outcome of interest, an OA is strengthened if there can be some comparison with findings from previous studies. For example, in a study of physical restraints, we measured prevalence and incidence, although earlier studies had relied almost exclusively on the latter. We were thus able to ascertain that the lower usage we documented was in fact a

decline based on comparisons with earlier reports, as well as demonstrate that there were very great differences between incidence and prevalence. Consult the Agency for Health Care Policy and Research (AHCPR) websites listed at the end of the chapter to learn how outcomes of interest to your project have been defined and measured.

Tracing Cause and Effect

Challenges

As students of traditional research know, a well-executed, double-blind, randomized pretest–posttest design is effective when one seeks to establish that a particular intervention produces measurable effect(s). In OA projects, this approach is usually not an option because of real-life issues. For example, it is often not possible to randomize patients or blind providers to treatment. It is rare to find a project that seeks to measure only one outcome. The science of improvement drives the desire to identify variables associated with the outcome. Seven challenges to the ability to make conclusions about causation and to identify interventions that might result in outcome improvement are common. These seven challenges are:

1. **Patient autonomy.** The patient may be following the recommended treatment on a continuum ranging from "entirely" to "not at all." The patient may be following one aspect of the treatment entirely and another not at all. The patient may follow a treatment plan one day and not at all the next.

2. **Multiplicity of health problems in a single individual.** Almost no patient presents with a single health challenge. Multiple system failures are common and the simultaneous presence of physical and mental disorders has been well-documented. This makes assessment of a single outcome related to a particular disorder difficult.

3. **Nonclinical characteristics.** Income, education, insurance coverage, geographical location, exposure to violence, and many other variables can influence outcomes.

4. **Multiplicity of health providers.** This includes known as well as unknown providers who, in turn, use many different types of treatments. Some of these treatments may have been obtained from ethnic healers. Some medications may have been obtained illegally. Other providers might be recognized in foreign countries and their advice obtained by the autonomous patient through the Internet. Even if the providers are known, their skill in providing a specific treatment may vary. Depending on the schedule, the patient may have received each treatment in a repetitive series from different providers.

5. **Unknown time delay between intervention and expected outcome.** The classic example of this challenge is the difficulty in determining the outcomes of providers' health-promotion activities because many years (and many intervening messages and experiences) will often pass before a condition manifests itself.

6. **Lack of baseline measurements.** Patients often change providers, and accumulating good baseline measures of health status, quality of life, and other variables are expensive to collect de novo. Even if there is support for de novo measures, it is often impossible to collect a full record that captures the rich and complex changes in human life that may influence an outcome.

7. **The complexity of nonpatient, nonindividual provider variables.** These variables include labor (overall staffing quantity and quality) and capital inputs (e.g., equipment),

as well as conditions of employment and leadership. In studies of whether or not a particular activity influences outcomes, these types of variables rather than the activity itself may be paramount. For example, staff may have the same beliefs and knowledge about ways to avoid extubation accidents, but a shortage of supplies or staff may make the execution of these steps impossible. Merely assessing extubations by practice group or before and after an educational session with the staff will not assist in tracing why an outcome is occurring.

Solutions

All of the solutions depend on the outcome assessor having a broad knowledge of patients, providers, and system variables. Consultants for each of these areas during the design phase can be worthwhile. They may ensure that the potential effects of these variables are at least considered.

Through interviews with providers and patients as well as review of clinical documents, such as medical records, determine what the potential is that aspects 1 through 4 may influence the OA. During this process, attempt to determine if these aspects are evenly distributed across cases or if only select groups are influenced. For example, many patients at one clinic site may visit a traditional healer down the street, and patients at another site might not. As with the issue of defining outcomes, patients and providers will not necessarily think that their situations are unique. During the project-planning phase, you will need to ask questions that will provoke a wide-ranging discussion, such as "Tell me about some of the things you do for your arthritis besides coming to the clinic."

Plan on multiple measurement over time. Multiple measures over time will help to ascertain any change/attenuation of effect on outcomes. This is especially important if the OA is part of an intervention effort. An outcome may at first seem to be favorably influenced, but there may be rapid attenuation. Conversely, it may take an unknown period of time for full effects to be realized.

After reviewing the availability of baseline data, recognize that significant OA resources may need to be assigned to build a database. The project budget needs to reflect this expense. Make it a priority to explore how to maintain the elements of these data after the assessment project is complete. Experience has shown that once providers and institutions have access to such a database, they are willing to devote the resources necessary for its maintenance because a well-designed database can be used for many OA projects, as well as to meet accreditation demands.

Use a framework such as the one in Figure 4.1 to ascertain that you have assessed the system variables that are most likely to influence outcomes. Many times the key to improving outcomes is to attempt to modify system—rather than individual provider or patient—variables. For example, in the past century, anesthesia outcomes were improved significantly when the tubing connection ends of various gases provided during surgery were made compatible only with the appropriate delivery device.

Analytic Issues

Challenges

As can be deduced from the discussion of the many variables that need to be accounted for in an OA project, multivariate analysis becomes a necessity. Any outcome may be

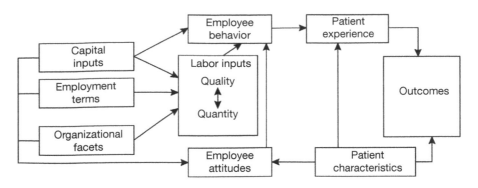

FIGURE 4.1 A framework of variables influencing patient outcomes.

Source: Developed in preparation of Minnick, Roberts, Young, Kleinpell, and Marcantonio (1997).

affected by attribute variables, contextual variables, and specific treatment effects. The problem in executing such an approach is that one usually does not know at the beginning of a project if the variables of interest are orthogonal to one another (an assumption of many statistical techniques). This problem is known as *collinearity*. A second problem is the definition and treatment of attribute and contextual variables. More analytic problems occur when an outcome is rare or infrequent. Finally, the third problem is that data of interest are drawn from different levels. For example, an outcome may be drawn from individual patient records, but variables such as staffing may be unit based with others drawn from an institutional level. Special techniques are needed for the analysis.

Solutions

Few practitioners are equipped to deal with these problems. The following steps are advisable for practitioners who do not have advanced statistical and design expertise:

1. Recognize what one does not know and consult experts during the design phase. The timing is essential because many of the solutions to these problems are rooted in selecting the proper design and definitions. For example, in the case of rare outcomes, a case–control approach may be advised.
2. The practitioner should, however, be knowledgeable enough to recognize the possibility that all three problems exist and to ask a statistician how the problems can be addressed. In asking the statistician for advice, the practitioner should inquire about the advantages and disadvantages of each proposed solution.

ADDRESSING OA PROJECT IMPLEMENTATION CHALLENGES

Challenges

Having considered the complexity of the design issues described previously, thoughtful practitioners may be tempted to run from the very idea of launching a systematic

OA. This section is devoted to providing "doable" solutions for the four major implementation challenges: (a) assembling a competent and productive team, (b) securing the resources to complete the project, (c) obtaining institutional cooperation, and (d) enlisting the cooperation of providers and patients.

Solutions

The solutions are based on the belief that the process of getting this type of project done is no different than the steps one would take in any type of project, from remodeling one's home to opening a new clinic. You would neither attempt to do either of these projects alone nor would you attempt to go forward without adequate resources.

1. Assemble a team of people who are as interested in the idea as you are. If no one is interested, begin building interest one person at a time. Put yourself in that person's position. What responsibilities or needs would this type of project help that person address? Use these points in discussion. Try to include formal resource allocators as well as informal opinion makers in this effort.

2. Consider all sources of support, including those outside of your institution. Your well-designed project and its findings could serve as a model for others. Foundations as well as federal agencies are interested in models and in projects that are large enough to produce generalizable findings about the outcomes. Once you have ascertained why your institution or an outside agency should be interested, prepare a short (no more than three pages) discussion paper that explains the need for the project, the answers it will produce, and why the results will be valuable to the funder. Include an estimate of the general costs. This is a major marketing tool. People who are asked for resources need to know what they are buying, why they need it, and what it is going to cost.

3. Build alliances with the database, statistical, and design experts whose help you will be able to afford once step 2 is accomplished. You will need to begin building these alliances before approaching resource holders to get a general idea of costs and to amass the technical expertise that will make the proposal a solid one.

4. Consider banding together with like-minded providers, institutions, professional associations, or health care systems. This cooperation can drive down costs by spreading the fixed expenses (e.g., statistical help) over a greater number of supporters. It also is a wonderful way to gather data on rare events and to develop a database that allows for exploration of multiple factor influences on outcomes. For example, if you are in Nebraska, you may not have sufficient population to explore the effect of a specific ethnicity on patient outcomes. A project that includes sites in Illinois, New York, or California may make this possible.

As noted in the beginning of this chapter, OAs are important sources of information on which public policies and private actions are based. Given this fact and the expense of these assessments, an OA can truly be said to be one of those activities in which "if it is worth doing, it is worth doing well." A poor OA can be worse than none at all because it will lead to poor decisions. With an awareness of the design pitfalls and access to solutions and experts, practitioners can help ensure that OAs are truly worth the investment.

▥ SUMMARY

Several design and implementation challenges exist when conducting an OA project; however, various solutions, as described in this chapter, can be used to ensure that an OA is rigorous and produces optimal results. OAs are important sources of information on which public policies and private actions are based. Given this fact and the expense of these assessments, an OA can truly be said to be one of those activities in which "if it is worth doing, it is worth doing well." A poor OA can be worse than none at all because it will lead to poor decisions. With an awareness of the design pitfalls and access to solutions and experts, practitioners can help ensure that OAs are worth the investment.

Answers to Chapter Discussion Questions

1. (a) Write the *questions* your project seeks to answer and, for each, indicate how answering it will lead to actions that improve outcomes for patients, the practice or institution, and the public. (b) For each project question, identify who cares about the answer and the level at which each person/agent functions when making decisions that might influence changes your project might suggest. (c) If in the preceding step you could not identify more than one audience of interest, reconsider the questions. (d) Verify through literature review and consultation at each specified level that these are the most important questions. (e) Consult with others to ensure that an assessment can be designed that produces data that can answer the questions.

2. (a) Check that the same outcome is used throughout the questions. (b) Discuss definitions at sites to determine if data are amassed using these definitions. (c) Complete a literature review of the definitions.

3. (a) Patient autonomy, (b) provider multiplicity, (c) nonclinical characteristics, (d) multiplicity of health problems, (e) unknown time of delay between interventions and expected outcome, (f) lack of baseline measurements, and (g) complex system variables.

4. Your answer should include assessment of the likelihood that the following issues might arise: collinearity, treatment of attribute and contextual variables, and how multiple levels of data will be addressed.

5. Your answer should revolve around specifics individualized to your project steps to address: (a) assembling a competent and productive team, (b) securing resources, (c) securing institutional cooperation, and (d) enlisting the cooperation of providers and patients.

▥ RESOURCES—BOOKS AND WEBSITES

AHRQ (http://www.ahrq.gov) is the nation's lead federal agency for research on health care quality, costs, outcomes, and patient safety and is a key source for information about national outcome assessment efforts.

CAHPS, the AHCPR's Consumer Assessment of Healthcare Providers and Systems program (http://www.ahrq.gov/cahps/index.html), is "a public–private initiative to develop standardized surveys of patients' experiences with ambulatory and facility-level care." The CAHPS website provides free information and AHRQ tools to measure consumers' assessments of their health care experiences. Survey tools can be downloaded and technical advice is available.

Doran, D. M. (Ed.). (2011). *Nursing outcomes: The state of the science*. Sudbury, MA: Jones & Bartlett. (This work reviews outcome categories, their measurement and use within the framework of nursing accountability.)

Kane, R. L., & Radosevich, D. M. (2011). *Conducting health outcomes research* (2nd ed.). Sudbury, MA: Jones & Bartlett. (Although aimed at researchers, this classic work points out many issues that could influence outcome assessments.)

Medical Care Research and Review. (2007). In April 2007, this journal sponsored a special supplement (Vol. 64, No. 2. Suppl.) on Performance Measurement and Outcomes of Nursing Care. The contents for this supplement, with downloadable PDFs of separate articles, can be retrieved from http://mcr.sagepub.com/content/vol64/2_suppl

Moorhead, S., Johnson, M., Maas, M. L., & Swanson, E. (Eds.). (2013). *Nursing outcomes classification (NOC): Measurement of health outcomes* (5th ed.). St. Louis, MO: Mosby.

Muennig, P., & Bounthavong, M. (2016). *Cost-effectiveness analyses in health: A practical approach* (3rd ed.). San Francisco, CA: Jossey-Bass. (Although assessing cost-effectiveness as an outcome requires specialized skills, this book is a good basic primer toward understanding this complex outcome.)

Wachter, R. M. (2012). *Understanding patient safety* (2nd ed.). New York, NY: McGraw Hill. (The chapters on defining errors, safety, and values as outcomes will help the reader in defining and constructing measurable variables for projects. It has the added benefit of reviewing interventions that have been tested to improve these outcomes.)

REFERENCE

Minnick, A. F., Roberts, M. J., Young, W. B., Kleinpell, R. M., & Marcantonio, R. J. (1997). What influences patients' reports of three aspects of hospital services? *Medical Care, 35*(4), 399–409.

CHAPTER 5

Locating Instruments and Measures for Advanced Practice Nursing Outcome Assessments

Marilyn Wolf Schwartz and Roger Green

Chapter Objectives

1. Provide a guide for finding instruments, including questionnaires, scales, and tools, to measure treatment outcomes
2. Discuss the value of using both print and web-based library resources, rather than public Internet search engines. There is value in consulting a professional medical librarian to find the appropriate instruments in a timely manner
3. Explain the importance of requesting permission to use instruments, whether standard or unpublished. Permission to use an instrument is an ethical issue related to copyright and proper research method

Chapter Discussion Questions

1. What two databases are appropriate to start a search for an instrument to use for diabetes primary care outcomes? What terms and strategy were used to do the search? List a measurement tool found in the database search that an advanced practice registered nurse (APRN) could use in practice.
2. In what reference books would you find a review and description of the Minnesota Multiphasic Personality Inventory (MMPI)? Search a local medical, nursing, or university library's online catalog to see if any of the books listed in the Resources section at the end of this chapter can be found in a local library.
3. What are two university websites that can serve as resources to learn about requesting permission to use an instrument? List an instrument on pain assessment and describe

where to request permission to use it, whether training is required to use it, and if there is a cost.

4. What mobile applications could be used to access resources discussed in this chapter when seeking information on an instrument that could be used to measure the physician–nurse professional collaboration?

5. What are the most promising resources for an outcome assessment, nursing problem, or medical problem that needs to be studied?

This chapter is intended to help APRNs find the instruments that measure the impact of APRN care and interventions. APRNs and researchers must know how to find surveys, questionnaires, or other measurement instruments to determine if a treatment is effective. In this evidence-based health care era, APRNs as well as researchers should study, measure, and report significant changes in interventions. When APRNs report evidence-based findings in the literature, they are improving the quality of health care and contributing to the profession.

Providing information on finding instruments would not be complete without mentioning the responsible use of tests and measures. Many university library websites explain the ethical use of measurement tools or instruments. Authors doing authentic research must prove validity and reliability. Textbooks on developing measurement tools emphasize the importance of testing and validating tools. Consequently, respected instruments are copyrighted, costly to develop, and need to be used appropriately. In the section Resources (University Library Websites) at the end of this chapter, several of the listed websites note the importance of requesting permission, and how to make such inquiries. To read a summary of ethics of use and why permission should be requested, please refer to the website info.library.okstate.edu/tests. The authors present major resources that librarians and clinicians can use to find instruments. The terms *instruments, questionnaires, surveys,* and *tools* are used interchangeably. "Instrument" is the preferred term and is used by the database Cumulative Index to Nursing and Allied Health Literature (CINAHL) when indexing the field. The descriptor "instrument" is used for the tools mentioned in articles.

In this chapter, five types of resources are explored:

1. **Books:** The books described herein are standard reference texts regarded as the first sources to check in finding instruments.

2. **Bibliographic databases:** These are defined in the order of importance to nursing applications. Examples are given for the kinds of instruments that might be found in the CINAHL and the Health and Psychosocial Instruments (HaPI) databases. Some suggestions are given regarding fields in which to search these databases for the instruments. The reader may then apply some of the same techniques to searching other databases. Using the controlled vocabulary or thesauri for retrieval in databases is important, and medical librarians are adept at using them effectively. It is important to consult a medical librarian, when available, to process searches, especially when doing an evidence-based study or publishing or presenting papers.

3. **Internet resources:** Those listed include professional organizations and governmental sites as well as library guides to tools. Library websites are good places to check for mobile apps to access literature databases and electronic books. University librarians, especially in medical settings, are placing descriptions of mobile applications (apps) used on iPads, iPhones, tablets, and other handheld devices to access literature searching tools. Note the Internet resources and University Library resources sections for more details on apps. The Internet resources listed are by no means exhaustive but considered selective.

4. **International literature and databases:** APRNs who work together and publish research findings with colleagues in other countries have access to sources worthwhile delving into. These databases contain information about health issues in countries other than the United States. Allow plenty of time to follow links, which may prove to have gems in them providing information about instruments used, and sometimes making instruments available to those outside their countries. Three such sources are described in this chapter: Hinari produced by the World Health Organization (WHO); Patient-Reported Outcome and Quality of Life Instruments Database (ProQolid) from the Mapi Trust; and the Global Health Exchange maintained by the Institute for Health Metrics and Evaluation (IHME) in Seattle.

5. **Open access resources:** The open access movement began so that researchers could share their work and findings with colleagues before formally publishing them. This sharing enables others to provide comments and suggestions to the authors. Open access is practiced internationally. Open access for journals is called *gold* open access; and open access for institutional repositories is called *green* open access. Universities and corporations often maintain repositories containing the preserved, published, and unpublished work of their staff. Finding and using the open access resources is time-consuming but may lead the reader to authors working on studies of interest.

The resources described in entries 4 and 5 are new to this edition. Because URLs change frequently, the sites listed in this chapter may no longer be current. However, a general Internet search using a standard browser such as Google may provide a newer link.

STANDARD BOOKS

In this age of technology, using standard textbooks is not the most popular source of information. However, following are some tried and true measurement tool books. Note the additional books listed in Resources at the end of this chapter, many of which are more specific to nursing and medicine. The books to consult are too numerous to describe individually. Many nursing and medical libraries own the books listed in Resources. Of course, most books may be purchased from online book vendors.

Mental Measurements Yearbooks (MMYBs) by Buros Institute of Mental Measurements

Check the website (www.buros.org) to see that this group has been around for 78+ years and are experts. MMYB has been published since 1938.

This standard reference text is available in most university and public libraries on reference shelves. It is updated annually and may be accessed online through many library database menus. The book lists tests in alphabetical order including descriptive information with purpose, intended population, acronyms, authors, scores, time, prices, publishers, and cross references. Each volume provides information on reliability, validity, and includes reviews of tests and test materials. Many libraries have access to this book online. Buros also publishes *Test Reviews Online*. To find the link for *Test Reviews Online*, use Google search with "Buros Test Reviews." This particular Buros site contains only review tests, which the user can decide to purchase.

Tests in Print (TIP) by Buros Institute of Mental Measurement

TIP lists target audience, length, score(s), and cost and is a companion to the Buros MMYB. The TIP and the MMYB are the main sources for finding information on published tests.

- *Tests: A Comprehensive Reference for Assessments in Psychology, Education, and Business, edited by Taddy Maddox. PRO-ED, Inc.,* **published from 1983 to the present, with a 2008 edition**
  Descriptions are brief and contain information on test population, purpose, format, scoring, and cost and do not include reviews or evaluations of tests.
- *Test Critiques, Kansas City, Missouri, Test Corporation of America,* **published since 1984**
  This multivolume set is the companion to *Tests* and includes reliability and validity information.
- *Directory of Unpublished Experimental Mental Measures, edited by B.A. Goldman and D.F. Mitchell,* **published by the American Psychological Association since 1970 (latest volume 9 published 2008)**
  Volume 9 lists tests published in the 2001 to 2005 issues of the 36 journals covered. This directory includes information on recently developed or noncommercial, experimental tests in 24 categories. The entries cover 36 relevant professional journals published in the United States. The measures described in dissertations are not included. Volumes do not include reviews. Check the category index. However, the volumes do not have title indexes. Some of the categories of measures are achievement, adjustment, aptitude, attitude, behavior communication, concept meaning, development, motivation, perception, personality problem solving and reasoning, values, vocational interest and evaluation, and trait measurement.

Please note the many additional books listed in Resources at the end of this chapter. The McDowell book, with a guide to rating scales and questionnaires is an excellent source for finding health-related instruments and is cited in Resources. University libraries usually have the books listed, some of which are in reference sections. Remember that most university libraries now have their catalogs available online. If a library has a collection of tests or instruments, the information on the tests may be found through the catalogs. Library staff can request interlibrary loans for books not owned. Reference and selection librarians usually welcome requests for purchase of instrument resource books when not owned by the library.

BIBLIOGRAPHIC DATABASES

Although searching bibliographic databases retrieves references to articles about instruments, the articles do not always print copies of the instruments. Remember that searching databases may provide references to articles that occasionally include the instruments. Finding full-text journal articles online in databases may show instruments in the articles. The Resources (Internet) section of this chapter provides a description of how to find dissertations, which usually include instruments used in doctoral or PhD work.

LEVELS OF EVIDENCE

The Medical Literature Analysis and Retrieval System Online (MEDLINE) and the Cochrane databases contain references to the highest quality journals or peer-reviewed literature as do the CINAHL, PsycINFO, and Educational Resources Information Center (ERIC). The database producers, especially MEDLINE, publish on their websites statements of the criteria required for the journals to be indexed. APRNs need to critically appraise the literature to verify that the evidence presented is sound and that the measurement tools used were appropriate.

CINAHL is available from the EBSCO Publishing database vendor and journal subscription agency. EBSCO and other vendors now provide tutorials, offered on YouTube or other media formats, to explain the use of search strategies for their databases. For access information, go to www.ebscohost.com.

A starting point for finding any instrument is the CINAHL because instruments may be searched directly in the instrumentation field of the bibliographic record. Log into CINAHL, and search directly on the "instrumentation" field from the "indexes" on the main screen. If you search the "publication type" field and choose "research instrument," you may actually find the full text of an instrument. This database is not free to the public, and users must request codes from institutional libraries, ask a librarian, or pay for a service to process searches. Remember that as technology changes for the vendors, screens may change. Call the technical support number or e-mail the vendor to learn how to search the indexes or "fields" as some vendors call them.

HEALTH AND PSYCHOSOCIAL INSTRUMENTS

HaPI is produced by Behavioral Measurement Database Service (BMDS). This database lists evaluation and measurement tools, questionnaires, and test instruments. HaPI is available through database vendors including Ovid, a Wolters Kluwer Publishing division (www.ovid.com), or EBSCOHost (www.ebscohost.com). University and medical school libraries pay for access to these databases for library patrons. Contact the HaPI publisher for direct access, and to find other database vendors who provide access.

The HaPI database does not provide copies of instruments. However, this database shows information on where to find the tool/instrument and often gives the address and phone number. This database is bibliographic, meaning that it retrieves references to articles about the instrument. The references are indicated as secondary sources, then below the citation the primary sources tell where the instruments were originally described and usually where to call or write to get a copy. Consult a librarian to find free access.

MEDLINE/PUBMED

PubMed.gov is the National Library of Medicine's database, which includes MEDLINE. This database is free to the public at pubmed.gov. Check with local medical resource libraries and librarians for instructions in using PubMed. Note that this database has brief tutorials with links to them on the home page. The time invested in looking at the tutorials usually pays off in terms of saving time in using the database.

APRNs may search this database for reference to articles on a specific instrument. The references often discuss the reliability and validity of the instrument. The articles, at times, provide a copy of the instrument discussed. In MEDLINE, e-mail addresses are provided with the authors' names making it easier to find an author to contact for further information about an instrument that may have been discussed in the article. One of the limiters available for searching is the publication types, including questionnaires.

COCHRANE DATABASES

The Cochrane databases are excellent sources to find the highest level evidence-based studies that describe instruments used. These databases are usually available through libraries or institutions, such as hospitals or drug companies. Ovid and EBSCO are two vendors providing access to many of the databases, including:

- Cochrane Database of Systematic Reviews
- Cochrane Database of Abstracts of Reviews of Effects
- Cochrane Central Register of Controlled Trials
- Cochrane Methodology Register
- Health Technology Assessment
- ACP Journal Club

The website of the Cochrane collaboration, www.cochrane.org gives free access to a few references containing reviews. Many university library sites have information on the databases and how to search them. The Cochrane databases are international in scope and some have mobile apps. The Cochrane Collaboration groups have had a nonvoting representative in WHO meetings since 2011. As of February 2013, Cochrane reviews allow open access 12 months after publication. Wiley is the publisher of the Cochrane Library and provides some items in open access.

When searching the Cochrane databases, you can limit the topics by filtering, using the terms "instrument(s)," "questionnaire(s)," "scale(s)," or "survey(s)." Use the truncation symbols identified by the various vendors. Usually, a dollar sign ($) or asterisk (*) at the ends of root words retrieves various spellings. For example, type in Instrument$ or instrument* to retrieve instrument, instruments, or instrumentation. Results in searching the systematic reviews will provide fewer references than in literature searches because the subject may not have been studied. In retrieving actual reviews, load up the printer with plenty of paper because reviews often can be more than 50 pages, or download the review onto a thumb drive.

EDUCATION RESOURCES INFORMATION CENTER

ERIC is produced by the Institute of Education within the U.S. Department of Education in Washington, DC. This database is free to the public at www.eric.ed.gov. The Educational Testing Service (ETS) of ERIC also has tests in microfiche. This database lists evaluation and measurement tools, questionnaires, and test instruments. ERIC's Clearinghouse on Assessment and Evaluation has a test locator at ericae.net/testcol.htm, which includes free tests. This site also has a link to Buros Institute of Mental Measurements and allows shopping and purchase of tests. The *Test Reviews Online* is on this link (buros.unl.edu/buros/jsp/search.jsp).

APRNs often participate in educating patient or staff about treatments or procedures. The challenge in the educational process is to show that what was presented caused a change in knowledge and practice. Although the ERIC database contains a limited amount of health or medical literature references, it does provide references to general educational concepts that may be applied to measure whether educational interventions are working.

PSYCINFO

PsycINFO is produced by the American Psychological Association and contains references to articles about various psychological instruments. Many database vendors offer PsycINFO, including Ovid, EBSCO, and ProQuest (formerly Dialog Knight-Ridder), and each has its own search engine

Depending on what the APRN is studying, the PsycINFO database may include references to articles relevant to measure psychological changes. This database covers professional and academic literature in psychology and related disciplines, including medicine and nursing. PsycINFO is international in scope and includes abstracts for citations in over 2,563 (in 2016) journals, dissertations, books, and book chapters. Some university libraries allow access to this database for users in the library or for students and staff to access remotely. Some libraries may require you to access via a professional librarian.

The strategy for using PsycINFO is different from CINAHL or HaPI. A search hint in using PsycINFO is to use the thesaurus and the "measurement" heading to find related topics. In PsycINFO, retrieval may be limited to "test & measures" using the limit button on Ovid. Retrieval will be for article references, and the possibility of the full instrument being in the article may occur occasionally. Rely on PsycINFO to find articles on validity or reliability of particular measures. Articles may be found on various measures used for a particular health or psychological issue.

Note: The American Psychological Association website listed in Resources under Internet is an excellent source for finding the actual instruments.

DISSERTATION ABSTRACTS INTERNATIONAL

Dissertation Abstracts is the index used for doctoral dissertations and master's theses written at most North American graduate schools. The CINAHL database also contains dissertations. The dissertations may be searched and ordered through UMI/Proquest company. Go to the website www.proquest.com to order a dissertation online and click on "Dissertations and Theses." On this database, the user may order a dissertation as an individual for the stated fee, or if your library/institution subscribes to this database, library service may request it for you. This site's name is Dissertations Express and in 2016, the cost for a dissertation varied with the format. The PDF format costs $38.00; unbound, $39.00; and microfiche, $55.00 for a 357-page dissertation. Pricing is given for soft cover, hard cover, and microfilm when ordering.

If a dissertation is not available through Dissertations Express, check with a local medical librarian to request an interlibrary loan from the institution from which the dissertation was required and published.

PROQUEST DIALOG

ProQuest Dialog provides access to hundreds of databases used by most universities and many hospitals to conduct searches. Individuals may want to use these databases through their libraries or institutions because of the expense. To view descriptions of databases that might be relevant to use, go to the ProQuest.com website. Click on "Products and Services" at the top of the page, which has a drop-down menu for databases.

INTERNET RESOURCES AND ONLINE LIBRARY RESOURCES

Use Resources at the end of this chapter to find the links to library websites that have guides for finding instruments. This list is not extensive but does contain quality sites. Use Google to find other websites that may be helpful: Google (www.google.com) and Google Scholar (scholar.google.com).

Google may be used as a starting point or last resort. In using Google, try to use advanced search if the basic search does not retrieve information needed. Use Google Scholar (scholar.google.com) for articles about an instrument. A Google Scholar search on the Visual Analog Pain Scale Faces retrieves several articles discussing uses of the scale, some with pictures of faces rating pain. This is only one of many pain scales that are visual.

UNIVERSITY LIBRARY WEBSITES

Regarding sites listed in Resources, some of the university sites have charts and tables describing databases and step-by-step methods for finding instruments. The majority of these websites include most of the information in this chapter.

MOBILE/HANDHELD DEVICES AND MEDICAL APPLICATIONS (APPS)

Practitioners often use mobile devices for medical "apps" to access patient records, drug information, and bibliographic databases, to name a few. To see lists of databases or other medical apps, many university libraries are providing information in chart format on their websites to make it easy for users to see what is available. For example, Texas A&M University Libraries has a list of mobile databases that are accessible through various devices. The guide shows that "CINAHL Plus with Full Text Mobile" is available from EBSCO. Check msl.library.tamu.edu/services/mobile_resources.html. With the latest handheld technology, APRNs could check CINAHL in a patient setting or when not near a laptop to look up information on an instrument. Another well-presented example of mobile apps is from the University of Washington Health Sciences Library, titled "Mobile Accessible Resources," available at guides.lib.uw.edu/hsl/mobile. San Jose State University library staff, in 2010, used the term "appography" to describe a bibliography for apps.

Many popular mobile or "handheld" (the term used by the National Library of Medicine) devices are utilized to access databases and websites when searching outcome measures. The APRN can access CINAHL, Medline/PubMed, HaPI, MMYB, TIP, and PsycINFO with mobile devices. The reader may do a Google search on each resource followed by the term "mobile" or "handheld" to retrieve university or vendor sites that describe how to access. Sometimes apps are free through local universities.

To learn about the National Library of Medicine's Gallery of Mobile Apps, go to www .nlm.nih.gov/mobile.

PROFESSIONAL ASSOCIATION SITES

American Nurses Association publishes books and pamphlets that may help in finding instruments. Other specialized, advanced practice nursing sites may have clues to instrument information. For example, check the sites for the American Academy of Nurse Practitioners, the American Academy of Clinical Nurse Anesthetists, National League for Nursing, American Nephrology Nurses, Emergency Nurses Associations, or others. If an APRN is part of a special professional association, encourage the website manager to include dissertations or articles of members who may have used or developed instruments.

The Sigma Theta Tau International Honor Society of Nursing Virginia Henderson Library may be another source of information for instruments. The website describes their evidence-based practice publication (www.nursinglibrary.org/vhl).

Many professional health and medicine associations now publish reports that may contain measurement tools. A well-respected site described in the previous edition of this book was the Institute of Medicine, which has been renamed Health and Medicine Division (HMD) of the National Academies of Sciences, Engineering, and Medicine. The new URL is www.nationalacademies.org/hmd/about-HMD.aspx. This website has a plethora of reports, projects, and publications of global interest, many of which pertain to nursing. When looking through the publication lists, consult the abstracts of some of the projects that describe measurement tools that might be available for use.

The Medical Library Association continuing education programs offers information for librarians who publish guides for finding measurement tools on library websites. Readers are advised to check local medical library websites for such guides.

CORPORATE WEBSITES

ProQolid is the acronym for Patient-Reported Outcome and Quality of Life Instruments Database. Go to eprovide.mapi-trust.org to learn about this database. Two access points are available on this website. A free-access section shows an alphabetical list of instruments available and listed by author's name, targeted population, and pathology/disease. There is a member charge to subscribe and is priced in euros because of its Lyon, France, origin. There is an online payment option.

Survey Monkey is a site that helps you develop your own survey and lists other programs available to help do your surveys. Go to www.surveymonkey.com to learn about this program.

The Rand Corporation website publishes many summaries of research projects and reports with a special section on health instruments. Check Rand Health Surveys and Tools at www.rand.org/health/surveys_tools.html. Note the "underline" character between "surveys" and "tools" in the URL.

GOVERNMENT SITES

Some governmental agencies have sections on their sites that contain useful instruments. Instruments developed by governmental agencies may be found in the "government document" departments of university and law libraries. Tax dollars pay for these agencies' work; they are free to use; and sites can be searched using the terms "surveys," "questionnaires," "measures," "tools," and "instruments." Check with the librarians to help find the publications cited. Please note the following:

- Agency for Healthcare Research and Quality (AHRQ): Tools and Resources for Better Health Care (www.ahrq.gov)
- Health Resources and Services Administration (HRSA) U.S. Department of Health and Human Services: The HRSA provides a wealth of information on a search of its website www.ahrq.gov with terms "measures," "tools," and "instruments." At the site www .hrsa.gov, the reader may click on "clinical quality measures" and find information on screening for various conditions.
- National Guideline Clearinghouse published by the AHRQof the U.S. Department of Health and Human Services: The site, www.guideline.gov, has a section on outcome measures relevant to specific health problems.
- National Technical Information Service (www.ntis.gov), Springfield, Virginia, Department of Commerce: This database is free and contains many reports of government-supported research. Searching the site using the terms "health surveys" or

"health questionnaires" combined with specific health conditions retrieves citations to reports that may contain measurement tools. Unlike other literature search results, the system displays older references first. Reports may be ordered at a cost, and summaries are free. This database is a stretch for finding a copy of an instrument but is worthwhile to check.

INTERNATIONAL LITERATURE AND DATABASES

A global perspective is important in advanced clinical practice, research, and publishing. As nurses and other health care providers travel to other countries to teach, practice, or attend conferences, it is useful to be aware of free resources from the WHO. The most commonly used service is Hinari, which the WHO defines as Access to Research in Health Programme. To learn details on Hinari do a Google search using "WHO Hinari." The Hinari service provides developing countries with free or low-cost access to medical databases including full-text articles, books, and reports of clinical research.

Notice, within the WHO website, that many other resources are listed. Examples include the International Clinical Trials Registry Platform (ICTRP), International Agency for Research on Cancer (IARC), Institutional Repository for Information Sharing (IRIS), and Global Index Medicus. These resources may be explored to find measurement tools used internationally. American nurses need to be aware of the resources of the WHO so that they may advise colleagues in other countries of the Hinari services provided by WHO.

The IHME produces the database Global Health Data Exchange, which is maintained by the University of Washington, Seattle (ghdx.healthdata.org). One of the data types that are searchable includes results of surveys. Some other data types are census, demographic surveillance, and Epi surveillance (data on suspected notifiable diseases). An example showing references of global significance is posttraumatic stress disorder. The summaries describe measurement tools used.

More resources providing references of global issues can be found at Sigma Theta Tau described in the section on professional associations. Global initiatives of Sigma Theta Tau are described in detail on its website, found by a Google search using "Sigma Theta Tau nursing library resources." One of the databases emphasized is EMBASE (Excerpta Medica) which is the European version of the American Index Medicus. EMBASE includes indexing of many non-English medical journals not found in Index Medicus.

Awareness of the previously described international resources is important even if not used in all searches for instruments. There is the possibility of finding relevant references to tools or perhaps copies of them.

OPEN ACCESS TO JOURNALS AND INSTITUTIONAL REPOSITORIES

As previously mentioned, open access to journals is referred to as gold open access while open access to institutional repositories is referred to as green open access. Searching in open access resources for measurement tools may be time-consuming. Practitioners and researchers should be aware of the open access movement taking place internationally. Academic libraries have been leaders in offering free access to articles written by their institutions' staffs. Open access is intended to encourage health care providers and scientists to share information as the research is being done, and to allow quicker access to treatments and information on health issues. For clinicians and researchers looking for tools being used by others, open access is a possible resource.

Open access has been controversial because of funding, copyright, and how standard publishers are involved. Authors of nursing, medical, and scientific articles and books usually do not receive remuneration for their work, but the publishers make a profit. The open access proponents address the problem of authors retaining copyright for their materials. An overview of open access may be found by a Google search using the term "Open Access Legacy."

To find out if a reader's institution has an institutional repository or other open access resources, check with librarians or departments known as *scholarly communications*. Another term often used by academic institutions with open access is *digital commons*. Knowledge of these resources is necessary in clinical practice or publishing research.

An excellent example and prototype of open access is PubMed Commons. References retrieved in PubMed often have the term "PubMed Commons" at the end of the citations. Authors have the opportunity to comment on the research presented. Authors need to register for this service and be willing (or not) to share remarks.

The Cochrane Collaborative plans to have open access to its reviews by 2020 and already has many open access publications on its website. As mentioned earlier in this chapter, Cochrane has always had a global perspective. The Cochrane Collaboration has a representative who is a nonvoting member of the WHO.

The "Global Nursing e-Repository" is on the heading of the home page for the Sigma Theta Tau Virginia Henderson website. This honorary nursing society is keen on encouraging nurses to share and allow feedback on nursing research. This is a good example of a green open access (institutional repository).

Awareness of the previously described international and open source information is important even if not used in all searches for instruments. There is the possibility of finding relevant references to tools or perhaps copies of them.

SUMMARY

In locating instruments, a search on Google may occasionally retrieve a copy of an instrument or scale. Librarians refer to such searches as a "quick and dirty" way of finding what is needed. Searching through the print books suggested is a good starting point for standard instruments. Many of the books cited in the text and in Resources are readily available in major university libraries with some providing full text online.

The databases suggested (CINAHL, HaPI, PubMed, Cochrane databases, PsycInfo, and ERIC), may all need to be searched methodically to find articles on validity and reliability. It is hoped that with the suggested terms given in this chapter, the APRN can practice basic search strategies and use the techniques in other databases to construct meaningful strategies. Luckily, some authors include the instrument in the article. If a dissertation contains an instrument, the document may be ordered online or through library service.

In using the Resources (Internet) section, take time to look at the university library websites to supplement the information in this chapter. It is worthwhile looking at these for more step-by-step approaches that are not covered here. And finally, medical librarians are good resources to help find measurement instruments.

Answers to Chapter Discussion Questions

1. The two best databases to start searching are CINAHL and HaPI. In CINAHL, when doing a search use the "Select Field" drop-down menu and choose "instrumentation" from the list. Type in the term "diabetes" in the box to the left of "instrumentation." Using the limiters on the left of the screen, under "Publication Type," scroll down to choose both "questionnaire/scale" and "research instrument." Other limiters were English and references published within the past 6 years. In CINAHL, the strategy retrieved: Kiblinger, L. (2007) Tool chest. Diabetes Risk/Improvement Scale, *Diabetes Educator, 33*(4), 628, 630, 632 passim. In the HaPI database, using the strategy of entering diabetes in the box and selecting the field "measure," and then "and-ing" nursing in all text fields allowed many references to be retrieved. Limits included 2000 to 2012 publication years. One of the references retrieved was: Lin, C., et al. (2008). Diabetes Self-Management Instrument, *Research in Nursing & Health, 31*, 370–380. EBSCO and some university websites have videos on their own players or on YouTube that explain how to use the CINAHL database.

2. To find details about the MMPI, check MMYB as well as test critiques. If in a library, check the other books in the reference collection around the MMYB to become familiar with these standard sources. This reference is also online in many libraries. Details on the MMYB are found in this chapter under Standard Books. To check which local library has these books, the online catalog may be found by conducting a Google search of the name of the university or public library. A good source to check is WorldCat at www.worldcat.org. This amazing site provides information on the libraries that own the book in the area where the reader lives. For example, search WorldCat for *Handbook of Disease Burdens and Quality of Life Measures*; scrolling down shows several locations in the state. WorldCat also has a mobile app for a fee.

3. In the Resources (University Library Websites) section, check different sites to see which ones have information on responsible use of tests. Dan Chaney, librarian at Oklahoma State University, offers succinct descriptions: "Suggestions for Getting a Copy of That Test or Measurement." Also listed are three points about "Responsible Use of Tests and Measures." The URL for this work is given in Resources at the end of this chapter. Permission was granted by Dan Chaney to use the link for this chapter. Article references often have the author's e-mail address, which can be used to find details about using the test/instrument described. Many instruments cannot be used except by social workers or psychology professionals or by special training. In the HaPI database is a primary source article titled "Worst Pain Intensity Scale," in *Oncology Nursing Forum, 38*(1), 33–42 by M. J. Dodd. When PubMed is checked for a recent article by M. J. Dodd, the e-mail address is listed as she is the first author. To find

out about the scale and how it is used, e-mail the author. Researchers are flattered that their work may be used and duplicated with their knowledge. The assumption might be made that this author would explain use and could give permission and training for use of the instrument.

4. For information on physician–nurse professional collaboration, the PsycInfo, CINAHL, HaPI, and PubMed Handheld are all available on mobile/handheld devices.

   ▪ PsycINFO app is available from EBSCOhost and the American Psychological Association site. CINAHL and HaPI are also available through EBSCOhost.
   ▪ The CINAHL database keywords for searching might be "work environment, nurse–physician relations, collaboration, occupational stress, professional autonomy, questionnaires, psychological tests, and theoretical nursing models."
   ▪ PubMed Handheld is available from the National Library of Medicine. A search of PsycINFO provides many references on nurse–physician professional collaboration using keywords, such as "practice environment, nurse physician communication, job satisfaction, nursing role effectiveness model, teamwork, and interprofessional education." In PubMed, medical subject headings to use are "attitude of health personnel, physician–nurse relations, cooperative behavior, questionnaires, medical staff, hospital, and nursing staff, hospital."

5. The most promising resources for the reader are subjective. The most promising databases are CINAHL, PubMed, HaPI, PsycInfo, and ERIC. All university websites listed at the end of this chapter are relevant. For books, many library catalogs can be searched online, and university libraries assign passwords to students and faculty enabling access to electronic books.

WEB LINKS

▪ Most bibliographic databases charge a fee and are accessed via universities, hospitals, or other places of employment. Following are some free-access databases:
   o National Library of Medicine's Medline. Pubmed.gov
   o Education Resources Information Center. www.ERIC.ed.gov
   o Cochrane Collaboration for evidence-based medicine free summaries. www.Cochrane.org
   o Google often retrieves references from Medline and other databases and provides some full-text articles. scholar.google.com
   o The American Psychological Association's site on tests provides information about ethical research and the proper use of psychological tests. www.apa.org
   o ETS database with descriptions of 25,000 tests and research instruments. www.ets.org

▪ Additional websites are provided at the end of this chapter in the section Resources (University Library Websites). MMYB has free Test Reviews Online (buros.unl.edu) for all publications by the Buros Institute (buros.org).
▪ To check a local library collection, consider using www.WorldCat.org. An added feature when using the mobile app, WorldCat Mobile, allows typing in the zip code to

locate the nearest library. In conjunction with WorldCat Mobile, the app RedLaser uses the mobile phone's camera to scan the ISBN to check on books in bookstores and to discover the books in library locations. Libraries are beginning to develop their own handheld apps so that users may access their catalogs.

RESOURCES

Books

Aday, L., & Cornelius, L. J. (2006). *Designing and conducting health surveys* (3rd ed.). San Francisco, CA: Jossey-Bass.

American Psychiatric Association. (2000). *Handbook of psychiatric measures*. Washington, DC: Author.

Anderson, N., Schlueten, J. E., Carlson, J. F., & Geisinger, K. F. (Eds.). (2016). *Tests in print* (9th ed.). Lincoln, NE: Buros Center. (Designed to be a companion to Mental Measurements Yearbook.)

Bowling, A. (2001). *Measuring disease: A review of disease-specific quality of life measurement scales* (2nd ed.). Philadelphia, PA: Open University Press.

Bowling, A. (2005). *Measuring health: A review of quality of life measurement scales* (3rd ed.). New York, NY: Oxford University Press.

Clayton, G. M. (1989). *Instruments for use in nursing education research*. New York, NY: National League for Nursing.

Corcoran, K., & Fischer, J. (2013). *Measures for clinical practice: A sourcebook* (5th ed., Vol. 2). New York, NY: Oxford University Press.

Cunningham, C. J. L., Weathering, B. L., & Pittenger, D. J. (2013). *Understanding and conducting research in health sciences*. Hoboken, NJ: Wiley.

Dana, R. H. (2005). *Multicultural assessment: Principles, applications, and examples*. Mahwah, NJ: Lawrence Erlbaum.

Frank-Stromborg, M. (2004). *Instruments for clinical health-care research*. Boston, MA: Jones & Bartlett.

Goldman, B. A., & Mitchell, D. F. (Eds.). (2007). *Directory of unpublished experimental mental measures*. Washington, DC: American Psychological Association.

Kane, R. L., & Radosevich, D. M. (2011). *Conducting health outcomes research*. Sudbury, MA: Jones & Bartlett.

Lewis, C. B. (1997). *The functional tool box: Clinical measures of functional outcomes* (Vol. 2). McClean, VA: Learn. (Tools to aid in measuring patient outcomes in rehabilitation interventions. Each tool has simplified instructions with population, descriptions, completion time, interpretation, reliability, validity, and complete references. [2000 edition out of print].)

Maddox T. (Ed.). (2008). *Tests: A comprehensive reference for assessments in psychology, education and business* (6th ed.). Austin, Texas: Pro-Ed. (Includes descriptions of tests, purpose of tests, cost, and availability. Does not contain evaluative critiques of data on reliability and validity.)

McDowell, I. (2006). *Measuring health: A guide to rating scales and questionnaires* (3rd ed.). New York, NY: Oxford University Press.

Measurement of nursing outcomes. (2nd ed.) (3 vols.) [Vol. 1: Waltz, C.F., & Jenkins, L. (Eds.). (2001). *Measuring nursing performance: Practice, education and research*; Vol. 2: Strickland, O. L., & Dilorio, C. (Eds.). (2003). *Client outcomes and quality of care*; Vol. 3: Strickland, O. L., & Dilorio, C. (Eds.). (2003). *Self-care and coping*]. New York, NY: Springer Publishing.

Miller, D. C., & Salkind, N. J. (2002). *Handbook of research design and social measurement* (6th ed.). Newbury Park, CA: Sage.

Murphy, L. L., Spies, R. A., & Plake, B. S. (Eds.). (2014). *Mental measurements yearbook* (19th ed.). Lincoln, NE: Buros Institute of Mental Measurements.

Peterson, K. W., Travis, J. W., Dewey, J. E., Framer, E. M., Foerster, J. J., & Hyner, G. C. (Eds.). (1999). *SPM handbook of health assessment tools*. Pittsburgh, PA: Society of Prospective Medicine, & Irving, Texas: Institute for Health and Productivity Management (published jointly). (This book discusses and lists various types of scales; also has addresses and validity/reliability remarks about them; contains life-style tools.)

Preedy, V. R., & Watson, R. R. (Eds.). (2010). *Handbook of disease burdens and quality of life measures* (Vol. 6). New York, NY: Springer. (Note: This is a $3,000.00 set, available in medical and university libraries; some have the electronic version. See website under Resources [Internet].)

Redman, B. K. (2003). *Measurement tools in patient education* (2nd ed.). New York, NY: Springer Publishing.

Schutte, N. S., & Malouff, J. M. (1995). *Sourcebook of adult assessment strategies*. New York, NY: Plenum. (2014 software reprint of original 1st ed. 1995.)

Shelton, P. J. (2000). *Measuring and improving patient satisfaction*. Gaithersburg, VA: Aspen. (Appendices include: Appendix A – Focus Group Moderator's Guide; Appendix B – Patient Satisfaction Survey Instrument; Appendix C – Principles of Continuous Quality Improvement: Presentation slides.)

Streiner, D. L., Norman, G. R., & Cairney, J. (2015). *Health measurement scales: A practical guide to their development and use* (5th ed.). New York, NY: Oxford University Press. (Note Appendix A: Where to find tests. This appendix contains 16 categories including general, online sources, health and clinical conditions, quality of life, and nursing and patient education.)

Test critiques (Vol. 10). (1984–present). Kansas City, MO: Test Corporation of America (This multi-volume set is the companion to *Tests* and includes reliability and validity information.)

Thompson, C. (1989). *Instruments of psychiatric research*. Somerset, NJ: John Wiley (This is a $595 book.)

Waltz, C. F., Strickland, O. L., & Lenz, E. R. (2016). *Measurement in nursing and health research* (5th ed.). New York, NY: Springer Publishing.

Internet

American Psychological Association (APA) has an excellent section on their home page entitled: Frequently Asked Questions (FAQ) on Psychological Tests. Retrieved from http://www.apa.org/science/testing.html

Educational Testing Service (ETS) Test collection database. www.ets.org contains descriptions of over 10,000 tests and research instruments with information indicating either a person or institution to contact or a journal citation for an article describing or including the test.

University Library Websites

Consider checking your favorite local university website when starting your search for instruments. Many librarians have created extensive, detailed guides to finding instruments because this is a common question asked of librarians. The following is a list of some good sites, but by no means is this a complete list. These may be starting points, and a Google search may retrieve many other university sites. *These sites were all active when accessed/retrieved October 15, 2016.* The year given after the titles on the sites refers to the last update of the page. If websites have gone inactive by the time you access them, try to do a Google search of the university library.

Bardeen, A. (2011). *Finding tests, surveys and measurements.* Chapel Hill, NC: University of North Carolina, Chapel Hill. Retrieved from http://www.lib.unc.edu/subjectguides/FindingTests

Hough, H. (2012*). Tests and measures.* Arlington, TX: University of Texas at Arlington. Retrieved from http://libraries.uta.edu/tmdb (Helen Hough, who put together this guide available on its own special server, is a good supplement to the material in this chapter. The library websites linked on this library guide are more comprehensive than the list provided here. Allow a large amount of time for browsing this guide because it is full of amazing open access books about scales, tests and instruments.)

San Diego State University Library has a website that has a section *SDSU Test Finder.* It was developed by librarian M. Stover and may be retrieved from http://www-rohan.sdsu.edu/~mstover/ tests (On this site, you will find an index of complete tests and instruments found in scholarly journal articles.)

Teno, J. M., Okun, S. N., Casey, V., & Welch, L. C. (2001). *Toolkit of instruments to measure end of life care resource guide (TIME). Resource guide: Achieving quality of care at life's end.* Retrieved from https://nts122.chcr.brown.edu/pcoc/resourceguide/resourceguide.pdf (The author was listed in 2001 as being from the Center for Gerontology and Health Research, Brown University. This text, which includes many appendices with tools, is considered free to use but not to publish. In searching for this website, Google may need to be used instead of the URL provided.)

University of Maryland Libraries. (2011). *Tests and measurements guide.* Retrieved from http://lib .guides.umd.edu/srch.php?q=tests+measures (This guide is designed to serve as a tool to help obtain information about published and unpublished educational, psychological, and vocational tests and measurements. This site has a step-by-step description of the process of finding tests.)

University of Michigan Taubman Medical Library. (2012). *Finding tests and measurement instruments.* Retrieved from http://guides.lib.umich.edu/tests (Note: This site provides a reference to a textbook on responsible test use.)

University of Pennsylvania. *Tests and measurements guides.* Retrieved from http://guides.library .upenn.edu/tests/tests (Note: Includes good section on getting tests.)

University of Washington has a library guide with some tutorials. (2016). *Measurement tools/ research instruments.* Seattle, WA: University of Washington. Retrieved from http://libguides.hsl .washington.edu/measure

CHAPTER 6

Measuring Outcomes in Cardiovascular Advanced Practice Nursing

Anna Gawlinski, Kathy McCloy, Virginia Erickson, Elizabeth Vandenbogaart, and Anna Dermenchyan

Chapter Objectives

1. Identify outcomes of concern to advanced practice registered nurses (APRNs) and compare these to the outcomes currently being measured in your institution and your patient population
2. Discuss advantages and disadvantages of each of the methods that are used for outcome measurement projects (e.g., research, research utilization, evidence-based practice [EBP], and quality improvement [QI] frameworks)
3. Analyze the relative effectiveness of interventions that have been shown to decrease medication discrepancies
4. Discuss the role of the APRN in working with interdisciplinary teams to improve outcomes in patients with cardiovascular disease

Chapter Discussion Questions

1. How does the medication reconciliation process defined in this chapter compare with the interventions implemented by the APRNs in the exemplar medication reconciliation outcome measurement project?
2. How do the outcomes of concern to APRNs listed in Exhibit 6.1 compare with outcomes currently being measured in your institution and your patient population?
3. Identify two to three clinical issues and related outcomes in your practice. Which research designs or other frameworks would be most appropriate to use in an outcome measurement project? Why?

4. How effective are the interventions described in the literature in decreasing medication discrepancies? Design a study to address the medication discrepancy issue for your patient population and discuss why you chose that design.

5. Discuss the interdisciplinary team's project to improve outcomes in patients with heart failure (HF). What aspects of the project could be beneficial to your own patient population?

EXHIBIT 6.1   **Select Outcomes for Advanced Practice Nursing**

Clinical (Care-Related) Outcomes

Mortality

Morbidity

   Infection: hospital associated, urinary tract infection, ventilator or catheter related

   Hand hygiene compliance rates

   Developing medical conditions such as acquiring heart failure from uncontrolled hypertension

   Loss of motor function

   Physiological response

      Blood pressure, heart rate

      Temperature

      Lung sounds

      Hemodynamic pressures

      Weight and weight management

      Serum/urine level of glucose

      Wound healing, skin integrity

   Symptom management

      Pain

      Fatigue

      Nausea, vomiting

Nutritional status/management

Sleep maintenance

Restraint use

Smoking cessation

Substance use/abuse (illicit or prescriptive)

Low birth weight, preterm infants

Rates of adherence to best practices

Psychosocial Outcomes

Coping, stress management

Mentation

Return to work

Role functioning

Family functioning/coping

Anxiety

(continued)

EXHIBIT 6.1   Select Outcomes for Advanced Practice Nursing (*continued*)

Depression
Sexual functioning
Caregiver strain/burden
Knowledge patient/caregiver: disease/condition, medications, diet, treatment regime, psychomotor skills
Health literacy
Cultural sensitivity
Underserved populations
Staff nurse knowledge
Functional Outcomes
Quality of life
Self-care: bathing, eating, dressing self, administration of nonparenteral medication
Mobility
Communication
Return to
Work
School
Normal activity/social interaction
Symptom control
Fiscal Outcomes
Length of stay (hospital and/or intensive care unit)
Readmission rates to hospital, home care, other services
Emergency department visits
Health care services utilization
Cost per episode of care
Resource utilization: ancillary services, community/other services
Patient flow, improve throughput
Access and barriers to health care
Disparities in care received and outcomes
Savings from APRN practice
Staff nurse retention rates
Satisfaction
Patient experience
Care provided
Services provided
Care provider
Family
Care provided to family member
Services provided/available
Payer
Provider

APRN, advanced practice registered nurse.

Source: Adapted from Urden (1999); Kleinpell-Nowell and Weiner (1999); and Newhouse et al. (2011).

National health care policy makers and health care professionals have increasingly advocated for the measurement and monitoring of patient safety, QI, and health care outcomes. The development and implementation of national practice guidelines that are based on the best available research have provided clinicians with interventions that can improve patients' outcomes (McClellan, McGinnis, Nabel, & Olsen, 2007). Yet these practice guidelines are not consistently used, and practices vary from clinician to clinician and from institution to institution, resulting in poor outcomes for patients (Centers for Medicare & Medicaid Services [CMS], 2012; Institute of Medicine, 2001; Melnyk & Fineout-Overholt, 2015).

This emphasis on EBP has resulted in increased focus and incentives for those institutions and providers that perform well on indicators of safety and quality, with measurable outcomes. For example, the CMS and The Joint Commission (TJC) have set standards for performance measurement for patients hospitalized with HF that include measures of use of research-based therapies, such as angiotensin-converting enzyme inhibitors and beta-blockers, as well as reduction in hospital readmission rates (CMS, 2011; TJC, 2012).

Cardiovascular disease in particular lends itself to measurement of such quality indicators and outcomes. Cardiovascular disease is the leading cause of mortality and health care cost for men and women in the United States (Mozaffarian et al., 2016). These statistics, along with the high acuity and chronicity of cardiovascular disease and the availability of published national guidelines outlining "best practices," contribute to the pressing need for outcome measurement in the field of cardiovascular nursing (Mozaffarian et al., 2016).

Although a great deal of effort has been devoted to developing EBP guidelines for cardiovascular disease, more data are needed to demonstrate how these guidelines can be translated into practice and what their subsequent effect is on outcomes in everyday clinical settings. Cardiovascular APRNs are in a key position to use their expert knowledge of research-based practices and outcome measurement to generate data that demonstrate successful translation of these guidelines into the clinical setting.

The purpose of this chapter is to provide an overview of outcome measurement in advanced practice nursing, discuss methods that can be used for outcome measurement, and describe the role of the cardiovascular APRN in outcome measurement. An outcome measurement project is presented to demonstrate the unique role of the APRN in using an EBP approach to implement changes that result in positive measurable outcomes. A discussion follows that demonstrates how the APRN-initiated outcome project provided important preliminary data for a system-wide QI initiative to improve outcomes in patients with HF. The contributors' aim is to present exemplars of outcome projects and share processes that can be replicated to reduce variations in practice and improve outcomes in cardiovascular patients.

CLINICAL OUTCOMES

Clinical and patient outcomes are defined as the end results of care that can be attributed to the health care services provided, such as treatments, procedures, and planned interventions (Kleinpell & Alexandrov, 2014). Outcomes are the consequences of treatment or interventions (Finkelman & Kenner, 2012; Kleinpell & Alexandrov, 2014). They can be used to characterize the results (effect) of an intervention, treatment, or system-level process of care. Clinical outcomes demonstrate the value and effectiveness of care and can be assessed for individuals, populations, and organizations (Kapu & Kleinpell, 2013).

Outcomes are often quantified or measured through the use of indicators, which are referred to as *metrics*. Outcome indicators or metrics provide estimates that reflect the degree to which patients are affected by their care (Stanik-Hutt, 2012). Indicators must be valid and reliable measures that are related to the outcome of interest. For example, to measure the adequacy of cholesterol management (a clinical outcome) in a patient with coronary artery disease, indicators of this outcome would include levels of various components of a patient's blood lipid panel such as the total cholesterol, the low-density lipoprotein (LDL), and the high-density lipoprotein (HDL). Indicators provide a picture of the progress toward achievement of the outcome, whereas outcomes can be considered predictors of end performance (Finkelman & Kenner, 2012).

Indicators or metrics that are reported to agencies outside the internal organization are referred to as *performance measures* (Finkelman & Kenner, 2012). In the past two decades, a wide array of standardized health care performance measures have been developed, and a large number of these have been endorsed by the National Quality Forum (NQF). The NQF is a private, not-for-profit membership organization whose purpose is to develop a national strategy for health care quality measurement and reporting. The NQF currently develops, reviews, and measures performance standards for health care, and promotes national standardization of these quality performance measures (Finkelman & Kenner, 2012).

A substantial growth has occurred in the number of entities using health care performance measures for a variety of purposes. For example, quality and efficiency performance measures are now embedded throughout the U.S. health care system. The purposes for their widespread use are (a) QI, (b) public reporting, (c) regulation (e.g., accreditation, certification, credentialing, and licensure), and (d) payment applications (e.g., financial incentives, tiered payment; Damberg et al., 2012).

Recently, the Patient Protection and Affordable Care Act (2010) authorized the Hospital Value-Based Purchasing (VBP) program as an initiative focused on improving hospital performance for quality measures related to clinical processes of care, hospital-acquired conditions, outcomes of care, and the patients' experience of care. In this program, CMS withholds a portion of hospital reimbursement each year and redistributes these funds as incentive payments to hospitals on the basis of their performance on these measures (CMS, 2011).

Performance measures are often benchmarked or compared with other institutions. *Benchmarking* is a process to identify best practices, which, when implemented, can lead to superior performance (DesHarnais, 2013). It is the use of external comparisons to understand how one is doing compared to one's peers and/or one's competitors (practitioners or institutions). Data of performance measures are compared between health care systems or within a single health care system (DesHarnais, 2013). These comparisons allow APRNs to identify areas of strengths and weaknesses in relation to best practice.

NURSING OUTCOMES

The care of patients often requires the expertise of several health care professionals. When many health care providers interact with patients and contribute to their care, it may be difficult to attribute successful clinical patient outcomes to any one provider or treatment. Thus, identifying outcomes that can be attributed only to nursing care can be a challenge, because attribution requires a high level of confidence that the outcome is a direct result of that provider's care (Dennison & Hughes, 2009).

For example, an HF patient who was discharged and begins to experience symptoms of increasing dyspnea and weight gain at home may be treated by several health care providers (RN, APRN, and registered dietitian [RD]). At hospital discharge, the RN provided the patient with detailed discharge instructions regarding the important aspects of HF management, including specific instructions regarding symptoms to immediately report to his or her health care provider (i.e., dyspnea and/or weight gain, 2 pounds in 24 hours or 5 pounds in 4 days). The RD counseled the patient in-hospital, reviewed the recommended guidelines for a low-sodium diet, and provided instructions about reading labels and interpreting sodium content.

The cardiovascular APRN was notified of the new onset of the patient's symptoms and asked the patient to schedule a clinic appointment. During the clinic appointment, the APRN assesses for contributing factors, such as physiologic changes in cardiac function, medication nonadherence issues, and dietary indiscretion. On the basis of the assessment, the APRN orders additional diagnostic tests (e.g., brain natriuretic peptide, echocardiogram), reinforces education regarding the need for the patient to adjust diuretic therapy on the basis of daily weight, and reinforces specifics about medication and dietary regimens. A referral is also made to the RD. The RD reviews the recommended low-sodium diet and helps the patient make better food selections. Upon follow-up, when the patient reports less dyspnea and decreased weight, the question arises as to which health care professional was responsible for the achievement of these positive outcomes. Was it the RN, the APRN, or the RD, or the whole team (Stanik-Hutt, 2012)?

Attempts to measure outcomes that can be attributed to nursing care have resulted in a definition of *nurse-sensitive outcomes*. Nurse-sensitive outcomes are defined as outcomes that are sensitive enough to measure the effect of nursing practice (Finkelman & Kenner, 2012; Joseph, 2007). They represent the impact of nursing interventions and describe the effect of what nurses do in response to the patient's condition. Several nursing care outcomes that reflect nursing performance have been selected for national reporting. These nursing care outcomes include measures of patient-centered outcomes such as mortality among surgical inpatients with treatable serious complications, prevalence of pressure ulcers, falls (with and without injury), use of restraints, and hospital-associated infections such as catheter-related urinary tract infections, central-catheter-associated bloodstream infections, and ventilator-associated pneumonias. Additional measures include nursing-centered intervention processes, such as smoking-cessation counseling, and system-centered structures and processes such as nursing staff skill mix and nursing care hours per patient day (Finkelman & Kenner, 2012; Kurtzman & Corrigan, 2007; Stanik-Hutt, 2012).

Researchers at the University of Iowa have provided leadership in the area of nurse-sensitive outcomes by creating the nursing interventions classification (NIC) and nursing outcomes classification (NOC), which link nursing interventions to diagnoses and outcomes. This research team has contributed to identifying outcomes and related measures at the individual patient, family, and community levels, which can be used to evaluate nursing care across the patient care continuum. Individual patients' outcome data can be aggregated in a number of ways to assess the effectiveness of nursing care within an organization and across various settings (Moorhead, Johnson, Maas, & Swanson, 2008). This research team is disseminating and publishing their work to facilitate more consistent documentation of nursing interventions and outcomes.

CLASSIFICATION OF OUTCOMES

Historically, the classification of health care outcomes has used medical definitions known as the "five Ds": death, disease, disability, discomfort, and dissatisfaction (Gawlinski et al., 2013; Lohr, 1988; Urden, 1999), but classification of outcomes varies. For example, outcomes can be categorized as generic and broad-based outcomes that pertain to all patients and health care providers (e.g., quality of care, access, cost, patients' satisfaction, and utilization of service). Outcomes have also been categorized in other ways, such as patient/care related, system related, practitioner or performance related, and cost/financial related (Kleinpell & Alexandrov, 2014). Other categories of outcomes are clinical, psychological, functional, and satisfaction related (Kleinpell & Alexandrov, 2014; Urden, 1999).

OUTCOME MEASURES USED IN ADVANCED PRACTICE NURSING

APRNs are often faced with the dilemma of what constitutes an outcome and which outcomes should be measured. The outcomes that best reflect clinical practice and the goals of treatment are the most meaningful and most amenable to measurement (Gawlinski, 2007; Gawlinski et al., 2013). Several websites (Table 6.1) and publications provide APRNs with excellent resources on selected health outcome information and specific outcome measures and instruments (Academy Health, 2011; Gawlinski et al., 2013; Moorhead et al., 2008). For example, Fulton and Baldwin (2004) published an annotated bibliography reflecting clinical nurse specialist practice and outcomes (Fulton & Baldwin, 2004). Urden (1999) published a list of a broad spectrum of outcomes using clinical, physiological, psychological, functional, fiscal, and satisfaction categories (Urden, 1999). Newhouse et al. (2011) presented a systematic review of APRN outcomes from 1990 to 2008 examining patient satisfaction, patient self-reported perceived health, functional status, glucose, lipid and blood pressure control, duration of mechanical ventilation, emergency department (ED) or urgent care visits, hospitalizations, length of stay, cost, complications, and mortality (Newhouse et al., 2011). This systematic review demonstrated that APRN care promotes patient access to care, reduces complications, and results in improved patient knowledge, self-care management, and patient satisfaction. Kleinpell (2003) provided a list of sources for identifying outcome

TABLE 6.1 Selected Health Outcome Information Websites

Organization	Website
Academy for Healthcare Research and Quality	www.ahrq.gov/clinic/outcomix.htm
Centers for Disease Control and Prevention (CDC)	www.cdc.gov/nchs/hus.htm
Centers for Medicare & Medicaid Services	www.cms.gov
Health Resources and Services Administration (HRSA)	www.hrsa.gov/index.html
Healthy People 2020	www.healthypeople.gov/2020/default.aspx
Institute for Healthcare Improvement (IHI): Transforming Care at the Bedside	www.ihi.org/engage/initiatives/completed/TCAB/Pages/default.aspx
Institute for Healthcare Improvement	www.ihi.org
Institute of Medicine of the National Academies	www.nationalacademies.org/HMD
International Society for Quality of Life Research (ISOQOL)	www.isoqol.org
The Joint Commission on Accreditation of Healthcare Organizations	www.jointcommission.org
National Academy of Medicine (formerly Institute of Medicine)	http://nam.edu
National Database of Nursing Quality Indicators®	www.pressganey.com/solutions/clinical-quality/nursing-quality
National Guideline Clearinghouse (NGC)	www.guideline.gov
National Committee for Quality Assurance	www.ncqa.org
National Quality Measures Clearinghouse (NQMC)	www.qualitymeasures.ahrq.gov
National Patient Safety Foundation	www.npsf.org
Nursing Quality Forum	www.qualityforum.org/Home.aspx
Patient-Reported Quality of Life Instruments Database	www.proqolid.org
Registered Nurses Association of Ontario—"Clinical Practice Guidelines Program"	http://rnao.ca/bpg/guidelines/clinical
University of Alberta—"Evidence-Based Medicine Toolkit"	www.ebm.med.ualberta.ca/ebm.html
University of Iowa College of Nursing	www.nursing.uiowa.edu/cncce/nursing-outcomes-classification-overview
U.S. Department of Health and Human Services—Hospital Compare	www.medicare.gov/hospitalcompare
U.S. National Library of Medicine (NLM)/HTA 101: Introduction to Health Technology Assessment	www.nlm.nih.gov and www.nlm.nih.gov/nichsr/hta101/ta10101.html

measures and outcome instruments for analyzing the impact of APRN care (Kleinpell, 2003). Exhibit 6.1 provides a listing of select outcome measures that can be used by APRNs according to these published literature reviews.

In 2011, Academy Health issued a list of publications (books and journals) and electronic resources (bibliographic databases and websites) that provides health care professionals with a comprehensive library of core and essential health outcome resources. This comprehensive list of health outcome resources can be accessed at www.nlm.nih.gov/nichsr/corelib/houtcomes-2011.html and has been reviewed and revised.

APRNs are at the forefront of improving care through outcome measurement. They serve as critical members of the health care team. Because of their key role in the health care system, APRNs frequently lead outcome measurement and QI initiatives. By virtue of their graduate education preparation, clinical knowledge, and critical thinking skills, APRNs have an essential role in evaluating outcomes for improvement efforts. Additionally, APRN core competencies demonstrate expertise and provide additional areas for measuring outcomes. These core competencies include expert coaching and advice, consultation, research skills, clinical and professional leadership, collaboration, and ethical decision making (Hamric, Hanson, Tracy, & O'Grady, 2012). For these reasons, as well as the APRNs' consistent presence with patients and their patient advocacy role, APRNs frequently possess an integrated, holistic, and broader view of what constitutes an important outcome. Using this view, APRNs not only measure traditional physiologic outcomes, but also include outcomes related to psychosocial, functional, behavioral, symptoms, quality of life (QOL), knowledge, and satisfaction. Because a change in one outcome may influence changes in another outcome, APRNs are interested in the interaction and relationship of these outcomes. For example, exacerbation of a patient's symptoms can interfere with a patient's physiologic, psychosocial, and functional status and with QOL. APRNs are especially interested in the management and control of symptoms.

In APRN practice, examples of physiologic outcomes of concern may include pulse, blood pressure, lipid levels, blood glucose levels, weight, and other physiologic parameters. Relevant psychosocial outcomes may include the patient's mood, attitudes, and abilities to interact with others. For functional outcomes, a patient's mobility, physical independence, and ability to participate in desired activities of daily living would be considered important. Behavioral outcomes of significance may include adequacy of coping with health care needs or a patient's ability to follow (adhere to) recommended care. Symptoms, such as pain, dyspnea, and fatigue would require an assessment and evaluation independent from the diseases that cause them. QOL is another natural outcome of interest for APRNs. QOL is defined as a patient's general perception of his or her physical and mental well-being that can be affected by many factors including disease and injury, stress and emotions, symptom control and functional status, as well as others. Finally, the patient's knowledge level would be a valuable outcome to measure for APRN practice. This measure could include an individual patient's understanding of health-related information such as his or her disease/condition, medications, diet, and aspects of treatment regime. Although patient satisfaction is a quality indicator for all health care providers, patient satisfaction with the care, communication, and compassion provided by the APRN would be particularly meaningful feedback for the individual practitioner (Stanik-Hutt, 2012).

Outcomes specific to the role of the APRN are also of interest. These types of role-based outcomes are frequently related to the health care system and to cost. They may include clinic wait times, hospital length of stay, bed occupancy rate, timely discharge, cost per adjusted discharge, and so forth.

Typically, the APRN is part of a larger entity, where multiple clinicians work as a health care team. Consequently, identifying outcomes specific to the impact of APRN care may not be a standard component of an institution's outcome measurement program. For example, Moote, Krsek, Kleinpell, and Todd (2011) reported that health care organizations that employed 200 or more APRNs did not consistently collect focused outcomes to assess the specific contribution of APRN care (Moote et al., 2011). However, researchers in some studies (Albert et al., 2010; Moote et al., 2011; Newhouse et al., 2011) have evaluated APRN utilization and/or comparability with other health care providers. Results of these studies indicate that patients' outcomes of care provided by APRNs in collaboration with physicians are similar and in some ways better than care provided by physicians alone for the populations and settings included (Newhouse et al., 2011). Albert et al. (2010) examined the influence of care by APRNs and physician assistants (PAs) on the delivery of guideline-recommended therapies for outpatients with HF (Albert et al., 2010). Compared to no APRNs or PAs, a cardiology practice with more than 2.0 APRNs or PAs was associated with greater use of implantable cardioverter defibrillator therapy, delivery of HF education, and equivalent use of drug and cardiac resynchronization therapies. Utilization of APRNs and PAs in academic health centers was initially cited as primarily for resident duty hour restrictions. However, secondary reasons for employing APRNs and PAs included improving patient throughput, increasing patient access, improving patient safety, reducing length of stay, and improving continuity of care (Moote et al., 2011). To date, further research is needed that identifies and tests metrics specific to the measurement of APRN practice. With the development of further regulatory agency requirements, such as CMS pay for performance initiatives (CMS, 2011), and the TJC practice standards (TJC Resources, 2011), measuring and highlighting APRN-specific outcomes is an important and essential component of advanced practice nursing (Kapu & Kleinpell, 2013).

Generally, outcome measures in the cardiac population have focused on phenomena such as the effect of an aggressive cholesterol management program implemented by an APRN, the effect of applying EBPs to manage HF, the effect of APRN practice on management and prevention of postoperative complications, interventions to promote QOL, and evaluation of a spectrum of physiological responses to APRN interventions (e.g., blood pressure, heart rate, hemodynamics, urine output, daily weight, nutrition, and symptom control; Becker et al., 2005; Bergenson & Dean, 2006; De la Porte et al., 2007; DeWalt et al., 2006; Kutzleb & Reiner, 2006; Meyer & Miers, 2005; Paez & Allen, 2006; Paul, 2000). Sample outcome measures that are of concern in the cardiovascular population are listed in Exhibit 6.2.

In an era of high-quality, safe, effective, and cost-containing health care, several professional organizations have taken the lead to form expert panels that identify EBPs and associated quality and performance measures for select high-volume and high-risk patient populations. This is especially true in the area of prevention, diagnosis, and treatment of patients at risk or patients with cardiovascular disease. For example, in 2010, the American Heart Association (AHA) identified Strategic Impact Goals for cardiovascular disease and stroke. These goals include that by 2020, cardiovascular health of all Americans will improve by 20%, while simultaneously reducing deaths from cardiovascular diseases and stroke by 20%. To help achieve this goal, the AHA created Life's Simple 7 Metrics. Four of the metrics are related to health behaviors (i.e., diet quality, physical

EXHIBIT 6.2   Selected Outcomes for the Cardiovascular Population

Reduction of Cardiac Risk Factors

Control of hypertension (blood pressure)

Diabetes control (blood glucose, glucose $A1_c$)

Body mass index, obesity, weight loss

Lipid (cholesterol, high- and low-density lipoproteins, triglycerides)

Physical activity

Diet quality (e.g., low fat, low sodium, low sugar intake)

Knowledge: medications, diet, treatment regimen, motor skills, condition specific

Smoking cessation

Alcohol intake

Obstructive apnea screening

Family history/genetic screening and counseling

Self-care interventions

Patient adherence

Acute Coronary Syndrome

Guideline-directed therapy (i.e., cardioprotective medication regimen)

    Frequency prescribed

    Frequency of reaching target goals for lipid levels

Presence or absence of chest pain

Presence or absence of arrhythmias

Resuscitation outcomes: CPR/defibrillation bystander/EMS/in hospital; time to treatment, survival

Time to BCLS, defibrillation, ACLS (bystander, EMS, in-hospital)

Time to hypothermia treatment intervention protocol

Time to reperfusion

Access and barriers to care

Gender/disparity differences

Depression

Resource utilization

    Echocardiograms, EKGs, blood tests, chest radiographs, etc.

    Pharmacist, case manager, home health, dietician, social services, physical therapy, etc.

Length of stay (hospital, cardiac care unit)

Cost per case

Functional status

Cardiac rehabilitation referral and attendance (or participation in exercise program)

In addition to those in *Reduction of Cardiac Risk Factors*

Heart Failure

Readmission rates

Symptom management

(continued)

EXHIBIT 6.2 Selected Outcomes for the Cardiovascular Population (*continued*)

Guideline-directed management therapy
Frequency prescribed
Adherence to medication regimen
Daily weight monitoring
Fluid limit
Adherence to low-sodium diet
Obstructive sleep apnea screening
Referral for implantable cardioverter defibrillator and device management
Pulmonary artery pressure sensor measurements (referral for implant effect of monitoring)
Functional status
Referral to cardiac rehabilitation and attendance (or participation in exercise program)
Anxiety
Depression
Mortality rates
Referral for palliative care
Referral for mechanical assist device and device management
Referral for advanced therapies such as heart transplant
Resource utilization
Echocardiograms, EKGs, blood tests, chest radiographs, etc.
Pharmacist, case manager, home health, dietician, social services, physical therapy, etc.
In addition to those mentioned previously in *Reduction of Cardiac Risk Factors*
After Percutaneous Transluminal Angioplasty/Stent Placement
Reocclusion rates
Hematoma rates
Bleeding requiring transfusion
Other vascular complications
Guideline-directed management therapy
Antiplatelet and antilipid therapy
Functional status before and after
Sheath removal techniques and products
In addition to those mentioned previously in *Reduction of Cardiac Risk Factors*
After Coronary Artery Bypass Graft
Pain control
Sedation
Hemodynamic stability
Early extubation
Blood transfusion
Early mobility

(continued)

EXHIBIT 6.2   **Selected Outcomes for the Cardiovascular Population (*continued*)**

Infections

  Surgery related (e.g., sternal, saphenous vein graft)

  Hospital associated

Wound healing, skin integrity

Cardioprotective meds

  Prescribed

  Adherence

Functional status

Referral to cardiac rehabilitation and attendance (or participation in exercise program)

Quality of life

Depression

Cognition

ACLS, advanced cardiac life support; BCLS, basic cardiac life support; CPR, cardiopulmonary resuscitation; EMS, emergency medical services.

activity, smoking cessation, body mass index [BMI]) and three of the metrics are related to health factors (i.e., serum level cholesterol, blood pressure, blood glucose level). These metrics include targets for individual patients and clinicians to achieve. Thus, APRNs are in a unique position to focus on these goals to improve overall cardiovascular health and reduce risk. APRNs are now challenged to develop and test novel and robust strategic interventions for individual patients, populations, and the health care system that aid in achieving these goals. Organizations and their related website links to these performance outcome measures can be found in Table 6.2; sample outcomes of concern for select cardiovascular populations can be found in Exhibit 6.2.

INSTRUMENTS AND APPROACHES TO OUTCOME MEASUREMENT

The use of valid and reliable measures and instruments is important in an outcome project and contributes to the level of confidence that one can have in the results (Polit & Beck, 2017a). Many valid and reliable instruments can be used to measure common health care outcomes such as QOL and functional status (Polit & Beck, 2017a); such instruments include self-report questionnaires or scales, symptom checklists, visual analog scales, and numeric rating scales (Nolan & Mock, 2000; Polit & Beck, 2017b).

In general, three major approaches can be used for outcome measurement: (a) outcome measurement evaluation, (b) outcome management, and (c) outcome research. *Outcome evaluation* is the monitoring and/or measuring of the extent to which providers meet the clinical or cost outcome goals of their patients or institutions. *Outcome management* is a systematic improvement of outcomes by acting on information gained from outcome measurement, often using the tools of continuous QI. *Outcome research* is a type of controlled, empirical assessment of the effect of a given intervention, product, or technology on patient, cost, or service outcomes (Polit & Beck, 2017c). The determination of which approach is used is dependent on the outcome of interest, available resources, and

TABLE 6.2   Selected Organization Websites and Quality Measures for Cardiovascular Populations

Organization Guideline and Website	Quality Measures for Selected Populations
AHA Heart Disease and Stroke Statistics 2016 Update: Chapters 1–13 http://circ.ahajournals.org/content/circulationaha/early/2015/12/16/ CIR.0000000000000350.pdf	Quality measures for cardiovascular risk reduction
AHA Heart Disease and Stroke Statistics 2016 Update: Chapters 17, 19, and 20 http://circ.ahajournals.org/content/circulationaha/early/2015/12/16/ CIR.0000000000000350.pdf	Quality measures for acute myocardial infarction
2014 AHA/American College of Cardiology (ACC) Guideline for the Management of Patients with Non-ST-Elevation Acute Coronary Syndromes: Chapter 8 http://content.onlinejacc.org/article.aspx?articleid=1910086	Quality measures for non-ST-elevated acute coronary syndrome
AHA Get With the Guidelines ACTIONS Registry, and GWTG Resuscitation www.heart.org/HEARTORG/Professional/GetWithTheGuidelines/Get-With-The-Guidelines_UCM_001099_SubHomePage.jsp	Quality measures for after resuscitation
American College of Cardiology Foundation (ACCF)/AHA/American Medical Association (AMA)–Physician Consortium for Performance Improvement (PCPI) 2011 Performance Measures for Adults with Heart Failure http://circ.ahajournals.org/content/125/19/2382	Quality measures for heart failure
AHA Heart Disease and Stroke Statistics 2016 Update: Chapters 20 and 23 http://circ.ahajournals.org/content/circulationaha/early/2015/12/16/ CIR.0000000000000350.pdf	Quality measures for heart failure
AHA Get With the Guidelines ACTIONS Registry, and GWTG Resuscitation www.heart.org/HEARTORG/Professional/GetWithTheGuidelines/Get-With-The-Guidelines_UCM_001099_SubHomePage.jsp	Quality measures for heart failure
ACC/AHA/SCAI/AMA-Convened PCPI/NCQA 2013 Performance Measures for Adults Undergoing Percutaneous Coronary Intervention http://circ.ahajournals.org/content/129/8/926	Quality measures for adults undergoing percutaneous coronary intervention
The Society of Thoracic Surgeons—Quality Performance Measures www.sts.org/quality-research-patient-safety/quality/quality-performance-measures	Quality measures for thoracic surgery

AHA, American Heart Association; GWTG, Get With the Guidelines; SCAI, Society for Cardiovascular Angiography and Interventions.

feasibility. Within these three major approaches, several methods can be used for outcome measurement projects, and these are discussed in the following section.

METHODS FOR OUTCOME MEASUREMENT

There are several methods that can be used for outcome measurement in advanced practice nursing using research, EBP, or QI frameworks. The APRN can use any of these methods to evaluate the impact of a new intervention on patient, system, and fiscal outcomes. Each of these methods has its advantages and disadvantages. No single set of research designs or methods is uniquely appropriate for outcome studies. The design and methods used will depend on the state of knowledge about a particular phenomenon and the resources available to the investigator. The APRN will choose among these methods depending on the variables under study, the outcome measures under study, the instruments used for measurements, and the feasibility in terms of time and resources (Gawlinski et al., 2013).

This section first reviews the most common research designs used by APRNs for outcome measurement projects (Figure 6.1) and discusses the strengths and weaknesses of each of these methods (Table 6.3). A discussion follows that describes other methods for outcome measurement, such as the research utilization process, EBP models, and QI frameworks.

Designs

Randomized Controlled Trials

The "gold standard" for evaluating the efficacy of drugs and other treatments and interventions in health care is the randomized controlled trial (RCT), or true experiment. RCTs must meet the following three criteria: (a) random assignment to the treatment or control group, (b) manipulation of the independent variable (treatment), and (c) a control or comparison group (Polit & Beck, 2017d). RCTs are concerned with efficacy, that is, with the question of whether a treatment works under ideal conditions. Because efficacy is most easily determined in a homogeneous study sample, RCTs typically have strict inclusion and exclusion criteria and are conducted under highly controlled conditions (O'Mathúna & Fineout-Overholt, 2015; Stevens, 2015). However, the same homogeneity that allows the researcher to determine the

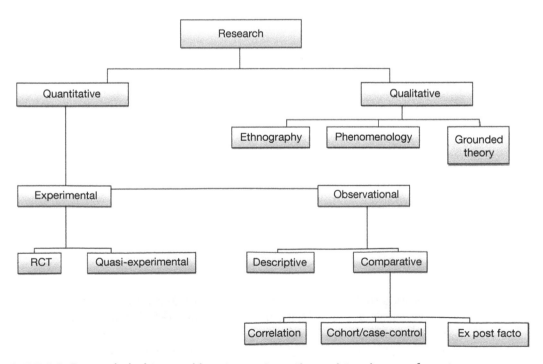

FIGURE 6.1 Research designs used by advanced practice registered nurses for outcome measurement projects.

RCT, randomized controlled trial.

TABLE 6.3   Research Designs: Advantages and Disadvantages

Design and Description	Advantage	Disadvantage

Randomized controlled trial (RCT) Requires:
    Randomization
    Manipulation of independent variable
    Control group
Aim: Determine causation
	Strong internal validity (confidence that effect was caused by manipulated variable)
	Most powerful design to test cause-and-effect relationships
	Provides strong evidence of a cause-and-effect relationship
	Confounding variables controlled for by randomization
	Clear measure of efficacy of intervention
		Poor external validity (generalizability)
		Can study only a limited number of variables
		Complicated and time-consuming
		Expensive
		Difficult to maintain integrity of intervention unless done by the research team
		Ethical and/or logistical issues with randomization
		May not be able to manipulate variables of interest
		Does not measure effectiveness of intervention in clinical practice

Quasi-experimental Lacks either: Randomization or control group Aim: Determine causation	More amenable to real-life clinical situations Practical, inexpensive, feasible Strong external validity (generalizability) Confounding variables may be able to be controlled by statistical means	Weaker internal validity (less causal attribution; i.e., less confidence that outcome was caused by manipulated variable) Confounding variables may be unknown or unable to be controlled for If there is no control group, alternative explanations cannot be ruled out
Descriptive Complete picture of current state Aim: Description	Simple Relatively unlimited number of variables	Does not address relationships between or among variables High risk of confounding and bias
Correlation Examine relationship(s) between and among variables Aim: Comparison/association	Test relationships between and among variables Can collect a large amount of data Can predict, as well as describe, association(s) Relatively simple Can study the relationship between many variables	Unable to determine cause–effect relationship Due to complex interactions of patient characteristics, tendency for variables to be related to one another (e.g., anxiety, coping, compliance)
Case–control "Case" has outcome of interest, "control" does not Aim: Retrospective comparison over time	Can use with relatively small sample sizes Time saving because design is retrospective: Research begins with outcome and searches for antecedent variable ("cause"), which has already occurred	May be difficult to select an appropriate control group Confounding variables may be unknown Limited to one outcome Confounding variables and bias are a concern Need to demonstrate comparability between cases and controls
Cohort Follow groups of subjects over time—exposure of interest Aim: Prospective comparison over time	Can assess several outcomes Temporal sequence is known Can be used to evaluate effectiveness in other populations of interventions found to be efficacious in RCT Stronger than retrospective comparison	Requires large sample size More resources needed to follow up subjects over time, especially if lengthy follow-up Results may not be identified for years Danger of attrition/dropout of subjects Confounding variables may be unknown
Ex post facto Evaluate effect of a naturally occurring event on subsequent outcome Aim: Identify possible causation	More realistic setting Can be used where a more rigorous experimental approach is not possible Can be a valuable exploratory tool to identify possible cause-and-effect relationships for further study	May be unable to identify all relevant variables, unknown if the causative factor has been identified Poor internal validity if unknown or unidentified variables provide an alternative explanation of relationship

(continued)

TABLE 6.3   Research Designs: Advantages and Disadvantages (*continued*)

Design and Description	Advantage	Disadvantage
	May be able to control for some antecedent variables with statistical procedures	The antecedent variable may be a combination of multiple factors Outcome may result from different antecedents on different occasions

Qualitative
  Develop concepts and themes
  Use words to explain phenomena
  Natural setting and context
  Inductive process (use specific data to elaborate theory and concepts)
Aim: Explanation/understanding
	Used when phenomena are poorly understood
	Requires a small number of subjects compared with quantitative studies
	Richness of understanding lived experiences
	Can complement quantitative research
	Used to explore complex phenomena
		Unable to determine causality or comparison
		Requires extensive training
		Time-consuming

impact of the intervention in a well-defined population also limits the extent to which the findings of an RCT apply to the diverse patients usually seen in clinical practice (O'Mathúna & Fineout-Overholt, 2015; Stevens, 2015). Thus, these studies have strong internal validity (attribution of causality), but weak external validity (generalizability).

Despite their significant strengths, RCTs also have important limitations. They are typically expensive, time-consuming, and designed to answer a single research question or test a small number of hypotheses. Additionally, the intensive follow-up necessary for most study protocols often bears little resemblance to follow-up patterns in usual clinical practice (O'Mathúna & Fineout-Overholt, 2015; Stevens, 2015). Finally, the importance of clinical significance versus statistical significance cannot be overlooked. Results that do not reach statistical significance do not exclude the possibility of a clinically important relationship (Gaskin & Happell, 2014; Polit & Yang, 2015). Thus, although rigorous RCTs establish the efficacy of a specific therapy in a limited patient population receiving close follow-up, they often leave remaining questions about the impact of therapy in populations not resembling those enrolled in the trial.

Quasi-Experimental

In some situations, a true experimental design is not feasible because of ethical or logistical constraints. In such circumstances, nonrandomized quasi-experimental studies are often the most appropriate design with which to test cause-and-effect relationships (Polit & Beck, 2017d). Quasi-experimental designs are differentiated from experimental designs by lack of random assignment and/or lack of a control or comparison group. However, they are similar to an experiment in that a variable is manipulated and comparison is made to a group not receiving the intervention.

Quasi-experimental designs do not have the rigor created by random assignment and control groups for comparison; rather, comparisons are made with nonequivalent groups or with periodic measurement of the same group (Polit & Beck, 2017d). Quasi-experimental designs are at risk for threats to internal validity, that is, factors that provide an alternative explanation for associations between the independent and dependent variables, and therefore have limited ability to make cause-and-effect statements (Polit &

Beck, 2017d). Attributing causation is strengthened if the researcher is able to account for alternative explanations of intervention–outcome relationships.

Many nursing outcome studies use a pretest/intervention/posttest method. These research designs can collect data from the same subject over time (within subjects), or from different participant groups (between subjects) at the same or different times. A within-subject design, also known as a repeated-measure design, tests the same subject at two or more time points. In between-subject designs, each participant participates in one and only one group.

Nonexperimental/Observational

Many studies measuring health care outcomes are observational in nature, in contrast to studies that recruit patients in a controlled fashion, as with RCTs. The advantage of an observational method is that patients' circumstances and outcomes of interventions are studied in a heterogeneous population, which better reflects actual practice environments. The obvious disadvantage is that without the controls imposed by an experimental study, observational results are subject to error and can be misleading or misinterpreted (Polit & Beck, 2017d). Threats to validity, such as bias, or confounding or random error, can provide an alternative explanation other than the effect of the independent variable for changes in the dependent variable after intervention.

Bias is any factor or influence that produces a systematic distortion or error in the study results (Polit & Beck, 2017e). Selection bias is especially problematic in nonrandomized studies; that is, such studies have the concern that subjects who elect to participate are systematically different from those who decline participation. Two main factors that can contribute to selection bias are self-selection, when the sample selects itself, and convenience sampling, when individuals are selected because they are easy to obtain (Polit & Beck, 2017e). For example, in a study of caregivers of terminally ill patients, the researcher may choose a sample of subjects who responded to a recruitment flyer (self-selection) or a sample of caregivers who attend a support group (convenience sample). Either sample is probably not representative of the total population of caregivers of terminally ill patients.

Confounding variables are variables that are associated with both the independent and the dependent variable in such a way that the relationship between the intervention and outcome is actually due to a third (known or unknown) variable, and the nature of the association between the independent and dependent variable is misrepresented (O'Mathúna & Fineout-Overholt, 2015). The effect of a confounding variable can offer an alternative explanation for a relationship between an intervention and an outcome (Carson, 2010). For example, researchers may find an association between consuming a vegetarian diet and lower BMI and draw the conclusion that the diet is the cause of lower BMI. However, this association may be confounded by the fact that vegetarians are perhaps more health conscious in general and exercise more regularly. Thus, exercise may be the true cause of the difference in BMI. The use of multivariate statistical models such as linear or logistic regression may be able to "adjust" for confounding variables in some situations (Carson, 2010).

Random error is essentially nonsystematic bias; that is, the factor or influence that produces error is as likely to influence results in one way as another (Polit & Beck, 2017e). Random error is due to variability in the data that occurs purely by chance. Because of random error, one cannot unequivocally state that the results obtained in a study are real rather than arising by chance. The probability that the outcome variable has occurred purely by chance is expressed as the p value. The most effective way of minimizing random error in a study is to increase the sample size (Polit & Beck, 2017e). The classic example of correcting random error is the coin toss. When tossing a coin, we expect heads to occur 50% of the time. If the coin were tossed 10 times, it is likely that the number of heads–tails would not be 5–5, but may be for example 6–4 or 3–7. However, if the coin were tossed 1,000 times, we would be more likely to approach 50–50 (or actually 500–500) on heads coming up.

Descriptive

The descriptive research design is the most basic. It simply describes the nature of the phenomenon of interest. Data are gathered for descriptive research in three ways: observation of actions, appraisal of records or documents, and results of surveys specifically designed to measure variables of interest. Descriptive research involves observing, describing, and documenting events or phenomena and then organizing, tabulating, depicting, and describing the data elements. Descriptive studies also report summary data such as measures of central tendency (mean, median, mode) and measures of dispersion (range and standard deviation). These designs describe what actually exists, determine the frequency with which it occurs, and categorize the information (Polit & Beck, 2017d). Descriptive statistical techniques allow very large amounts of data to be made meaningful to the researcher.

Descriptive data are the foundation of any quantitative study and can serve as a foundation for theory generation or hypothesis testing in a quantitative study (Polit & Beck, 2017d). The fact that descriptive studies are "simple" and one cannot infer causality from them does not diminish the value of the descriptive study design. An example of an important, purely descriptive research is the decennial U.S. Census, the purpose of which is to accurately and precisely describe the population of the entire country.

Correlation

Correlation determines whether, and to what degree, a relationship exists between two or more variables. This design is used to determine if changes in one or more variables are related to changes in another variable (Melnyk, Morrison-Beedy, & Cole, 2015). Correlation can tell you only that two or more phenomena are related, not that a causal relationship exists. The degree of the relationship between variables is expressed as a correlation coefficient. The correlation coefficient indicates the strength of relationship (strong, weak, or none) as well as the direction of the relationship, that is, positive, in which variables move in the same direction, or negative, in which variables move in opposite directions. Correlation coefficients range in value from –1.0 (strongly negative) to +1.0 (strongly positive), with 0 indicating no relationship.

Correlation designs can be either descriptive or predictive. *Descriptive* correlation simply describes the variables under study and the relationship(s) between and among them. *Predictive* correlation predicts the amount of variance in one or more variables based on the amount of variance in other variable(s), given that the predictor variable occurs earlier in time (Melnyk et al., 2015).

Case-Control and Cohort

In the case–control study design, "cases" with a disease or condition are identified within a population of patients, and investigators go back a period of time before onset of the disease or condition and assess the presence of potential risk factors or other influences preceding the disease or condition (Melnyk et al., 2015). For example, K. D. Burns et al. (2009) conducted a case–control study to identify risk factors for delirium in patients undergoing elective heart surgery (K. D. Burns et al., 2009). The "cases" were the 11 patients (29%) who had developed postoperative delirium and the "controls" were the 27 patients (71%) who did not. Numerous preoperative, intraoperative, and postoperative variables were included in the analysis to determine risk factors for delirium. The factors most strongly associated with delirium were recent alcohol use, intubation time, time in the intensive care unit (ICU), and postoperative creatinine levels (K. D. Burns et al., 2009).

In the cohort study design, the presence of risk or predictor variables is measured at baseline within a selected population. Investigators then follow subjects over time to determine which patients have the disease or developed the condition of interest. Typically, cohort studies are prospective in nature, that is, subjects are followed forward in time (Melnyk et al., 2015). Perhaps the most famous cohort study in the United States is the Framingham Heart Study, begun in 1947 by the U.S. Public Health Service, and continued under the auspices of the National Heart, Lung, and Blood Institute (NHLBI) of the National Institutes of Health (NIH). The study initially enrolled a random sample of 5,209 subjects, aged 30 to 59 in the town of Framingham, Massachusetts (Dawber, Meadors, & Moore, 1951). Since 1948, the subjects have continued to return to the study every 2 years for a detailed medical history, physical examination, and laboratory tests. In 1971, the study enrolled a second generation, 5,124 of the original participants' adult children and their spouses, to participate in similar examinations. In 2002, enrollment of a third generation of participants was begun. Since 1951, investigators have published 2,346 studies based on Framingham Heart Study data in peer-reviewed medical journals.

Ex Post Facto

Literally translated, *ex post facto* means "from what is done after." In ex post facto studies, the researcher retrospectively examines the effects of a naturally occurring event on a subsequent outcome for the purpose of establishing a causal link between them. Ex post facto studies are similar to case–control studies in that they begin by observing an existing condition or state of affairs. Subsequently, the researcher searches back in time for plausible causes, relationships, or associations between the variables (Giuffre, 1997). The study begins with preexisting groups that are already different in some respect(s) and searches in the past for the factor(s) that brought about the differences (Cohen, Manion, & Morrison, 2000).

By convention, the antecedent variable is often referred to as the "independent variable" or "cause," and the outcome variable is also called the "dependent variable" or "effect" (this despite the fact that ex post facto designs can only weakly predict cause and effect). For the purposes of clarity, the authors use the terms "antecedent" and "outcome" variable.

Ex post facto designs are used when the researcher is interested in cause-and-effect relationships, but it is not possible to manipulate variables (i.e., to conduct an experimental study). Results of these ex post facto studies can provide a beginning sense of cause-and-effect relationships that can subsequently be tested with more rigorous research methods. It is an inexpensive study design in that the phenomena of interest have already occurred and no interventions are performed.

One of the major challenges for researchers in using an ex post facto design is to identify preexisting groups that are comparable to a randomly assigned group, that is, the challenge is to ensure that the only difference in the groups is the presence or absence of the outcome or "effect" variable (Giuffre, 1997). One of the most common means of achieving this comparability is to match the subjects in the "effect" and "no effect" groups on variables known or believed to influence the outcome variable. The difficulty with this strategy is that it assumes that the investigator knows what all the relevant factors are that may be related to the outcome variable. Similarly, factors that could influence the antecedent variable must be accounted for; again, there is the assumption that the investigator can identify all the relevant factors (Cohen et al., 2000).

Finally, the researcher must recognize that no single antecedent variable may be the "cause" of the outcome. Many antecedent variables may be interrelated or the result of more than one variable interacting with others. Likewise, a particular outcome may result from different antecedents on different occasions.

Qualitative

Qualitative studies describe human responses in a particular situation and context and the meaning that human beings bring to the situation (Powers, 2015a). Qualitative studies are often exploratory in nature and seek to generate new insight or understandings, using inductive (starting with data and developing hypotheses) rather than deductive (starting with hypotheses and testing them with data) approaches (Powers, 2015a).

The three most often used qualitative designs are ethnography, phenomenology, and grounded theory (Powers, 2015a). *Ethnography* is the direct description of a group, culture, or community—the culture as experienced by its members. Although ethnographic methods originated in cultural anthropology, they can also be used to describe the culture of a health care organization or patient care unit. *Phenomenology* uses in-depth interviews and open-ended discussion to describe and interpret the lived experience or phenomenon under study and to derive a depth of understanding and meaning from the experiences of participants.

Grounded theory uses data points (verbatim quotations) to generate or modify a theory. Data are collected from in-depth interviews and open-ended discussion to understand processes and behaviors as individuals move through experiences over time. The purpose of this design is to generate a theory that is "grounded" in real-life empirical data (Corbin & Strauss, 2008). The developing theory evolves during data collection and analysis as a part of the research process and the sample of participants is constantly developed to explore insights that emerge from the data (Corbin & Strauss, 2008).

The application of grounded theory is illustrated in a landmark study (Conrad, 1985) using data from 80 in-depth interviews of people with epilepsy. The study analyzed the meaning of medications in the lives of the subjects to determine why people did or did not take their medications. From the interview data, it was found that, from the patients' perspective, the issue was more of controlling dependence, and the practicalities of frequent medication administration. Conrad developed the theory of self-regulation from his belief that what appeared to be noncompliance (from a medical perspective) was actually a form of asserting control over a disorder.

Qualitative research designs are often used in areas in which data or knowledge is inadequate or in which conventional theories may not be applicable. Qualitative methods can be used to understand complex social processes to capture essential aspects of a phenomenon from the perspective of study participants, and to uncover beliefs, values, and motivations that underlie individual health behaviors (Powers, 2015b).

Qualitative research can be distinguished from quantitative research in several ways. First, quantitative research uses numbers (e.g., frequency or magnitude of variables) to describe phenomena, whereas qualitative research uses words to describe and understand the complexity and depth of phenomena or experiences. Second, quantitative research *tests* hypotheses with statistical methods to determine statistical significance, whereas qualitative research seeks to *generate* hypotheses about a phenomenon, its antecedents, and its aftermath. Third, quantitative research is performed primarily in experimental settings and generates numeric data using valid and reliable instruments to measure predetermined variables. In contrast, qualitative research occurs in natural settings and produces word-based data through open-ended discussions, in-depth interviews, focus groups, observation, and document review (Powers, 2015b).

Mixed Methods

Mixed methods, in which quantitative and qualitative research designs are combined, are increasingly recognized as appropriate and important in health care research because they capitalize on the respective strengths of each approach (Curry, Nemhard, & Bradley, 2009). The NIH published a useful resource in their report "Best Practices for Mixed Methods Research in the Health Sciences" (Creswell, Klassen, Plano Clark, Smith, & the Office of Behavioral and Social Sciences Research, 2011). The report provides practical recommendations for researchers seeking to incorporate mixed-methods research into their applications for NIH "R" series research grants as well as fellowship, career, training, and center grants.

Qualitative studies can generate theories and identify relevant variables to be studied subsequently in quantitative studies. They can also be used in a complementary fashion to yield findings that are broader in scope and richer in meaning than those derived from quantitative data alone (Powers, 2015b).

In the seminal work by Greenhalgh (2002), three ways are described in which qualitative research designs interact with quantitative methods: exploratory, explanatory, and evaluative. First, an exploratory process can be used to generate hypotheses and often serves as the first step in a sequence of research that includes a quantitative stage. Second, qualitative data can be used in an explanatory fashion to further inform relationships between or among variables in a quantitative study. Although a quantitative study could answer the question of whether an intervention is efficacious, a qualitative study could answer the question of *why* the intervention was successful. Finally, after a quantitative study has demonstrated the efficacy of a particular intervention, qualitative data can be used to evaluate why this evidence may not become incorporated into practice or may be incompletely incorporated.

Approaches to mixed-methods studies can vary based on the sequence of studies and the relative emphasis placed on each approach. The qualitative and quantitative elements may be performed concurrently or sequentially and, depending on the phenomena under investigation, one approach or the other may dominate the study design. For example, if a quantitative study yields unexpected or conflicting results, a qualitative follow-up study may help to ascertain important relationships that inform interpretation of the results. Likewise, qualitative studies may be performed to generate hypotheses or characterize a phenomenon about which little is known, which are then further studied using one or more quantitative methods. Strategies to enhance the validity of mixed-methods studies include recognizing the role of each strategy and adhering to the methodological assumptions of each design (Creswell et al., 2011).

Methods

Research Utilization and EBP

APRNs may opt to use existing research to make a practice change and evaluate the effects of implementing a new innovation on specific outcomes. This type of project would use a research utilization approach or framework. Research utilization refers to the "process by which specific research-based knowledge (science) is implemented in practice" (Estabrooks, Walling, & Milner, 2003, p. 5). A disadvantage to using strictly research utilization methods is that traditional researchers use inclusion and exclusion criteria that restrict the subjects to a homogeneous sample, in order to decrease possible biases and variance and to increase the probability of identifying a statistically significant difference (N. Burns & Grove, 2015). Application of research findings to a population other than that studied may be problematic. One of the important steps in research utilization is to critique and synthesize research findings to determine relevance and feasibility in the APRN's particular practice setting (Stetler, 2001). Increasingly, research utilization is being integrated into the larger concept of EBP.

EBP represents a broader concept than research utilization. When clinicians use the EBP approach, they can incorporate additional levels of evidence and consider the nurse's clinical expertise as well as the patient's preferences and values. Sackett et al. originally defined EBP as "the conscientious, explicit and judicious use of current best evidence in making decisions about the care of the individual patient. It means integrating individual clinical expertise with the best available external clinical evidence from systematic research" (Sackett, Rosenberg, Gray, Haynes, & Richardson, 1996, p. 71). Consideration of the individual patient's values and preferences was considered as part of the health care provider's clinical expertise (Sackett, Richardson, Rosenberg, & Haynes, 2000). Ingersoll (2000) proposed that EBP should also consider the importance of using theoretical foundations in the evidence-based decision-making process.

There are a number of models for implementing an EBP method for outcome research. Common elements of all EBP models include (a) identifying a clinical problem, (b) gathering evidence, (c) critiquing and synthesizing evidence, (d) implementing practice change, and (e) evaluating the impact of practice change on outcomes. These models can assist nurses to systematically approach clinical practice problems and proceed toward actual implementation in a specific practice setting. Use of an EBP model can prevent incomplete or unsuccessful implementations of the practice change, promote timely evaluation, and maximize use of time and resources (Gawlinski & Rutledge, 2008). EBP models that have specific stages or phases that can guide the APRN in an outcome measurement project are described in Table 6.4. EBP models that do not have specific stages or phases, but help describe and conceptualize the many variables and interactions that can occur when making an EBP change, are described in Table 6.5.

Quality Improvement

Finally, a QI process can be chosen to guide an outcome measurement project. The QI method involves systematic processes of data collection and inquiry and refers to activities that use data-based methods to bring about rapid improvements in health care delivery (McLaughlin & Kaluzny, 2013). A basic premise of QI is that measures of good performance reflect good-quality practice and that comparing performance among providers and organizations will encourage better performance (McLaughlin & Kaluzny, 2013).

The QI process includes developing indicators to assess progress toward certain predefined goals and reviewing performance against these measures. Data for

TABLE 6.4   Selected Evidence-Based Practice Nursing Models and Their Key Components

	Iowa	Stetler	Rosswurm and Larrabee	Johns Hopkins	Academic Center for Evidence-Based Practice (ACE) ACE Star
Emphasis	Organizational process	At individual nurse or organizational level	Organizational process	Organizational process	Knowledge transformation
Stages/ phases	1. Trigger: problem or new knowledge 2. Organizational priority? 3. Team formation 4. Evidence gathered 5. Research base critiqued and synthesized 6. Sufficient? 7. Pilot change 8. Decision? 9. Widespread implementation with continual monitoring of outcomes 10. Dissemination of results	1. Preparation 2. Validation 3. Comparative evaluation 4. Decision making 5. Translation/ application 6. Evaluation	1. Assess need for change in practice 2. Link problem interventions and outcomes 3. Synthesize best evidence 4. Design practice change 5. Implement and evaluate change in practice 6. Integrate and maintain	1. Practice question identified 2. Evidence gathered 3. Translation: plan, implement, evaluate, communicate	1. Knowledge discovery 2. Evidence summary 3. Translation into practice recommendations 4. Integration into practice 5. Evaluation

Source: Adapted from Gawlinski and Rutledge (2008).

TABLE 6.5   Select Evidence-Based Practice Frameworks

	ARCC Model	PARIHS Framework
Key focus	Organization of department or unit	Understanding key components of EBP
Key concepts	EBP mentor—an individual who has proficient knowledge and skills in EBP and the passion to help others practice daily from an evidence-based care	Evidence Context Facilitation
Major proposition	The development of APRNs and other nurses as EBP mentors facilitates an organizational culture change toward evidence-based care	Practice changes are most likely when based upon robust evidence, conducted in a context "friendly" to change, and facilitated well
Utility—practical implications	Need to . . . Assess and organize culture and readiness for EBP Identify strengths and major barriers to EBP implementation Implement ARCC strategies Develop and use of EBP mentors Interactive EBP skill-building workshop EBP rounds and journal clubs EBP implementation Improve patient, nurse, system outcomes	Need to . . . Critically appraise evidence Thoroughly understand the practice arena before implementing a change Make a strategic plan for facilitation of any practice change—from development through implementation and evaluation

ARCC, Advancing Research and Clinical Practice through Close Collaboration; EBP, evidence-based practice; PARIHS, Promoting Action on Research Implementation in Health Services.
Source: Adapted from Gawlinski and Rutledge (2008).

QI investigation are derived internally and usually reported only internally. QI evaluates work processes in a cyclic fashion, benchmarks practice against established indicators, and provides a means to continually evaluate and improve established practice (McLaughlin & Kaluzny, 2013).

QI methods enable organizations to make change in a systematic way, measuring and assessing the effects of a change, feeding the information back into the clinical setting, and making adjustments until they are satisfied with the results (McLaughlin & Kaluzny, 2013). The APRN is in an ideal position to implement and participate in QI activities through the roles of practitioner, teacher, researcher, and consultant. A thorough knowledge of the institution's QI method as well as skillful implementation of the QI process is required for the APRN to monitor unit-based quality indicators of care, the performance of practitioners, and the overall quality of care provided (Altmiller, 2011).

No one "right" QI method can be applied that will be effective in all organizations. Individual organizations have their own networks, structures, organizational histories, and challenges, which need to be considered in relation to the choice and implementation of QI methods. The specific approach (or combination of approaches) may be less important than the thoughtful consideration of the match and "best fit" for the particular circumstances (Seidl & Newhouse, 2012). A number of QI methods have been adapted to the health care setting (Nicolay et al., 2012). A brief description of these methods is provided in Table 6.6.

TABLE 6.6   Quality Improvement Models

Model	Description
Donabedian's Model of Quality Health Care Donabedian was one of the founders of quality improvement, and the model continues to serve as a unifying conceptual framework for quality improvement All steps are vital: process improvement is limited and temporary, when the structure is not also improved.	Structure: Availability, accessibility, and quality of resources Process: Delivery of health care services by clinicians Outcome: Final results of health care
Total Quality Management and Continuous Quality Improvement (Deming) Developed in Japan in the 1950s to rebuild and improve their manufacturing industry Terms are now also used to describe more general approaches to quality improvement Important concepts include: Continuous performance evaluation Involves management at all levels Quality is the responsibility of everyone Quality improvement is data driven	Process management: Focus on process and systems to improve, rather than individuals Problem solving: Use of structured approaches based on statistical analysis; data is a key tool Leadership: Management involvement at all levels Employee empowerment: Use of teams to identify problems and opportunities and to take the necessary action
PDCA (plan–do–check–act) Also known as rapid-cycle QI; promoted by the Institute for Healthcare Improvement (IHI) Repeated short-cycle small-scale changes Begin with easiest changes, repeat cycles to address more complex processes Cyclic and iterative	Plan: A change in process to improve quality Do: Implement the change with a strategic plan for implementation Check: Evaluate and analyze results Act: Adopt, adapt, or abandon
Six Sigma Developed by Motorola in the 1980s for QI Sigma is the statistical term for variance; 1 Sigma is one standard deviation, 6 Sigma is 6 standard deviations, which represents 99.99966% of possible events Goal is 3.4 failures per million "opportunities" Also cyclic and iterative	Define: Goal of improvement and key people involved Measure: Current system; may be challenging if data are not available for the processes of interest Analyze: Ways to close gap Improve: Implement and evaluate Control: Plans and process to maintain
Toyota Lean Developed by Toyota in 1940s Basic principle is to minimize waste, both in product and processes Focuses on value to the customer	Value stream map identifies exact steps of the work process and the value associated with the step Processes are aligned for continuous flow of work Create an environment of constant review Extensive use of visual cues to streamline processes and prevent error
Root Cause Analysis Began as a way to evaluate industrial accidents Systematic retrospective analysis to identify and understand the underlying cause of process failures Extensive use of tools and diagrams of process requires extensive training	Focus on systems and processes Goal is to understand contributory factors that create an environment where errors can happen Required by The Joint Commission (TJC) and other regulatory agencies for all sentinel events Extensive use of tools and diagrams of process requires extensive training
Failure Modes and Effects Analysis (FMEA) Prospective risk assessment tool developed by the military and National Aeronautics and Space Administration (NASA) to evaluate potential failures and unrecognized hazards. Can be used to evaluate both designs and processes	Identify the system to be analyzed and the individual processes within the system that are the most problematic or high risk Create a process map (diagram) to describe each individual step in the process Identify all potential failures in a process

(continued)

TABLE 6.6   Quality Improvement Models (*continued*)

Model	Description
Goal is to identify process failures that would be the most significant and design preventive or mitigating measures before failure occurs Flowcharts and brainstorming are useful tools	Define and anticipate effect of each failure, cause, degree of seriousness, and possible solutions Calculate a risk priority score for each potential failure System or process redesign Reanalysis

QI, quality improvement.

ROLE OF THE APRN IN OUTCOME MEASUREMENT

The role of the APRN is to integrate education, research, management, leadership, and consultation into his or her clinical practice, making the APRN well-suited to manage the complexities of HF patients and their evolving care needs. The following section describes an evidence-based outcome measurement project initiated by the APRNs employed in the Ahmanson University of California Los Angeles (UCLA) Cardiomyopathy Center, for the purpose of improving patient education and decreasing medication discrepancies during the high-risk transition from hospital to home. Through a detailed plan of interventions, the APRNs created a new process across the continuum from hospitalization to home. APRNs providing in-hospital patient education, facilitating and participating in the patient discharge process, and providing phone monitoring through to the outpatient follow-up clinic visit have resulted in a decrease in medication discrepancies after hospital discharge.

Background

HF continues to be a major public problem resulting in substantial morbidity and mortality. A rapidly increasing aging population coupled with the advancement of life-prolonging interventions has led to increasing rates of HF. HF prevalence increases with age, its incidence accelerates from 20 per 1,000 individuals 65 to 69 years of age to more than 80 per 1,000 individuals older than 85 years of age (Curtis et al., 2008; Yancy et al., 2013; American College of Cardiology Foundation [ACCF]/AHA HF guideline). A 2016 update from the AHA estimated that 5.7 million people older than 20 years of age in the United States have HF, with an incidence of 915,000 new cases diagnosed annually (Atherosclerosis Risk in Communities Study [ARIC] of the NHLBI, 2005–2012; Chang et al., 2014; Mozaffarian et al., 2016). Projections indicate that by 2030, more than 8 million people older than 18 years of age will have HF, a 46% increase in prevalence from 2012 (Heidenreich et al., 2013; Mozaffarian et al., 2016). Although survival after HF diagnosis has improved over time, the mortality rate remains unacceptably high. One in nine deaths in 2009 included HF as a contributing cause (National Center for Health Statistics, 2013; NHLBI, 2013) and approximately 7% of all cardiovascular deaths are due to HF (Go et al., 2013). Among Medicare beneficiaries, the overall 1-year HF mortality has remained high at 29.6% (Chen, Normand, Wang, & Krumholz, 2011; National Center for Health Statistics, 2011), with continued estimates that 50% of people with a diagnosis of HF will die within 5 years of diagnosis. Additionally, in the ARIC study, 30-day, 1-year, and 5-year case fatality rates after hospitalization for HF were 10.4%, 22%, and 42.3%, respectively

(Chang et al., 2014; Loehr, Rosamond, Chang, Folsom, & Chambers, 2008; Yancy et al., 2013 [ACCF/AHA HF guideline]).

HF also accounts for a large burden in rising health care expenditures, translating into 5 million office visits (National Hospital Ambulatory Medical Care Survey Data, 2009; Voigt et al., 2014), 553,000 ED visits, and 1.1 million hospitalizations per year (Roger et al., 2012). It is the most common diagnosis-related-group discharge in persons older than 65 years (Roger et al., 2012). The indirect and direct costs of HF treatment in the United States now exceed $30 billion annually, a sobering statistic, driving 5.4% of all health care costs (Go et al., 2013). The lifetime burden of hospitalizations in persons with a diagnosis of HF has been reported as 83% of patients hospitalized at least once and 43% of patients hospitalized at least four times (Dunlay et al., 2009). Although physician office visits accounted for $1.8 billion, more than half of the total costs for HF was spent on hospitalizations. Go et al. (2013) estimated the mean cost of an HF-related admission at $23,077 per patient (Go et al., 2013). With a mean 4.7-day length of stay, hospitalization is the predominant contributor to HF costs and is the largest single expense for Medicare. Unfortunately, nearly 25% of HF patients are readmitted within 30 days of discharge (Dharmarajan et al., 2013).

Quality and accountability of practitioners and organizations have become paramount in medical practice particularly in relation to the potential impact for the HF population. Performance measures for HF include process measures and outcome measures. The CMS, TJC, Hospital Quality Alliance, Agency for Health Research and Quality (AHRQ), and ACCF/AHA/Physician Consortium for Performance Improvement (PCPI) define quality metrics and performance measures for patient care and HF management. Process performance measures focus on the aspects of care delivered to a patient and are based on professionally developed and definitive clinical practice guideline recommendations. Performance measures are suitable for use for accountability whereas quality metrics are suitable for QI (Yancy et al., 2013). Medication safety, patient counseling and education, implementation of evidence-based HF guideline management, and adequate postdischarge follow-up are critical elements defined by these organizations. "Hospital Compare," created through the efforts of the CMS, the Department of Health and Human Services (DHS), and the Hospital Quality Alliance: Improving Care through Information initiative, provides objective and verifiable data regarding HF outcomes. CMS data identified HF as the most frequent diagnosis-related group with the highest readmission rate of any other common medical or surgical condition in Medicare beneficiaries. Thus, HF admission and mortality rates, and in particular, 30-day rehospitalization rates and 30-day mortality rates for HF are now key national outcome measures. These performance measures are now incorporated into the CMS VBP program. With an intended effort to have hospitals pay close attention to HF patients after discharge, the Patient Protection Affordable Care Act of 2010 created new incentives to reduce readmissions. Hospitals with high readmission rates would be penalized as much as 3% of their Medicare reimbursement by 2015 and beyond (Bradley et al., 2013). The VBP program focuses on a hospital's performance on 25 quality measures related to clinical process of care measures and patients' care experience. Patient satisfaction determines 30% of incentive payments while improved clinical outcomes generate 70% (CMS, 2011).

Because of the high mortality and tremendous costs associated with HF treatment, adherence to evidence-based therapy is critical. Literature supports the benefits of evidence-based guideline medical therapy and lifestyle modification in delaying disease progression and improving survival in patients with HF (Calvin et al., 2012; Fonarow et al., 2010). However, patients' adherence to these treatment regimens shows high variability, with rates ranging from 10% to as high as 85% (Calvin et al., 2012; Fonarow et al., 2010; Foust, Naylor, Bixby, & Ratcliffe, 2012; Yancy et al., 2013). The most common factors associated with patient nonadherence to HF treatment recommendations and rehospitalization include complicated medical regimens, inappropriate medication reconciliation, poor discharge instructions, lack of patient understanding, lack of health literacy, poor communication among health care providers between sites of care, lack of a plan for appropriate medical follow-up after discharge, lower socioeconomic status, minority status, psychosocial variables, and age (Calvin et al., 2012; Fonarow et al., 2010; Foust et al., 2012; Wiggins, Rodgers, DiDomenico, Cook, & Page, 2013; Yancy et al., 2013). A significant proportion of hospital readmissions are caused by medication-related adverse events. An estimated 19% of discharged patients experienced an adverse event after discharge, of which two thirds were attributed to medications. Additionally, lack of adherence to medications prescribed at discharge is a driver of adverse drug events after discharge (Bristol Calvert et al., 2012; Hubbard & McNeil, 2012). Consequently, medication management is at the core of advanced discharge planning and transitional care for avoidable hospital readmissions.

Clinical Issue

Maximizing evidence-based HF guideline therapy is part of inpatient and outpatient HF management. Despite written hospital discharge instructions and prescriptions provided by the hospital's cardiac care unit service, a large number of patients had a significant knowledge deficit regarding what medications, purpose or indication, dose or frequency they were prescribed when interviewed at their 1-week hospital follow-up HF clinic visit. The patients and/or care providers were often confused about their medication regimens and changes made while in the hospital. Medication discrepancies can be detrimental to the control of HF symptoms for the patient, resulting in clinical HF progression, fluid overload exacerbation, hypertension, hypotension, hyperkalemia, hypokalemia, renal insufficiency, or liver dysfunction. It became apparent to the cardiomyopathy APRNs that there was a need to bridge the education gap at the transition from hospital discharge to home. The APRNs found that cardioprotective medications initiated, uptitrated, or changed in the hospital were often not continued after discharge. In an effort to improve the discharge transition to home, the APRNs identified the factors contributing to medication discrepancies, which included the following:

- New prescriptions not filled because of need for prior insurance authorization, high cost, or inability to go to the pharmacy
- Patients experienced side effects and discontinued medicines without consultation with a practitioner
- Patients used old prescriptions/medications available at home of the same drug but having a dose or strength different from what was prescribed
- Patients expressed that discharge paperwork was overwhelming and/or confusing

- Patients were uncertain whom to contact regarding medication questions (especially if discharged weekend/after hours)
- Elderly patients with functional impairments often had difficulty following and understanding dosing regimen
- Patients' lack of social support to assist with medication management
- Patients' knowledge deficit of the importance of their HF medications

REVIEW OF THE LITERATURE

To evaluate how to best improve the clinical problem, a focused review of evidence-based literature regarding the transition from hospital discharge to home and improving post-hospital medication discrepancies was essential. The APRNs began a literature-based patient improvement project to determine whether implementing a standardized in-hospital to outpatient transitional medication education and reconciliation process could improve the number of medication discrepancies at discharge.

Medication discrepancies at care transitions, such as from hospital discharge to home, are common and may lead to patient harm. A high burden of illness often accompanied by polypharmacy and variable health literacy creates greater vulnerability for medication discrepancies to occur during the transition from hospital discharge to home. The scope of this problem is well recognized with approximately 1.5 million preventable adverse medication events occurring annually at a cost of more than $3 billion per year (Institute of Medicine, 2006). The World Health Organization (WHO) Collaborating Centre for Patient Safety (2007) cites 46% of all medication errors occur at transition points such as hospital discharge and that medication reconciliation is a crucial component in ensuring prevention of adverse drug events at these transition times. Effective interventions to decrease medication discrepancies need to be implemented to decrease the potential for medication errors, especially at high-risk transition times. Medication reconciliation is a strategy that can reduce risk and ensure safe and effective medication use.

Medication reconciliation is a process that involves obtaining and maintaining accurate and complete medication information across the continuum of care (American Pharmacists Association, American Society of Health-System Pharmacists, Steeb, & Webster, 2012). The process requires members of the health care team to comprehensively evaluate a patient's medication regimen to avoid medication errors at all care transition points.

Gleason et al. (2010) reported medication reconciliation errors in 36% of their study population, primarily occurring with admission medication orders. Of these medication reconciliation errors that occurred with admission orders, the majority (85%) occurred during practitioners' gathering of patients' medication history during hospital admission. Both an age of 65 years or older and number of prescriptions were significantly associated with medication errors and the potential to cause harm. Cardiovascular medications were the most common classification of medications omitted in this study sample. The presence of a medication list or review of actual medication bottles was associated with fewer incidences of errors (Gleason et al., 2010).

In addition to hospital admission, the transition from hospital to home is an especially high-risk time because of changes in medication regimens that occur during an acute illness requiring hospitalization. Foust et al. (2012) performed a literature review to determine the rates and types of medication reconciliation problems among older adults hospitalized for HF who were discharged home. Investigators found medication discrepancies commonly occurred at hospital discharge (39.6%–70.7%) and during the posthospital transition (14.1%–94%). Among posthospital adverse events, medications were the most common cause (66%–72%), and nearly all posthospital adverse drug events involved a new medication or dosage change (Foust et al., 2012). Medication reconciliation, therefore, needs to be an integral part of the care transition process at hospital discharge.

In addition, Bell et al. (2011) reviewed records of all hospitalizations and corresponding outpatient prescriptions from 1997 to 2009 for more than 396,000 patients aged 66 or older to determine (a) continuous use of at least one of five medication classes and (b) failure to renew prescriptions within 90 days after hospital discharge. Investigators found that patients prescribed medications for chronic conditions were at higher risk for unintentional discontinuation following hospital discharge and that an ICU stay during hospitalization further increased the risk of medication discontinuation (Bell et al., 2011).

Medication reconciliation at hospital discharge is a complex process, which can involve a multitude of critical elements such as (a) case manager involvement, (b) use of discharge checklists that incorporate medication and disease-specific information, and (c) designating a specific health care provider to review and reconcile medications at the point of discharge. Mueller, Sponsler, Kripalani, and Schnipper (2012) provided a systematic review of 26 studies regarding medication reconciliation in the hospital setting from 1966 through 2010. These studies involved various interventions aimed at reducing medication discrepancies. The authors found that various interventions for medication reconciliation were associated with a decrease in adverse drug events. These interventions included involvement of a pharmacist, use of information technology, and the electronic medical record, as well as interventions such as use of a standardized medication reconciliation tool and staff education and feedback (Mueller et al., 2012).

A number of relevant studies within the review highlighted the effectiveness of a dedicated pharmacist in the medication reconciliation process at hospital discharge (Eggink, Lenderink, Widdershoven, & van den Bemt, 2010; Gillespie et al., 2009; Polinski et al., 2016). Gillespie et al. (2009) evaluated the effectiveness of focused interventions by hospital unit-based pharmacists on reducing morbidity and rehospitalization in 368 elderly patients who were randomized to either usual care or an intervention by a hospital unit-based pharmacist. The pharmacist performed medication histories and medication reconciliation at hospital admission and discharge, provided patient and health care provider counseling during hospitalization, communicated with the primary care physician at hospital discharge, and communicated with the patient via a follow-up phone call 2 months after hospital discharge. The pharmacist-based intervention group demonstrated an 80% decrease in drug-related readmissions, a 47% decrease in visits to the ED, and a 16% decrease in all visits to the hospital (Gillespie et al., 2009).

Eggink et al. (2010) randomized 81 HF patients to a pharmacist intervention or usual care. The pharmacists provided medication education and medication reconciliation at hospital discharge and at the first follow-up visit after hospitalization. Patients randomized to the pharmacist-guided intervention demonstrated a reduction of almost half in medication discrepancies and prescription errors (68% pharmacist group vs. 38% usual care; Eggink et al., 2010).

Polinski et al. (2016) demonstrated significant improvements in medication adherence, reductions in medication errors at hospital discharge and significant reductions in 30-day hospital readmission rates for more than 250 patients at high risk for HF by using a care transition program based on medication reconciliation as provided by outpatient pharmacists as compared with usual care. The intervention group received a medication reconciliation consultation visit within 3 days of discharge during in-home visits and/or via telephone following hospital discharge as well as personalized adherence education and coaching and a personalized care plan that was also shared with the patient's providers. The patient and pharmacist could initiate contact with each other for 30 days. During the 30-day follow-up period, patients in the control group were 50% less likely to be readmitted than were controls, for an absolute risk reduction of 11%. In addition, a cost savings was realized for each patient in the intervention group, with a savings of $2 for every $1 spent (Polinski et al., 2016).

Phatak, Prusi, Ward, Hansen, and Williams (2016) showed similar outcomes in that 30-day all-cause readmission rates were significantly lower when a pharmacy team was involved at discharge transitions utilizing a combination of face-to-face medication reconciliation, a patient-specific pharmaceutical care plan, counseling at the time of hospital discharge, and postdischarge phone calls at predetermined points in time, specifically days 3, 14, and 30. The study included 278 patients discharged from an internal medicine unit on three or more discharge medications or on at least one high-risk medication. The pharmacist-led study group showed a significant reduction in 30-day readmission rate to 24.8%, as compared with the usual-care group, which demonstrated a 39% 30-day readmission rate ($p = .01$). Despite the improvement in readmission rates, a statistically significant difference in medication-related events was not demonstrated in this study (Phatak et al., 2016).

In addition to pharmacists, nurses have been identified as positive factors in the medication reconciliation process. Discharge protocols and education by staff nurses at the time of discharge are recognized as important components of the medication reconciliation process in patients with HF (Foust et al., 2012).

Corbett, Setter, Daratha, Neumiller, and Wood (2010) described and classified medication discrepancies as identified by nurses when high-risk patients transitioned from hospital to home. High-risk patient diagnoses included HF, coronary artery disease, myocardial infarction, diabetes, and others. These nurse-identified medication discrepancies were classified as either patient level or system level. The most common patient-level medication discrepancies were intentional nonadherence, nonintentional nonadherence, and not filling a prescription. The most common system-level medication discrepancies were incomplete or inaccurate discharge instructions, conflicting information from different sources, and duplication of medications (Corbett et al., 2010).

A research group at Boston University developed Project Re-Engineered Discharge (RED) to promote patient safety and reduce rehospitalization rates (AHRQ, 2011). The project tested strategies to improve the hospital discharge process for high-risk patient populations including patients with HF. Results of this project included development of a guideline that provided targeted actions aimed at improving the hospital discharge process. As part of Project RED, Jack et al. (2009) randomized 749 medical patients to a nurse-led educational intervention with pharmacist follow-up, compared with usual care. The nurse-taught intervention group demonstrated significantly lower rates of hospital utilization after discharge compared with the usual-care group (22% vs. 27%, p = .028). The success of Project RED has led to development of a standardized approach to the discharge process in the form of a "toolkit" that has gained nationwide use (Jack, Paasche-Orlow, Mitchell, Foursythe, & Martin, 2013).

Foust et al. (2012) provide a retrospective chart review of nurse-identified rate and types of medication reconciliation problems in 162 older adults with HF. They found at least one type of medication reconciliation discrepancy 71.2% of the time, and 76% of these discrepancies involved a high-risk medication. The most common issues identified were medication discrepancies (58.9%), incomplete hospital discharge summaries (52.5%), and partial discharge instructions (48.9%).

Reducing hospital readmission rates in patients with HF is identified as a nationwide imperative set forth by the CMS (2011). Medication reconciliation is considered just one of multiple interventions targeted at preventing hospital readmission among high-risk populations such as patients with HF transitioning from one care setting to another (Feltner et al., 2014). In a review by Bradley et al. (2013), multiple strategies were identified that were associated with lower hospital risk-standardized readmission rates (RSRRs) for patients with HF by linking hospital survey data with hospital readmission rates. Six strategies were significantly associated with lower risk-standardized 30-day readmission rates; one of those strategies was having nurses responsible for medication reconciliation (0.18 decrease percentage point: p = .002). Additional strategies included partnering with community physicians or physician groups to reduce readmissions, partnering with local hospitals to reduce readmissions, arranging a follow-up appointment before discharge, having a process in place to send all discharge paper or electronic summaries directly to the patient's primary physician, and assigning staff to follow up on test results that return after the patient is discharged.

In a systematic review of 47 trials of adults with a mean age of 70 years with moderate to severe HF, Feltner et al. (2014) identified transitional care interventions that used patient education and self-care training before or at hospital discharge. They found that home-visiting programs employing a nurse or pharmacist to provide patient education and additional interventions such as medication reconciliation and interventions provided by interdisciplinary HF clinics after discharge were associated with reductions in all-cause readmissions and mortality at 30 days. In this review, structured telephone support after discharge was also associated with reduced HF-specific readmissions and mortality (Feltner et al., 2014).

Kutzleb et al. (2015) demonstrated improved outcomes in readmission rates of HF patients by implementing an APRN-led initiative. A pilot project called the Home Health Initiative (HHI) led to development of a hospital-wide Nurse Practitioner (NP) Model of Care. In the HHI cohort, 312 adult patients 20 to 89 years of age with HF who were considered at high risk for early readmission were randomized to the NP Model of Care employing an MD and NP team directing HF management versus usual care. The NP Model of Care focused on a variety of issues pertinent to the HF patient population, including patient education with daily weight charting, individualized medication administration schedules, and emphasis on the importance of lifestyle modification, which included a four-step approach to low-salt diet, daily exercise, smoking cessation, and elimination of alcohol. Thirty-day readmission rates in the NP Model of Care group were 8% as compared with the usual-care group with a readmission rate of 26%. Improvement in readmission rates for the NP Model of Care group was sustained over time with 60- and 90-day readmission rates at 4% and 3%, respectively, as compared with 27% and 29% in the usual-care group. Cost reductions at 30 days were significant for the NP Model of Care group, $311,818, versus $1,019,405 for the usual-care group. This translated to an approximate two-thirds reduction in overall costs for the study group as compared with the usual-care group (Kutzleb et al., 2015).

In summary, studies using specific interventions to improve the medication reconciliation process, such as use of pharmacists or nurse-led education, have shown beneficial outcomes. However, further testing of these interventions and other innovative strategies is needed in larger populations and with more diverse groups of patients. Medication reconciliation remains an essential component of transitional care interventions aimed at reducing the risk of adverse drug events and improving 30-day hospital readmission rates among high-risk HF patients. Continued evaluation of the effectiveness of APRNs in medication reconciliation is warranted as the APRN has a unique role in coordination of clinical care and oversight at times of care transitions, such as hospital discharge.

PROJECT FRAMEWORK, GOALS, AND CRITERIA

Using the Iowa Model of Evidence-Based Practice to Promote Quality Care (Titler et al., 2001), authors spearheaded an outcome project to improve the medication reconciliation process. The goals of the project were to increase patients' knowledge about their HF medications and to decrease discrepancies related to HF medications when patients transitioned from hospital to home. Patient selection criteria for the project included (a) being admitted with a primary HF diagnosis, New York Heart Association class II to IV HF, (b) having more than one hospitalization for HF within the past year, and (c) requiring enhanced HF patient education based on the assessment of the APRN.

Interventions for Project Development and Implementation

The first intervention was to implement a thorough HF education teaching session where the APRN met with the patient and caregiver(s) (pending caregiver availability), to review information in the *Heart Failure Handbook*. The contents of the handbook included important aspects of HF management, which are listed in Exhibit 6.3. The handbook was written at an eighth-grade reading level and was available in Spanish. Spanish-speaking patients constitute a large portion of the HF patient population at the health care facility. When needed, an interpreter was used for teaching sessions in other languages. The UCLA Health System has a robust interpreter service with 24-hour availability in all languages.

Based on APRNs' assessment, many patients/caregivers received more than one teaching session to reinforce information and to enhance adherence and compliance. If caretakers were not available in person, the teaching was completed with them over the phone, and then reinforced during the first follow-up phone call and at the first follow-up clinic visit. HF patients who would not be returning to the clinic under the care of

EXHIBIT 6.3   *Heart Failure Handbook*: Table of Contents

Introduction to Heart Failure
- What is the normal function of the heart?
- What is cardiomyopathy?
- What is heart failure?
- What are the signs and symptoms of heart failure?
- When do you call your doctor?

Prescribed Daily Routine
- Two-liter fluid restriction
- Daily weights
- Adjustment of diuretic dose

Important Changes to Your Diet
- Two-gram sodium diet
- Low-fat, low-cholesterol diet
- How to read a food label
- Alcohol
- Caffeine
- Cigarette smoking

Know Your Medications
- Medical regimen
- Commonly prescribed heart failure medications
- Warfarin (Coumadin) and your diet
- Safe cold, flu, and allergy medications
- Dental procedures and preventive antibiotic therapy
- Medications to be cautious with (e.g., NSAIDs)

Device Therapy for Heart Failure

Additional Patient Information
- Exercise and heart failure
- What about sex?
- Travel tips
- Advance directive

Diagnostic Tests
- Echocardiogram
- CPX
- Pulmonary artery catheter

Appendices
- Weight chart
- Chart of heart failure medications and doses
- Personal exercise schedule

CPX, cardiopulmonary exercise test; NSAIDs, nonsteroidal anti-inflammatory drugs; UCLA, University of California Los Angeles.
Source: Used with permission from the Ahmanson University of California Los Angeles Cardiomyopathy Center.

the HF service received all teachings and interventions for the medication reconciliation project. These patients, however, were excluded from the measurements of the project outcomes.

The second intervention included the development of an individualized typed medication list for each patient that included the name of each cardiac medication prescribed, the rationale for taking the medication, and the dose and frequency of the medication (Exhibit 6.4). The "frequency" section of the medication list included columns labeled breakfast, lunch, dinner, and bedtime. An "X" was used to indicate the time the patient was scheduled to take the medications. Other information on the medication list included patient's name, medical record number, the date last updated, the cardiomyopathy physician's name, and the next scheduled clinic appointment with office phone contact. Additionally, patients were reminded to bring their medication bottles and the medication list to the first cardiomyopathy clinic appointment.

Medication lists were also tailored to each patient's specific needs. For example, if the patient could read only Spanish, the list was typed in Spanish. If a patient had vision problems, then font size was enlarged and the font was bolded.

Patients were encouraged to view their medication list as an educational tool. The medication list included all HF-related medications but did not consistently include all of their other condition-specific medications. Patients were educated regarding the need to follow all instructions written on their discharge medication prescription bottles. They were also encouraged to continuously update their medication list by writing in any additional changes to their medication regimen. When the APRN identified that a patient was confused by the medication list or had difficulty understanding instructions, the medication list was provided to a family member. Detailed instructions were then reviewed with the family member, including all aspects of HF medication use and management.

The third intervention involved review of a form titled the "Heart Failure Medication Management Patient Information" (Exhibit 6.5) with the patients and caretakers. The purpose of the form was to enhance patients' understanding of their medications, to facilitate patients' adherence and responsibility for their medication regimen, and to encourage or foster self-care. The medication information sheet emphasized the importance of the following:

1. Ensuring all new discharge prescriptions were filled the day of discharge
2. Bringing an updated medication list and medication bottles to the patient's clinic appointments
3. Updating the patient's medication list with any changes in medications
4. Including all regularly taken medications (herbs, vitamins, over-the-counter medications, etc.) on the patient's medication list
5. Allowing at least a 2-day notice to his or her physician for any medication refills

A statement was also included to indicate that adhering to the preceding recommendations would expedite the patient's check-in time at the clinic.

After the APRN reviewed the medication sheet with the patient (or caregiver), the APRN requested the patient identify the primary person responsible for managing the medications. This person, typically the patient himself or herself, was asked to sign the medication

EXHIBIT 6.4 Sample Patient Medication List

Patient Name _____		Medical Record Number _____			Date _____	
			When to Take My Medications			
Drug name	**Indication/Why**	**Dose/How Much**	**Breakfast**	**Lunch**	**Dinner**	**Bedtime**
Coreg/Carvedilol	Protects heart/lowers heart rate and blood pressure	3.125 mg take twice a day	X		X	
Lisinopril/Zestril	Protects heart/lowers BP	10 mg take twice a day		X		X
Lasix/Furosemide	Diuretic/increases urination	80 mg take twice a day	X		X	
Potassium Chloride	Potassium replacement	20 mEq take twice a day	X		X	
Spironolactone/ Aldactone	Protects heart/potassium sparing mild diuretic	25 mg take once a day	X			
Fish oil	Lowers cholesterol	1 g twice a day	X		X	
Aspirin (baby)	Mild blood thinner	81 mg daily	X			
Coumadin/Warfarin	Thins blood/for LV clot	2 mg tabs—take daily as directed by clinic/doctor	Start Wed if labs okay 1 mg daily			X
Amiodarone/ Pacerone	Prevents heart arrhythmia	200 mg take once a day	X			
Digoxin/Lanoxin	Protects heart	0.125 mg take once a day			X	
Magnesium oxide	Supplement	400 mg take once a day	X			
As needed meds						
Tylenol/ acetaminophen	Mild pain/headache	500–650 mg as needed 3–4 times per day				
Docusate/Colace	Stool softener	100 mg twice a day				
Magnesium hydroxide/MOM	Laxative/relieves constipation	30 mL = 2 tablespoons as needed				
UCLA Cardiomyopathy	Clinic address	Clinic phone number				
Bring medication list AND bottles to clinic visit		**Cardiomyopathy physician name, and clinic appointment date/time**				

BP, blood pressure; LV, left ventricular; MOM, milk of magnesia; UCLA, University of California Los Angeles.
Source: Used with permission from the Ahmanson University of California Los Angeles Cardiomyopathy Center.

information sheet indicating agreement with the guidelines for self-managing medications. If patients were not able to perform the functions listed in the medication management information sheet, then the caregiver was asked to sign the form, indicating agreement with following the guidelines for managing the patient's medications.

EXHIBIT 6.5 **Heart Failure Medication Management Patient Information**

You have been provided a list of your medications, their doses, and why and when they need to be taken. As a patient, it is important that you have an understanding of your medications and take them as prescribed by your physician.

We request that you do the following:

- Have all new discharge prescriptions filled the day of discharge.
- Bring an updated medication list to all your appointments.
- Bring all medication bottles to your appointments.
- Keep a copy of your medication list in your purse or wallet.
- Whenever a medication change is made, update your medication list.
- Include all medications on your medication list (herbs, vitamins, and any over-the-counter medications, e.g., Advil, Tylenol) that you take regularly.
- Please allow 48 hours notice for all refills.

"Check-in" at your clinic appointment may be delayed if you do not have your updated medication list/medications with you.

Name of the person who helps organize your medications:

_____

_____

Contact number:

_____

I, _____, have read the information above and will educate myself about the medications I take and take them as prescribed by my physician.

Patient Signature:

_____

Date:

_____

UCLA, University of California Los Angeles.
Source: Used with permission from the Ahmanson University of California Los Angeles Cardiomyopathy Center.

The fourth intervention was initiation (incorporation) of a follow-up phone call to the patient by the APRN on the first business day after discharge to review medications and HF management instructions. During the phone call, the person responsible for managing medications was asked to read back pill strength and dosing directions on the discharge medication bottles. To verify that the patient was taking the correct prescriptions, the APRN cross-referenced the medications the patient had at home to the hospital's documented discharge summary. If a medication discrepancy was identified, it was documented and corrected with the patient. If a medication was missing, the APRN would immediately contact the patient's pharmacy to submit a new prescription. Additionally, the APRN asked about the patient's current weight, and compared it with the patient's discharge weight to determine if adjustments in diuretics were needed. Signs and symptoms of HF and daily weight monitoring were reinforced, as was the importance of following sodium and fluid restrictions. Last, the patient was reminded to bring the medication bottles and an updated medication list to the clinic appointment.

The fifth intervention occurred at the first clinic appointment. Initially, the nursing assistant documented whether the patient brought the medication list and bottles to the clinic visit. If the patient arrived without a medication list, the nursing assistant would provide a wallet-sized blank medication card for the patient to complete. After check-in procedures, the APRN performed medication reconciliation for each medication. If a discrepancy was encountered, it was documented in the clinic chart and corrected with the patient. If the APRN assessed that the patient required further clarification regarding a medication discrepancy, the patient was contacted the next day and asked to verbalize the corrected instructions on his or her list and on the medication bottle(s).

While the project was being implemented, the APRNs collaboratively discussed problems they encountered and shared ways of improving the project. Ideas for improvement included (a) having the administrative office staff remind patients to bring their medication list and bottles to their visit during appointment-confirmation calls, (b) having the APRNs update the patient's existing medication list at the first visit as needed, and (c) having the APRNs demonstrate the process of writing down medications on the wallet-sized blank card when patients did not bring their medication list to the clinic.

Other important aspects of the project included ongoing education and reinforcement of project details to all staff nurses caring for these patients. The APRN project leader attended unit staff meetings to discuss specific details of the outcome project. For example, the APRN described the purpose of the project, the rationale for providing patients with an individualized medication list, and the importance of the staff nurses in providing and reinforcing HF teaching during each interaction with a patient and the patient's family.

Outcomes Measured

The outcomes identified for this project were selected based on problems the APRNs observed related to patients' accurate and safe medication use during their transition of care (i.e., from hospital discharge to home and the follow-up clinic visit). These outcomes included the percentage of patients who (a) were provided with a medication list before discharge, (b) brought either their medication list or their medication prescription bottles to the clinic, (c) experienced medication discrepancies that were identified during the first follow-up phone call, and/or (d) experienced medication discrepancies identified at the first follow-up clinic visit.

Monthly, the APRN project leader performed an audit on all patient charts (Exhibit 6.6). The audit consisted of documenting the number of patients discharged each month and the number who received the interventions previously identified for this project. The audit tool tracked the important outcomes of the project such as the number of medication discrepancies, the type of discrepancies (e.g., correct drug, dose, frequency, or supply), and the number of patients who brought their medication lists and/or medication prescription bottles to their clinic appointment.

Results Before and After Project Implementation

After implementing the outcome project, the APRNs evaluated the changes in outcome measures from before to after implementation (Figures 6.2–6.4). Outcomes improved

EXHIBIT 6.6 **Medication Reconciliation: Monthly Audit Tool**

1. Number of patients discharged:
2. Number of patients who were provided:
   A. HF education/medication review/HF handbook: ____/____
   B. Medication list: ____/____
   C. Medication contract/copy in chart: ____/____
   D. Phone call s/p hospital discharge: ____/____
3. Number of patients with:
   A. Medication discrepancy identified on phone follow-up: total # ____/____

   Type of discrepancy

Drug	ACE/ARB	BB	AA	Diuretic	K+
Dose					
Frequency					
Supply					

   B. Medication list at first clinic visit s/p hospital discharge: total # ___/___
   C. Medications brought to first clinic visit s/p hospital discharge: total # ___/___
   D. Medication discrepancy at first clinic visit s/p hospital discharge: total # ___/___

   Type of discrepancy

Drug	ACE/ARB	BB	AA	Diuretic	K+
Dose					
Frequency					
Supply					

AA, aldosterone antagonist; ACE, angiotensin-converting enzyme; ARB, angiotensin-receptor blocker; BB, beta-blocker; HF, heart failure; K+, potassium; s/p, status post; UCLA, University of California Los Angeles.
Source: Used with permission from the Ahmanson University of California Los Angeles Cardiomyopathy Center.

over time in areas of (a) patients consistently receiving their medication list (before: approximately 10%; after: 71%–100%), (b) patients consistently bringing their medication list and/or prescription bottles to their first clinic visit (before: approximately 50%; after: 86%–100% for the majority of months), (c) medication discrepancies, which markedly decreased during the first follow-up phone call (before: approximately 38%; after: decreased with time to 0% for the majority of months), and (d) medication discrepancies, which also decreased markedly at the first follow-up clinic visit (before: approximately 50%; after: decreased with time to 0%). For the outcome related to patients bringing their medication list or medication bottles to the clinic, an improvement occurred from 10% before to 100% for the first 10 months after the intervention. During months 11 and 12, the percentage compliance of these measures decreased because a non-APRN health care professional who was unfamiliar with the new medication reconciliation processes was seeing the patient (Figure 6.3). The opportunity also was missed to

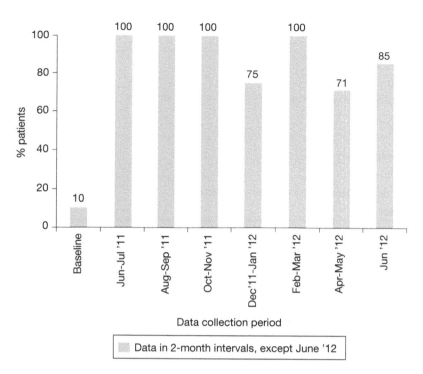

FIGURE 6.2 Percentage of patients provided with medication list before discharge.

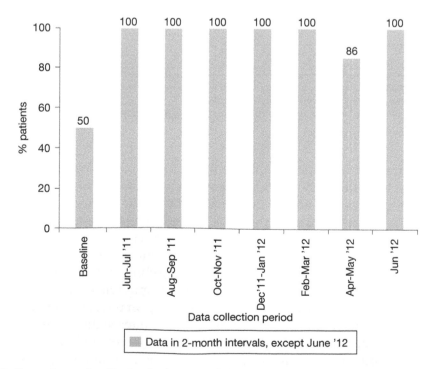

FIGURE 6.3 Percentage of patients who brought either medication list or prescription bottles to first clinic visit.

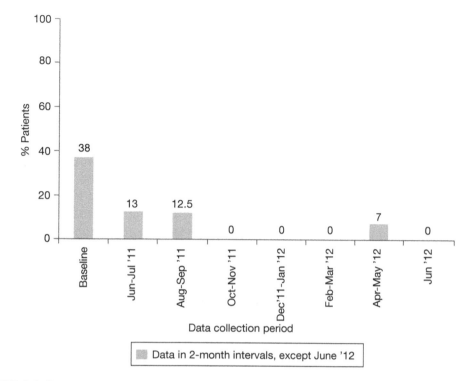

FIGURE 6.4 Percentage of patients with medication discrepancies at first follow-up phone call.

document whether a patient brought his or her medication list or bottles to the first follow-up clinic visit.

The overall improvements in project outcomes indicated an adoption of the new medication reconciliation processes by the patients, the caregivers, and the APRNs. However, additional strategies had to be identified for when non-APRN health care professionals assessed patients in the clinic. Additionally, project reminders were needed for documentation by nursing assistants regarding whether patients brought their medication list or bottles to the clinic.

Limitations

The design of the medication reconciliation outcome project was based on current best evidence and patient-, clinic-, and APRN-identified needs. Consequently, results and tools may be applicable only to similar patients, hospitals, and clinic settings. Although medication discrepancies were frequently identified by APRNs during patients' first postdischarge clinic visits, no standardized mechanism was available to consistently collect and summarize the frequency of medication discrepancies and other outcome variables during the preintervention (baseline) period. However, the newly standardized medication reconciliation processes developed for this outcome project have been effective in achieving project goals. Patients consistently received their medication list, brought their medication list or bottles to the clinic, and the medication discrepancies decreased.

PATIENT NAVIGATOR PROGRAM

The success of the APRN medication reconciliation project exemplified how the implementation of evidence-based interventions reduced medication discrepancies in patients with HF. Medication discrepancies have been associated with hospital readmission. With the potential reduction of hospital reimbursement by the CMS for HF patients readmitted within 30 days of discharge, leaders at the Ronald Reagan UCLA Medical Center (Ronald Reagan University of California Los Angeles [RR UCLA]) desired to implement strategies to improve care and patients' experience and reduce readmissions. To achieve this goal, UCLA accepted an invitation from the American College of Cardiology (ACC) to join the Patient Navigator Program. The program was developed in response to data that suggest that readmissions can be prevented by improving early follow-up and medication management and by empowering patients to take an active role in their recovery (i.e., improved self-care with self-management support).

The goal for the ACC Patient Navigator Program is for hospitals to establish a patient-centered focus that involves making hospitalization less stressful for patients by providing evidence-based QI strategies. These strategies include providing the right amount of information and resources while the patient is hospitalized, as well as supporting the patient during recovery and transition to home. These goals are achieved through an interdisciplinary plan of care, comprehensive interventions, the addition of home monitoring, and early follow-up appointments. Ultimately, the ACC Patient Navigator Program combines the power of available national data (e.g., registries) with team-based improvement strategies to reduce avoidable hospital readmissions (ACC, 2014).

The ACC Patient Navigator Program lasts 26 months and is organized in three phases: preimplementation (months 1–8), implementation (months 9–20), and evaluation (months 20–26). In the preimplementation phase, each hospital conducts a kick-off event and invites key leaders to learn about the goals of the program and identify areas of focus. Each team submits data to the ACC on baseline performance, conducts an online assessment to determine the hospital's performance data compared with national benchmarks, and develops strategies to achieve the specified goals and benchmarks. During this period, the team also identifies problems and selects interventions. During the implementation phase, the hospital develops and implements a plan for improvement and monitors progress through quarterly reporting of data to the ACC. Best practices and barriers are shared through monthly conference calls and quarterly webinars with other ACC Patient Navigator Program hospitals. During the evaluation phase, the team analyzes the data and summarizes the lessons learned. The team continues to track data and identify gaps for further areas of improvement.

At the first UCLA committee meeting, the interdisciplinary team (physicians, nurses, pharmacists, nutritionists, case managers, social workers, physical therapists, and administrators) identified the following goals:

- Develop a risk model to identify patients who are at high risk of readmissions before discharge
- Track performance and documentation of medication reconciliation
- Track documentation of all prescribed medications, instructions on when and how they should be taken, and any changes to medications
- Verify follow-up appointments in the medical record and documentation of the plan of care based on the health care encounter (called an after-visit summary [AVS])

- Refer to cardiac rehabilitation at discharge
- Individualize each patient's plan of care, including when to call health care providers
- Document teach-back with patient education
- Document referrals to community resources

Risk Model and Interventions

To identify patients who would benefit from specific interventions, the ACC recommended that ACC Patient Navigator Program hospitals use one of the evidence-based risk stratification tools to identify HF patients at risk for readmission within 30 days after hospital discharge. RR UCLA decided to adapt the LACE Index tool used by most ACC Patient Navigator Program hospitals. The LACE Index tool scores each patient from 0 to 19 on the basis of all the following parameters: length of stay (L), acuity of admission (A), comorbidity (C), and ED visits in the preceding 6 months (E). This tool has been used to predict the risk of unplanned readmissions as well as mortality within 30 days of hospital discharge in both medical and surgical patients (Wang et al., 2014). Based on the LACE criteria, a low (0–6), medium (7–10), or high (≥11) score is calculated for the HF patient. The UCLA Patient Navigator Program teams then identified bundled interventions for each level of risk. For example, an HF patient with a low risk score of 6 would receive a medication reconciliation from the pharmacist, an updated medication list from the nurse, and a standardized discharge summary from the discharging physician, as well as a follow-up appointment within 5 days (Table 6.7). In contrast, an HF patient with a high risk score

TABLE 6.7   **LACE Risk Stratification Score and Bundled Interventions at Ronald Reagan UCLA Medical Center**

Intervention Needed and Responsible Provider	LACE Score		
	Low (0–6)	Med (7–10)	High (≥11)
Standardized D/C summary (after-visit summary)	X	X	X
Medication reconciliation (MD/pharmacist)	X	X	X
Update medication list (RN)	X	X	X
Physical therapy consultation		X	X
Pharmacy 1:1 teaching		X	X
Social work (psychosocial issues/complex cases)			X
Care coordination: home health, community-based care transition program (case management)			X
Nutrition 1:1 teaching (dietician)			X
Post hospital follow-up visit with physician (Department of Medicine staff)	≤5 days	≤5 days	≤3 days/home health RN
Palliative care (PRN)			

D/C, discharge; LACE, length of stay, acuity of admission, comorbid conditions, and emergency department visits; MD, physician; PRN, as needed.

of 14 would receive the same interventions plus consultations by a physical therapist, a social worker, a case manager, and a dietician; one-to-one medication teaching by the pharmacist; and a follow-up appointment within 3 days.

Outcomes

The outcomes important to the organization and the ACC Patient Navigator Program program are listed in Table 6.8, along with descriptions of the outcomes and the data sources. Figure 6.5 illustrates preliminary results of 30-day unadjusted readmission rates for HF patients comparing UCLA and ACC Patient Navigator Program hospitals. Outcomes improved in 2015 quarter 1 and 2016 quarter 2, whereas in some quarters, readmissions were higher than at other ACC Patient Navigator Program institutions.

TABLE 6.8 **ACC Patient Navigator Program Heart Failure Outcome Measures, Description, and Data Source**

Outcome Measure	Description	Data Source
30-day risk-standardized readmission rate for HF	Hospital-specific 30-day all-cause risk-standardized readmission rate following hospitalization for HF among Medicare beneficiaries aged 65 years or older at the time of index hospitalization	Self-reported by hospital (quarterly) CMS claims data (annually)
30-day risk-standardized mortality rate for HF	Estimation of a hospital-level risk-standardized mortality rate for patients discharged from the hospital with a principal diagnosis of HF	Self-reported by hospital (quarterly) CMS claims data (annually)
Patient satisfaction	Hospital Consumer Assessment of Healthcare Providers and Systems (HCAHPS)	HCAHPS or hospital satisfaction survey data
Patient quality of life/health status (optional metric)	Quality of life assessment performed by health care team	Hospital QOL tool
(a) LVEF assessment, (b) ACE/ARB therapy for patients with LVSD, (c) beta-blocker therapy for patients with LVSD, (d) patient self-care education	Percentage of patients, older than 18 years of age with a diagnosis of HF documented within the past 12 months	Self-reported by hospital via chart abstraction/other method (hospital EHR/GWTG-HF)
HF patients are identified before discharge *and* risk of readmission is determined	Number of times medication reconciliation occurs in the hospital (ideally at admission and discharge)	Self-reported by hospital via chart abstraction/other method
Follow-up visit or cardiac rehabilitation referral within 7 days is scheduled, documented in the medical record, and patient is provided with documentation of the scheduled appointment	Number of patients with follow-up appointments made within 7 days of discharge from hospital and provided with documentation before discharge	Self-reported by hospital via chart abstraction/other method
HF patient arrives at follow-up appointment, within 7 days of discharge from hospital	Number of patients who see a clinician within 7 days of discharge	Self-reported by hospital via chart abstraction/other method

ACE, angiotensin-converting enzyme; ARB, angiotensin-receptor blocker; CMS, Centers for Medicare & Medicaid Services; EHR, electronic health record; HF, heart failure; GWTG-HF, Get With the Guidelines-Heart Failure; LVEF, left ventricular ejection fraction; LVSD, left ventricular systolic dysfunction; QOL, quality of life.

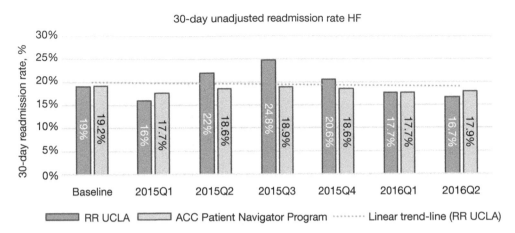

FIGURE 6.5 UCLA versus ACC Patient Navigator Program 30-day unadjusted readmission rate for heart failure.

Note: The graph shows linear trend line for variables that are increasing or decreasing at a steady rate over time.

ACC, American College of Cardiology; HF, heart failure; RR UCLA, Ronald Reagan University of California Los Angeles.

In this process, RR UCLA has learned that numerous factors contribute to hospital readmissions. RR UCLA is continuously working to identify best practices to reduce readmissions.

In the area of patient experience related to patients' understanding of medications, RR UCLA is consistently higher than other ACC Patient Navigator Program hospitals and has identified and shared best practices (Figure 6.6). In addition, RR UCLA has increased the number of HF patients consistently receiving a follow-up appointment within 7 days after discharge (Figure 6.7).

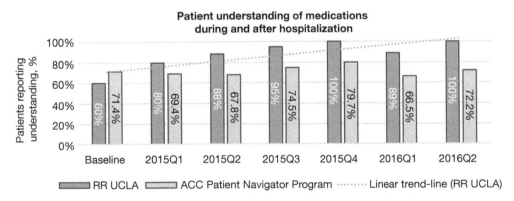

FIGURE 6.6 Percentages of heart failure patients reporting understanding of their medications during and after hospitalization.

Note: Patient satisfaction metrics from HCAHPS survey results. The graph shows linear trend line for variables that are increasing or decreasing at a steady rate over time.

ACC, American College of Cardiology; HCAHPS, Hospital Consumer Assessment of Healthcare Providers and Systems; HF, heart failure; RR UCLA, Ronald Reagan University of California Los Angeles.

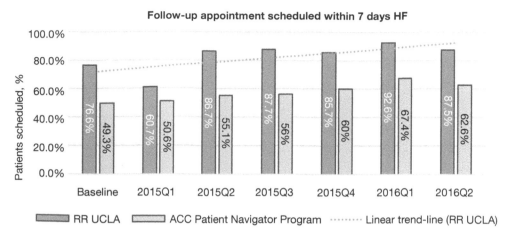

FIGURE 6.7 Number of heart failure patients with a follow-up appointment scheduled within 7 days.

Note: The graph shows linear trend line for variables that are increasing or decreasing at a steady rate over time.

ACC, American College of Cardiology; HF, heart failure; RR UCLA, Ronald Reagan University of California Los Angeles.

SUMMARY

Effective medication reconciliation is composed of multiple processes that together support safe medication use by patients. Medication reconciliation structures and processes can be improved by assessing current practices during transitions of care, developing an evidence-based process improvement intervention, and evaluating the impact on outcomes. In this project, cardiovascular APRNs found that implementing an evidence-based medication reconciliation process for HF patients has improved the process of medication reconciliation in several ways. These processes and tools have been effective in increasing the consistency with which patients received an accurate medication list and brought their medication list or bottles to the clinic. Additionally, medication discrepancies decreased during the first follow-up phone call and at the first follow-up clinic visit. This preliminary work by APRNs was incorporated into a component of the hospital-wide interdisciplinary initiative to reduce hospital readmissions for HF patients. Cardiovascular APRNs, at the point-of-care delivery, play a key role in developing and successfully implementing an effective medication reconciliation process for high-risk HF patients. They are also members of interdisciplinary teams and participate in the development and evaluation of hospital-wide performance improvement initiatives to improve care and outcomes.

Answers to Chapter Discussion Questions

1. Medication reconciliation is a process that involves obtaining and maintaining accurate and complete medication information across the continuum of care. The process requires members of the health care team to comprehensively evaluate a patient's medication regimen to avoid medication errors at all care transition points. The transition

from hospital to home is an especially high-risk time because of changes in medication regimens that occur during an acute illness requiring hospitalization. The interventions implemented by the APRNs in the exemplar provided in this chapter are consistent with this definition. Note: The APRN and/or student should expand on how the interventions in the exemplar are consistent with the definition.

2. The outcomes of concern to APRNs listed in Exhibit 6.1 are broad-spectrum outcomes in categories of clinical, physiological, psychosocial, functional, fiscal, and satisfaction outcomes. These outcomes may be similar, but may not include all nurse-sensitive outcomes that have been selected for national reporting. Nurse-sensitive outcomes represent the impact of nursing interventions and describe the effect of what nurses do in response to a patient's condition. These outcomes may be the result of direct care, non-APRN practices, and thus may not all be listed in Exhibit 6.1.

3. The APRN and/or student should review the advantages and disadvantages of various research designs illustrated in Table 6.2 and determine appropriate designs/frameworks in relationship to the clinical issue and outcomes they identify. The APRN and/or student may be able to use more than one research design or framework. Note: Have the students provide rationales and support for their selection of various research designs and frameworks.

4. The APRN and/or student should identify the relative effectiveness of interventions described in the review of literature section in this chapter. These interventions include, but are not limited to (a) case manager involvement, (b) use of discharge checklists that incorporate medication and disease-specific information, and (c) designating a specific health care provider to review and reconcile medications at the point of discharge. Review the advantages and disadvantages of various research designs and other methods for outcome measurement projects.

5. The APRN and/or student should discuss the role of the APRN in working with interdisciplinary teams to improve outcomes. APRNs are at the forefront of improving care through outcome measurement. They serve as critical members of the health care team. Because of their key role in the health care system, APRNs frequently lead outcome measurement and QI initiatives. By virtue of their graduate education preparation, clinical knowledge, and critical thinking skills, APRNs have an essential role in evaluating outcomes for improvement efforts. Additionally, APRN core competencies demonstrate expertise and provide additional areas for measuring outcomes. Note: Have students identify how APRN core competencies provide foundational knowledge and skills for outcome measurement.

REFERENCES

Academy Health. (2011). Health outcomes core library recommendations, 2011. Retrieved from https://www.nlm.nih.gov/nichsr/corelib/houtcomes-2011.html

Agency for Healthcare Research and Quality. (2011, October). Preventing avoidable readmissions: Improving the hospital discharge process. Rockville, MD. Retrieved from http://www.ahrq.gov/professionals/quality-patient-safety/patient-safety-resources/resources/impptdis/index.html

Albert, N. M., Fonarow, G. C., Yancy, C. W., Curtis, A. B., Gattis-Stough, W., Gheorghiade, M., . . . Walsh, M. N. (2010). Outpatient cardiology practices with advanced practice nurses and physician assistants provide similar delivery of recommended therapies (findings from IMPROVE HF). *American Journal of Cardiology, 105*, 1774–1779.

Altmiller, G. (2011). Quality and safety education for nurses' competencies for the clinical nurse specialist. *Clinical Nurse Specialist, 24*(4), 187–188.

American College of Cardiology. (2014). Patient navigator program. Retrieved from http://cvquality.acc.org/Initiatives/Patient-Navigator.aspx?_ga=1.7382962.124192929.1455129164

American Pharmacists Association, & American Association of Health System Pharmacists. (2012). Improving care transitions: Optimizing medication reconciliation. *Journal of the American Pharmacists Association, 52*(4), e43–e52. doi:10.1331/JAPhA.2012.12527

Aspden, P., Wolcott, J. A. J., Bootman, L., & Cronenwett, L. R. (2006). *Preventing medication errors.* Washington, DC: National Academies Press. Retrieved from http://www.nap.edu

Becker, D. M., Yanek, L. R., Johnson, W. R., Jr., Garrett, D., Moy, T. F., Reynolds, S. S., & Becker, L. C. (2005). Impact of a community-based multiple risk factor intervention on cardiovascular risk in Black families with a history of premature coronary disease. *Circulation, 111*(10), 1298–1304.

Bell, C. M., Brener, S. S., Gunraj, N., Huo, C., Beirman, A. S., Scales, D. C., & Urbach, D. R. (2011). Association of ICU or hospital admission with unintentional discontinuation of medications for chronic diseases. *Journal of the American Medical Association, 306*(8), 840–847. doi:10.1001/jama.2011.1206

Bergenson, S. C., & Dean, J. D. (2006). A systems approach to patient-centered care. *Journal of the American Medical Association, 296*(23), 2848–2851.

Bradley, E. H., Curry, L., Horwitz, L. I., Sipsma, H., Wang, Y., Walsh, M. N., . . . Krumholtz, H. M. (2013). Hospital strategies associated with 30-day readmission rates for patients with heart failure. *Circulation Cardiovascular Quality and Outcomes, 6*(4), 444–450. doi:10.1161/circoutcomes.111.000101

Bristol Calvert, S., Kramer, J. M., Anstrom, K. J., Kaltenbach, L. A., Stafford, J. A., & Allen LaPointe, N. (2012). Patient-focused intervention to improve long-term adherence to evidence-based medications: A randomized trial. *American Heart Journal, 163*, 657–665.

Burns, K. D., Jenkins, W., Yeh, D., Procyshyn, R. M., Schwartz, S. K. W., Honer, W. G., & Barr, A. M. (2009). Delirium after cardiac surgery: A retrospective case-control study of incidence and risk factors in a Canadian sample. *BC Medical Journal, 51*(5), 206–210.

Burns, N., & Grove, S. (2015). *Understanding nursing research: Building an evidence-based practice* (6th ed.). Philadelphia, PA: Saunders Elsevier.

Calvin, J. E., Shanbhag, S., Avery, E., Kane, J., Richardson, D., & Powell, L. (2012). Adherence to evidence-based guidelines for heart failure in physicians and their patients: Lessons from the heart failure adherence retention trial (HART). *Congestive Heart Failure, 18*(2), 73–78.

Carson, S. S. (2010). Outcomes research: Methods and implications. *Seminars in Respiratory Critical Care Medicine, 31*(1), 3–12.

Centers for Medicare & Medicaid Services. (2011). Hospital quality initiatives: Hospital value-based purchasing program. Retrieved from https://www.cms.gov/hospitalqualityinits

Centers for Medicare & Medicaid Services. (2012). Roadmap for quality measurement in the traditional Medicare Fee-for-Service Program. Retrieved from http://www.cms.hhs.gov

Chang, P. P., Chambless, L. E., Shahar, E., Bertoni, A. G., Russell, S. D., Ni, H., & Rosamond, W. D. (2014). Incidence and survival of hospitalized acute decompensated heart failure in four US communities (from the Atherosclerosis Risk in Communities Study). *American Journal of Cardiology, 113*, 504–510. doi:10.1016/j.amjcard.2013.10.032

Chen, J., Normand, S. L., Wang, Y., & Krumholz, H. M. (2011). National and regional trends in heart failure hospitalization and mortality rates for Medicare beneficiaries, 1998–2008. *Journal of the American Medical Association, 306*, 1669–1678. doi:10.1001/jama.2011.1474

Cohen, L., Manion, L., & Morrison, K. (2000). *Research methods in education* (5th ed.). London, England: Routledge Falmer.

Conrad, P. (1985). The meaning of medications: Another look at compliance. *Social Science Medicine, 20*(1), 29–37.

Corbett, C. F., Setter, S. M., Daratha, K. B., Neumiller, J. J., & Wood, L. D. (2010). Nurse identified hospital to home medication discrepancies: Implications for improving transitional care. *Geriatric Nursing, 31*(3), 188–196.

Corbin, J., & Strauss, A. (2008). *Basics of qualitative research: Techniques and procedures for developing grounded theory* (3rd ed.). Thousand Oaks, CA: Sage.

Creswell, J. W., Klassen, A. C., Plano Clark, V. L., Smith, K. C. (2011). Best practices for mixed methods research in the health sciences. Retrieved from https://obssr.od.nih.gov/training/mixed-methods-research

Curry, L. A., Nembhard, I. M., & Bradley, E. H. (2009). Qualitative and mixed methods provide unique contributions to outcomes research. *Circulation, 119*(10), 1442–1452.

Curtis, L. H., Whellan, D. J., Hammill, B. G., Hernandez, A. J., Anstrom, L. J., Shea, A. M., & Schulman, K. A. (2008). Incidence and prevalence of heart failure in elderly persons, 1994–2003. *Archives of Internal Medicine, 168*(4), 418–424. doi:10.1001/archinternmed.2007.80

Damberg, C. L., Sobero, M. E., Lovejoy, S. L., Lauderdale, K., Wertheimer, S., Smith, A., . . . Schnyer, C. (2012). An evaluation of the use of performance measures in health care. *RAND Health Quarterly, 1*(4), 3. Retrieved from http://www.rand.org/pubs/periodicals/health-quarterly/issues/v1/n4/03.html

Dawber, R. T., Meadors, F. G., & Moore E. F. (1951). Epidemiological approaches to heart disease: The Framingham Study. *American Journal of Public Health, 41*(3), 279–286.

De la Porte, P. W., Lok, D. J., vanVeldhuisen, D. J., van Wijngaarden, J., Comel, J. H., Zuithoff, N. P., . . . Hoes, A. W. (2007). Added value of a physician- and nurse-directed heart failure clinic: Results from the Deventer-Alkmaar heart failure study. *Heart, 93*(7), 819–825.

Dennison, C. R., & Hughes, S. (2009). Reforming cardiovascular care: Quality measurements and improvement, and pay-for-performance. *Journal of Cardiovascular Nursing, 24*(5), 341–343.

DesHarnais, S. I. (2013). The outcome model of quality. In W. A. Sollecito & J. K. Johnson (Eds.), *McLaughlin and Kaluzny's continuous improvement in health care* (4th ed., pp. 155–180). Burlington, MA: Jones & Bartlett.

DeWalt, D. A., Malone, R. M., Bryant, M. E., Kosnar, M. C., Corr, K. E., Rothman, R. L., . . . Pignone, M. P. (2006). A heart failure self-management program for patients of all literacy levels: A randomized, controlled trial [ISRCTN11535170]. *BMC Health Services Research, 2006*(6). doi:10.1186/1472-6963-6-30

Dharmarajan, K., Hsieh, A. F., Zhenqiu, L., Bueno, H., Ross, J. S., Horwitz, L., & Krumholz, H. M. (2013). Diagnoses and timing of 30-day readmissions after hospitalization for heart failure, acute myocardial infarction, or pneumonia. *Journal of American Medical Association, 309*, 4, 355–363. doi:10.1001/jama.2012.216476

Dunlay, S. M., Redfield, M. M., Weston, S. A., Therneau, T. M., Hall Long, K., Shah, N. D., & Roger, V. L. (2009). Hospitalizations after heart failure diagnosis: A community perspective. *Journal of the American College of Cardiology, 54*, 1695–1702. doi:10.1016/j.jacc.2009.08.019

Eggink, R. N., Lenderink, A. W., Widdershoven, J., & van den Bemt, P. (2010). The effect of a clinical pharmacist discharge service on medication discrepancies in patients with heart failure. *Pharmacy World & Science, 32*(6), 759–766. doi:10.1007/s11096-9433-6

Estabrooks, C. A., Walling, L., & Milner, M. (2003). Measuring knowledge utilization in health care. *International Journal of Policy and Evaluation, 1*(3), 3–12. Retrieved from http://hdl.handle.net/10755/153540

Feltner, C., Jones, C. D., Cené, C. W., Zheng, Z.-J., Sueta, C. A., Coker-Schwimmer, E. J. L., . . . Jonas, D. E. (2014). Transitional care interventions to prevent readmissions for persons with heart failure. *Annals of Internal Medicine, 160*(11), 774–784. doi:10.7326/M14-0083

Finkelman, A., & Kenner, C. (2012). *Learning IOM: Implications of the Institute of Medicine Reports for Nursing Education* (3rd ed.). Silver Spring, MA: Nursesbooks.org.

Fonarow, G. C., Albert, M. N., Curtis, A. B., Sough, W. G., Gheorghiade, M., Heywood, J. T., & Yancy, C. W. (2010). Improving evidence-based care for heart failure in outpatient cardiology practices: Primary results of the registry to improve the use of evidence-based heart failure therapies in the outpatient setting (IMPROVE HF). *Circulation, 12*, 585–596.

Foust, J. B., Naylor, M. D., Bixby, M. B., & Ratcliffe, S. J. (2012). Medication problems occurring at hospital discharge among older adults with heart failure. *Research in Gerontological Nursing, 5*(1), 25–33. doi:10.3928/19404921-20111206-04

Fulton, J., & Baldwin, K. (2004). An annotated bibliography reflecting CNS practice and outcomes. *Clinical Nurse Specialist, 18*(1), 21–39.

Gaskin, C., & Happell, B. (2014). Power effects, confidence and significance: An investigation of statistical practices in nursing research. *International Journal of Nursing Studies, 51*, 795–806.

Gawlinski, A. (2007). Evidence-based practice changes: Measuring the outcome. *AACN Advanced Critical Care, 18*(3), 320–322.

Gawlinski, A., McCloy, K., Erickson, V., Chaker, T. H., Vandenbogaart, E., Creaser, J., Livingston, N., & Rourke, D. (2013). Measuring outcomes in cardiovascular advanced practice nursing. In R. M. Kleinpell (Ed.), *Outcome assessment in advanced practice nursing* (pp. 129–185). New York, NY: Springer Publishing.

Gawlinski, A., & Rutledge, D. (2008). Selecting a model for evidence-based practice changes: A practical approach. *AACN Advanced Critical Care, 19*, 1–10.

Gillespie, U., Alassaad, A., Henrohn, D., Garmo, H., Hammarlund-Udenaes, M., Toss, H., & Morlin, C. (2009). A comprehensive pharmacist intervention to reduce morbidity in patients 80 years or older. *Archives of Internal Medicine, 169*(9), 894–900.

Giuffre, M. (1997). Designing research: Ex post facto designs. *Journal of Perianesthesia Nursing, 12*(3), 191–195.

Gleason, K. M., McDaniel, M. R., Feinglass, J., Baker, D. W., Lindquist, L., Liss, D., & Noskin, G. A. (2010). Results of the medications at transitions and clinical handoffs (MATCH) study: An analysis of medication reconciliation errors and risk factors at hospital admission. *Journal of General Internal Medicine, 25*(5), 441–447. doi:10.1007/s11606-010-1256-6

Go, A. S., Mozaffarian, D., Roger, V. L., Benjamin, E. J., Berry, J. D., Borden, W. B., . . . Turner, M. B. (2013). Heart disease and stroke statistics–2013 update: A report from the American Heart Association. *Circulation, 127*, e6–e245. doi:10.1161/CIR.0b013e31828124ad

Greenhalgh, T. (2002). Integrating qualitative research into evidence-based practice. *Endocrinology and Metabolism Clinics of North America, 31*(3), 583–601.

Hamric, A. B., Hanson, C. M., Tracy, M. F., & O'Grady, E. T. (Eds.). (2012). *Advanced nursing practice: An integrative approach* (5th ed.). St. Louis, MO: Elsevier Saunders.

Heidenreich, P. A., Albert, N. M., Allen, L. A., Bluemke, D. A., Butler, J., Fonarow, G. C., . . . Stroke Council. (2013). Forecasting the impact of heart failure in the United States: A policy statement from the American Heart Association. *Circulation Heart Failure, 6*, 606–619. doi:10.1161/HHF.0b013e318291329a

Hubbard, T., & McNeil, N. (2012). Improving medication adherence and reducing readmissions. Retrieved from http://www.nacds.org/pdfs/pr/2012/nehi-readmissions.pdf

Ingersoll, G. L. (2000). Evidence-based nursing: What it is and what it isn't. *Nursing Outlook, 48*(4), 151–152.

Institute of Medicine. (2001). *Crossing the quality chasm: A new health system for the 21st century*. Washington, DC: National Academies Press.

Jack, B. W., Chetty, V. K., Anthony, D., Greenwald, J. L., Sanchez, G. M., Johnson, A. E., & Culpepper, L. (2009). A reengineered hospital discharge program to decrease hospitalization: A randomized trial. *Annals of Internal Medicine, 150*(3), 178–187.

Jack, B. W., Paasche-Orlow, M. K., Mitchell, S. M., Foursythe, S., & Martin, J. (2013). *An overview of the re-engineered discharge (RED) toolkit* (Prepared by Boston University under Contract No. HHSA2902006000012i). Rockville, MD: Agency for Healthcare Research and Quality. AHRQ Publication No. 12(13)-0084

Joseph, A. M. (2007). The impact of nursing on patient and organizational outcomes. *Nursing Economics, 25*(1), 30–34.

Kapu, A. N., & Kleinpell, R. (2013). Developing nurse practitioner associated metrics for outcomes assessment. *Journal of the American Academy of Nurse Practitioners, 25*(6), 289–296.

Kleinpell, R., & Alexandrov, A. W. (2014). Integrative review of outcomes and performance improvement research on advanced practice nursing. In A. B. Hamric, C. M. Hanson, M. P. Tracy, & E. T. O'Grady (Eds.), *Advanced practice nursing: An integrative approach* (5th ed., pp. 607–636). St. Louis, MO: Elsevier Saunders.

Kleinpell, R. M. (2003). Measuring advanced practice nursing outcomes: Strategies and resources. *Critical Care Nurse, 23*(1, Suppl.), 6–10.

Kleinpell-Nowell, R., & Weiner, T. M. (1999). Measuring advanced practice nursing outcomes. *AACN Clinical Issues, 10*(3), 356–368.

Kurtzman, E. T., & Corrigan, J. M. (2007). Measuring the contribution of nursing to quality, patient safety and health care outcomes. *Policy, Politics & Nursing Practice, 8*(1), 20–36.

Kutzleb, J., & Reiner, D. (2006). Impact of nurse-directed patient education for improved quality of life and functional capacity in people with heart failure. *Journal of the American Academy of Nurse Practitioners, 18*(3), 116–123.

Kutzleb, J., Rigolosi, R., Fruhschien, A., Reilly, M., Shaftic, A. M., Duran, D., & Flynn, D. (2015). Nurse practitioner care model: Meeting the health care challenges with a collaborative team. *Nursing Economics, 33*(6), 297–304.

Loehr, L. R., Rosamond, W. D., Chang, P. P., Folsom, A. E., & Chambless, L. E. (2008). Heart failure incidence and survival (from the Atherosclerosis Risk in Communities study). *American Journal of Cardiology, 101*, 1016–1022. doi:10.1016/j.amjcard.2007.11.061

Lohr, K. N. (1988). Outcome measurement: Concepts and questions. *Inquiry, 25*(1), 37–50.

McClellan, M. B., McGinnis, M., Nabel, E. G., & Olsen, L. M. (2007). *Evidence-based medicine and the changing nature of healthcare*. Washington, DC: The National Academies Press.

McLaughlin, C. P., & Kaluzny, A. D. (2013). *Continuous quality improvement in healthcare: Theory, implementations, and applications* (4th ed.). Sudbury, MA: Jones & Bartlett.

Melnyk, B. M., & Fineout-Overholt, E. (Eds.). (2015). *Evidence-based practice in nursing & healthcare: A guide to best practice* (3rd ed.). Philadelphia, PA: Wolters Kluwer Health.

Melnyk, B. M., Morrison-Beedy, D., & Cole, R. (2015). Generating evidence through quantitative research. In B. M. Melnyk & E. Fineout-Overholt (Eds.), *Evidence-based practice in nursing & healthcare: A guide to best practice* (3rd ed., pp. 439–475). Philadelphia, PA: Wolters Kluwer Health.

Meyer, S. C., & Miers, L. J. (2005). Cardiovascular surgeon and acute care nurse practitioner collaboration on post-operative outcomes. *AACN Clinical Issues: Advanced Practice in Acute & Critical Care, 16*(2), 149–158.

Moorhead, S., Johnson, M., Maas, M. L., & Swanson, E. (2008). *Nursing outcomes classification (NOC)* (4th ed.). St. Louis, MO: Mosby.

Moote, M., Krsek, C., Kleinpell, R., & Todd, B. (2011). Physician assistant and nurse practitioner utilization in academic medical centers. *American Journal of Medical Quality, 26*, 452–460. doi:10.1177/1062860611402984

Mozaffarian, D., Benjamin, E. J., Go, A. S., Arnett, D. K., Blaha, M. J., Cushman, M., & Turner, M. B. (2016). Heart disease and stroke statistics–2016 Update: A report from the American Heart Association. *Circulation, 133*(4), e38–e360. doi:10.1161/CIR.0000000000000350

Mueller, S. K., Sponsler, K. C., Kripalani, S., & Schnipper, J. L. (2012). Hospital-based medication reconciliation practices. *Archives of Internal Medicine, 172*(14), 1057–1059. doi:10.1001/archinternmed .2012.2246

National Center for Health Statistics. (2011). *Mortality multiple cause micro-data files, 2011: Public-use data file and documentation: NHLBI tabulations*. Retrieved from http://www.cdc.gov/nchs/products/ nvsr.htm

National Center for Health Statistics. (2013). *Mortality multiple cause micro-data files, 2013: Public-use data file and documentation: NHLBI tabulations*. Retrieved from: http://www.cdc.gov/nchs/data_ access/Vitalstatsonline.htm#Mortality

National Hospital Ambulatory Medical Care Survey Data. (2009). Public use data file and documentation: NHAMCS tabulations. Retrieved from http://www.nber.org/data/national-hospital -ambulatory-medical-care-survey.html

Newhouse, R. P., Stanik-Hutt, J., White, K. M., Johantgen, M., Bass, E. B., Zangaro, G., & Weiner, J. P. (2011). Advanced practice nurse outcomes 1990–2008: A systematic review. *Nursing Economics, 29,* 230–250.

Nicolay, C. R., Purkayastha, S., Greenhalgh, A., Benn, J., Chaturvedi, S., Phillips. N., & Darzi, A. (2012). A systematic review of the application of quality improvement methodologies from the manufacturing industry to surgical healthcare. *British Journal of Surgery, 99*(3), 324–325.

Nolan, M. T., & Mock, V. (2000). *Measuring patient outcomes.* Thousand Oaks, CA: Sage.

O'Mathúna, P. D., & Fineout-Overholt, E. (2015). Critically appraising quantitative evidence for clinical decision making. In B. M. Melnyk & E. Fineout-Overholt (Eds.), *Evidence-based practice in nursing & healthcare: A guide to best practice* (3rd ed., pp. 87–138). Philadelphia, PA: Wolters Kluwer Health.

Paez, K. A., & Allen, J. K. (2006). Cost-effectiveness of nurse practitioner management of hyper-cholesterolemia following coronary revascularization. *Journal of the American Academy of Nurse Practitioners, 18*(9), 436–444.

Paul, S. (2000). Impact of a nurse-managed heart failure clinic: A pilot study. *American Journal of Critical Care, 9,* 140–146.

Phatak, A., Prusi, R., Ward, B., Hansen, L. O., Williams, M. V., Vetter, E., . . . Postelnick, M. (2016). Impact of pharmacist involvement in the transitional care of high-risk patients through medication reconciliation, medication education, and post discharge call-backs (*IPITCH* study). *Journal of Hospital Medicine, 11*(1), 39–44. doi:10.1002/jhm.2493

Polinski, J. M., Moore, J. M., Kyrychenko, P., Gagnon, M., Matlin, O. S., Fredell Shrank, W. H., . . . Shrank, W. H. (2016). An insurer's care transition program emphasizes medication reconciliation, reduces readmissions and costs. *Health Affairs, 35*(7), 1222–1229. doi:10.1377/hlthaff.2015.0648

Polit, D. F., & Beck, C. T. (2017a*).* Rigor and validity in quantitative research. In D. F. Polit & C. T. Beck (Eds.), *Nursing research: Generating and assessing evidence for nursing practice* (10th ed., pp. 216–235). Philadelphia, PA: Wolters Kluwer.

Polit, D. F., & Beck, C. T. (2017b). Data collection in quantitative research. In D. F. Polit & C. T. Beck (Eds.), *Nursing research: Generating and assessing evidence for nursing practice* (10th ed., pp. 266–298). Philadelphia, PA: Wolters Kluwer.

Polit, D. F., & Beck, C. T. (2017c*).* Specific types of quantitative research. In D. F. Polit & C. T. Beck (Eds.), *Nursing research: Generating and assessing evidence for nursing practice* (10th ed., pp. 240–244). Philadelphia, PA: Wolters Kluwer.

Polit, D. F., & Beck, C. T. (2017d*).* Quantitative research designs. In D. F. Polit & C. T. Beck (Eds.), *Nursing research: Generating and assessing evidence for nursing practice* (10th ed., pp. 189–235). Philadelphia, PA: Wolters Kluwer.

Polit, D. F., & Beck, C. T. (2017e*).* Planning a nursing study. In D. F. Polit & C. T. Beck (Eds.), *Nursing research: Generating and assessing evidence for nursing practice* (10th ed., pp. 160–181). Philadelphia, PA: Wolters Kluwer.

Polit, D. F., & Yang, F. M. (2015). *Measurement and the measurement of change: A primer for health professionals.* Philadelphia, PA: Wolters Kluwer.

Powers, B. A. (2015a). Critically appraising qualitative evidence for clinical decision making. In B. M. Melnyk & E. Fineout-Overholt (Eds.), *Evidence-based practice in nursing & healthcare: A guide to best practice* (3rd ed., pp. 139–165). Philadelphia, PA: Wolters Kluwer Health.

Powers, B. A. (2015b). Generating evidence through qualitative research. In B. M. Melnyk & E. Fineout-Overholt (Eds.), *Evidence-based practice in nursing & healthcare: A guide to best practice* (3rd ed., pp. 476–489). Philadelphia, PA: Wolters Kluwer Health.

Roger, V. L., Go, A. S., Lloyd-Jones, D. M., Benjamin, E. J., Berry, J. D., Borden, W. B., & Turner, M. B. (2012). Heart disease and stroke statistics 2012 update: A report from the American Heart Association. *Circulation, 125*, 2–220.

Sackett, D. L., Richardson, W. S., Rosenberg, W., & Haynes, R. B. (2000). *Evidence-based medicine: How to practice and teach EBM* (2nd ed.). Edinburgh, Scotland: Churchill Livingstone.

Sackett, D. L., Rosenberg, W. M., Gray, J. A., Haynes, R. B., & Richardson, W. S. (1996). Evidence based medicine: What it is and what it isn't. *British Medical Journal, 312*, 71–72.

Seidl, K. L., & Newhouse, R. P. (2012). The intersection of evidence-based practice with 5 quality improvement methodologies. *The Journal of Nursing Administration, 42*(6), 299–304.

Stanik-Hutt, J. (2012). Translation of evidence to improve clinical outcomes. In K. M. White & S. Dudley-Brown (Eds.), *Translation of evidence into nursing and health care practice* (pp. 61–76). New York, NY: Springer Publishing.

Stetler, B. C. (2001). Updating the Stetler model of research utilization to facilitate evidence-based practice. *Nursing Outlook, 49*(6), 272–279.

Stevens, K. R. (2015). Critically appraising knowledge for clincial decision making. In B. M. Melnyk & E. Fineout-Overholt (Eds.), *Evidence-based practice in nursing & healthcare: A guide to best practice* (3rd ed., pp. 77–86). Philadelphia, PA: Wolters Kluwer Health.

The Joint Commission. (2012). *Comprehensive accreditation manual for hospitals.* Medical staff standards MS.08.01.01, MS 08.01.03. Oakbrook Terrace, IL: The Joint Commission.

Titler, M. G., Kleiber, C., Steelman, V. J., Rakel, B. A., Budreau, G., Everett, L. Q., . . . Goode, C. J. (2001). The Iowa model of evidence-based practice to promote quality care. *Critical Care Nursing Clinics of North America, 13*(4), 497–509.

Urden, L. D. (1999). Outcome evaluation: An essential component for CNS practice. *Clinical Nurse Specialist, 13*(1), 39–46.

Voigt, J., John, M. S., Taylor, A., Krucoff, M., Reynolds, M. R., & Gibson, C. M. (2014). A reevaluation of the costs of heart failure and its implications for allocation of health resources in the United States. *Clinical Cardiology, 37*(5), 312–321. doi:10.1002/clc.22260

Wang, H., Robinson, R. D., Johnson, C., Zenarosa, N. R., Jayswal, R. D., Keithley, J., & Delaney, K. A. (2014). Using the LACE index to predict hospital readmissions in congestive heart failure patients. *BMC Cardiovascular Disorders, 14*, 97. doi:10.1186/1471-2261-14-97

WHO Collaborating Centre for Patient Safety. (2007). Assuring medication accuracy at transitions in care. *Patient Safety Solutions, 1*, 1–4.

Wiggins, B. S., Rodgers, J. E., DiDomenico, R. J., Cook, A. M., & Page, R. L. (2013). Discharge counseling for patients with heart failure or myocardial infarction: A best practices model developed by members of the American College of Clinical Pharmacy's Cardiology Practice and Research Network based on the hospital to home initiative. *Pharmacology, 33*(5), 558–580.

Yancy, C. W., Jessup, M., Bozkurt, B., Butler, J., Casey, D. E., Drazner, M. H., & Wilkoff, B. L. (2013). 2013 ACCF/AHA guideline for the management of heart failure. *Journal of the American College of Cardiology, 62*(16), 147–239.

CHAPTER 7

Ambulatory Nurse Practitioner Outcomes

Mary Jo Goolsby

Chapter Objectives

1. Review the purpose and importance of measuring and documenting outcomes of individual nurse practitioner (NP) practices
2. Briefly summarize some of the literature on NP outcomes
3. Describe the categories and examples of outcome measures relevant to ambulatory NPs
4. Discuss practical considerations for selecting outcomes and a measurement approach
5. Provide examples of how to approach outcome measurement in practice
6. Discuss available resources relevant to primary care outcome measurement

Chapter Discussion Questions

1. What are two potential measures in each of the following categories for a patient diagnosed with diabetes: physiologic, behavioral/knowledge, and resource utilization?
2. What two enabling factors support NP entry into outcome measurement?
3. Describe an outcome measure plan for a patient diagnosed with a chronic illness, based on a national evidence-based clinical recommendation.
4. How do performance measures and outcome measures differ? Provide a brief summary, with an example of each related to a specific condition.

The potential outcomes of ambulatory care match the broad range of conditions and patients encountered in these settings, whether primary or specialty care. NPs in primary care settings care for patients with both chronic and acute conditions. While they manage the range of well-defined acute to complex chronic conditions, they also address their patients' health promotion and disease prevention needs. The incidence of many chronic conditions, such as hypertension, chronic obstructive pulmonary disease (COPD), and diabetes, is increasing and many of these patients routinely seek care in primary care settings, along with patients with acute conditions, such as pneumonia, urinary tract infections, and upper respiratory infections. In both primary and specialty ambulatory care, NPs will want to measure outcomes of routine management, as well as acute illnesses and exacerbations.

This author's interest in ambulatory care outcome measurement stems from her first assignment as a new NP to a military internal medicine clinic in the early 1980s. The creation of a one-page form on each of her patients, most of whom had been referred for management of one or more chronic conditions, allowed quick access to patient-specific information, such as blood pressure, lipids, blood glucose, and weight, recorded immediately following each encounter because the patients' health records were maintained outside the clinic. Initially planned as a means of responding readily to patient needs when records were unavailable, before long, curiosity prompted comparisons of the data over time. As the primary care provider for adults with chronic conditions, such as hypertension, diabetes, COPD, and heart failure, these forms allowed for extraction of clinical comparison over time and the habit of outcome measurement was born. Summaries of the data trends soon found their way into administrative reports describing the practice and benefits associated with referrals to an NP. Over the years, technology and outcome measurement skills improved, allowing for enhanced analysis and reporting of practice outcomes.

It can be intimidating to contemplate establishing a formal process for measuring outcomes. However, it is increasingly expected that providers such as NPs measure and report their outcomes as an objective indication of their quality, safety, cost-effectiveness, and patient centeredness. This chapter builds on the early chapters of this textbook by providing a practical framework that ambulatory care NPs can use in implementing outcome measurement in their practices. It (a) reviews the purpose and importance of measuring and documenting outcomes of individual NP practices, (b) briefly summarizes some of the literature on NP outcomes, (c) describes the categories and examples of outcome measures relevant to ambulatory NPs, (d) discusses practical considerations for selecting outcomes and a measurement approach, (e) provides examples of how to approach outcome measurement in practice, and (f) discusses available resources relevant to primary care outcome measurement (see Table 7.1).

IMPORTANCE/PURPOSE OF PRIMARY CARE OUTCOME MEASUREMENT

As noted in earlier chapters, there are many reasons for conducting outcome measurement in practice. Outcome research should ultimately improve the health of our patients. Further, many stakeholders are interested in how and to what degree we improve the health of those we serve. These stakeholders include our current and potential patients,

TABLE 7.1   Ambulatory Outcome Measures

Outcome Category	Outcome Examples
Physiologic status	Vital signs
	Physical examination findings
	Laboratory studies
Psychosocial status	Mentation
	Mood and affect
	Coping status
	Social function
Functional status	ADL function
	IADL function
Behavioral activities and knowledge	Performance of therapeutics
	Problem-solving ability
	Knowledge test scores
Symptom control	Pain
	Fatigue
	Dyspnea
	Nausea
	Incontinence
Patient perception	QOL
	Satisfaction with care
Resource utilization	Hospital readmission rates
	Emergency department visits
	Unplanned office visits

	Health care costs
	    Diagnostic tests
	    Prescriptions

Performance measures	Availability of recommended resources
	Implementation of recommended practices

ADL, activities of daily living; IADL, instrumental activities of daily living; QOL, quality of life.

employers, colleagues, payers, policy makers, and others. They are interested in knowing how much NP care costs and saves, what precisely NPs do in their patient encounters, and the objective patient-centered benefits of that care. Ambulatory providers who receive fee-for-service payments from the Centers for Medicare & Medicaid Services (CMS) are increasingly expected to participate in the Physician Quality Reporting System (PQRS).

Not specific to physicians, PQRS reporting can result in incentive payments and/or payment adjustments. It is a major example of the increasing expectation for public reporting of data by health care systems, organizations, and providers in smaller practices. As practitioners of a relatively new role created in the mid-1960s, NPs must continue to document the outcomes of their care.

Evaluation of clinical outcomes is now an expectation of the NP role. The National Organization of Nurse Practitioner Faculties lists a number of competencies relative to outcome measurement in the 2012 NP Core Competencies (National Organization of Nurse Practitioner Faculties, 2012). Examples of outcome-related competencies are evident throughout the domains, including using evidence to continuously improve the quality of care; evaluating the relationships among factors, such as cost, quality, and so on; and improving outcomes through application of clinical investigative skills.

SUMMARY OF EXISTING PRIMARY CARE NP OUTCOME LITERATURE

The published research on NP outcomes has consistently supported the quality and cost-effectiveness of NP practice. In 1974, a classic report of the Burlington Trial documented outcomes in mortality, as well as physical, emotional, and social function, concluding that NP and physician outcomes were comparable (Spitzer et al., 1974). The Congressional Budget Office reviewed studies on NP practice and outcomes in 1979, with the conclusion that the NPs' outcomes, diagnoses, and management were at least as good as those of physicians. In 1986, the Office of Technology Assessment came to the same conclusions. Later, meta-analyses of NP care had similar findings (Brown & Grimes, 1995; Horrocks, Anderson, & Salisbury, 2002; Laurant et al., 2004), as have additional review articles (Cunningham, 2004). Mundinger et al. (2000) and Lenz, Mundinger, Kane, Hopkins, and Lin (2004) described primary care outcomes of patients assigned to either physicians or NPs, finding equivalent outcomes for both sets of patients. Regarding cost-effectiveness of NP care, studies have also consistently demonstrated that NPs provide quality care efficiently with reduced cost, compared with physicians (Burl, Bonner, & Rao, 1994; Chenowith, Martin, Penkowski, & Raymond, 2005; Office of Technology Assessment, 1981; Paez & Allen, 2006; Roblin et al., 2004). Newhouse et al. (2011) conducted a systematic review of the published literature (1990–2008) on NPs and other advanced practice registered nurses (APRNs), confirming that the evidence continues to support high-quality outcomes associated with NP care. More recent reports demonstrate similar outcomes. Virani et al. (2015) found similar outcomes among outpatient cardiovascular patients whether seen by a physician, NP, or physician assistant. Perloff, DesRoches, and Buerhaus (2016) analyzed large CMS data sets, reporting that the outpatient costs for Medicare beneficiaries assigned to NPs were 18% lower than the costs for beneficiaries assigned to physicians.

MEASURES RELEVANT TO AMBULATORY CARE PRACTICE

The outcomes selected by a given NP will depend on factors such as the type of practice, areas of interest, and available resources. Even in a focused subspecialty-type practice, there are several options to measure. Outcomes can be categorized in many ways. One categorization (Table 7.1) would classify outcomes as best demonstrating one of the following: physiologic status, psychosocial status, functional status, behavioral activities and knowledge, symptom control, patient perception, or resource utilization. Within each category, there are likely measures relevant to any area of practice. Another common area of measurement that does not fit the definition of *outcome* but which must be considered relevant to contemporary ambulatory care involves performance measures.

Physiologic status involves those biomarkers that are usually readily available in the course of routine patient care. They include routinely collected vital signs, such as blood pressure, pulse, and temperature; physical exam findings, such as lung sounds and weight; and laboratory values, such as glucose and lipid levels. Abnormal findings in these physiologic markers are often the defining characteristics of health problems and the targets of care; thus, they provide a means of later following response to and outcomes of treatment. For instance, the outcomes of diabetes, hypertension, or hyperlipidemia management should include measurement of blood glucose/glycosylated hemoglobin, blood pressure, or lipids, respectively. A feature of physiologic measures, such as vital signs and laboratory findings, is that they are objective and quantified. Laboratory studies, in particular, are usually validated against some control procedure. The quality of vital signs and physical examination findings is dependent on the quality of the equipment and technique used in obtaining the measures.

Although psychosocial status includes measures often included in the history and which are qualitative in nature, psychosocial measures can be quantified through use of validated tools. Examples of psychosocial outcomes include mentation, mood and affect, attitude, coping status, and general social functioning. While psychosocial status outcomes often involve some degree of subjectivity, there are a number of validated and quantitative scales available, depending on the focus of concern. For instance, there are validated scales to measure depression and anxiety, confusion, and dementia. Depending on the outcome of interest, sources are often available to discuss measurement options. For example, the Mini-Mental State Examination is a common tool for cognitive function, well published and validated. Harvan and Cotter (2006) review and compare a range of dementia-screening tools for use in clinical practice.

Specific functional status involves the ability to achieve routine activities of daily living (ADL) and instrumental activities of daily living (IADL), and can be measured with global functional scales or measures more specific to select abilities such as mobility and communication. A number of measures of functionality exist, including the physical activities of daily living and instrumental activities of daily living scales, as well as the 10-minute Screener for Geriatric Conditions. Others include the Functional Independence Measure Scale and the Barthel Scale.

Behavioral activities and knowledge include areas of both therapeutic competence and understanding of treatments. Therapeutic competence involves the ability to perform the skills necessary to carry out prescribed or recommended treatments, as well as the ability to solve problems related to therapeutic guidance. Understanding is related to basic knowledge regarding recommended diet, medications, and treatments without a behavioral component. Knowledge tests have been developed and described in the literature for select conditions. Measurement of behavioral activity competence is more complex to assess than knowledge, by comparison.

Symptom control is another area of outcomes where the history often includes the basic related details, but requires further quantification to serve as an outcome measurement. Examples of the symptoms that could be quantified as outcome measures include level of pain, fatigue, dyspnea, nausea, constipation, diarrhea, and incontinence. There are a number of validated scales to measure many symptoms, and pain scales are perhaps among the better known. One means of assessing specific symptoms would be to use a 10-centimeter visual analog scale (VAS), where the poles of the scale represent symptom extreme (complete absence of the symptom versus worst possible degree of the symptom), or having the symptom similarly rated using a numerical scale.

Patient perceptual category, relative to the patient centeredness of care, includes areas such as a patient's perceived quality of life (QOL) and expressed satisfaction with care. QOL refers to patients' satisfaction with their life circumstances and sense of well-being. It can further relate to a more narrowed focus of satisfaction with specific components of the patient's life, for instance, with how a specific symptom affects life quality. There are general and condition-specific QOL scales, and a VAS can also be used to measure perceived QOL. In contrast, satisfaction refers to satisfaction with the patient experience and care received. Patient perceptions also include a patient's determination of progress toward meeting goals. For instance, patients can identify their personal goals for treatment, and then subsequently rate the degree to which they are able to accomplish the goal over time.

Resource utilization involves a range of outcomes, such as numbers of hospitalizations or readmissions, length of stay for any admission, the cost of care, and unplanned office or emergency visits. In many cases, it is difficult to accurately identify all hospitalizations or emergency visits, along with the cost for each, as dependent on the patient's recall. However, within a well-defined system such as a managed care organization, accountable care organization, or hospital-anchored system, pulling electronic or paper records of other visits, admissions, and associated costs such as those related to diagnostic studies and prescription medications is more easily accomplished. In addition to identifying any change in resource utilization associated with care, cost analysis of the actual care provides another outcome indicator.

Recommendations for performance, quality, and outcome assessment measures are available through a number of national initiatives and repositories, such as the National Quality Forum (NQF), the National Committee for Quality Assurance (NCQA), and the National Quality Measures Clearinghouse (NQMC). These entities are generally engaged in interprofessional development, recommendation, and/or dissemination of quality measures for systems, organizations, and providers, so that it is critical to identify measures created for outpatient practice. An increasingly important source of outcome measures is available through the PQRS program.

Many recommended measures include a focus on performance, rather than the ultimate outcome. It is worthwhile considering the difference between performance measures and outcomes of care. Performance measures document what is performed or done, rather than the outcomes of that practice. Performance measures sometimes serve as surrogates for actual outcomes in various reporting programs. With the increasing availability of electronic health records, queries of coded procedures allow ready identification of completed clinical activities. Certainly, current "pay-for-performance" mandates are based primarily on documenting the resources available and the processes implemented, as opposed to actual outcomes, so that incentives are based on providers documenting activities such as making appropriate referrals, ordering and monitoring suggested laboratory studies, and administering or ordering recommended treatments (e.g., pneumonia vaccines for persons 65 years of age or older, or beta-blockers for patients experiencing a myocardial infarction) rather than the associated outcomes that are subject to a number of intervening influences. Although clinical recommendations often imply that specific activities should result in improved outcomes, it is ideal to document the results of the performance measures, as well as the performance, to validate the desired result.

SELECTING PRACTICAL OUTCOMES OF INTEREST

With the broad range of potential outcomes of primary care NP practice, the dilemma becomes determining what should and can be measured. It is advisable to start with an answerable question and then proceed to select the available measures and/or type of data that will contribute to the answer. Certainly one deciding factor should be the provider's own areas of interest and questions. Other considerations will include the context in which the care is delivered, the resources available to support outcome measurement, and anticipated patient variables.

The decision to measure outcomes of practice may be based on questions the NP has regarding how his or her practice outcomes compare to some benchmark or published report. In practices with an established performance improvement (PI) process, there may be baseline data that support the need for improvements and that trigger outcome measures. Just as PI activities typically focus on conditions of large volume, high cost, and high risk, these same three criteria are helpful in guiding decisions on where to expend energy in outcome measures.

The practice context is important, as practices vary in the range and quality of resources helpful to outcome measurement. The progress toward broad implementation of electronic health records in ambulatory practice offers great promise for increased ability to automate queries regarding specific outcomes or activities performed. Practices with a well-designed electronic health record have an advantage when it comes to identifying relevant patients and tracking and measuring outcomes and performance. When selecting outcome data to be collected from an electronic system, it is critical to ensure that data are accurately coded and entered. The use of narrative notations rather than precoded options limits the utility of pulling needed data once entered. It also remains critical that the language of the system accurately fits the data and the practice involved. Another organizational consideration involves a philosophical expectation or mission that could mandate select measures used for outcomes and collegial support for the effort. Because it is rare for a health care provider to be the sole provider in an ambulatory clinic, it is often helpful for the team of providers to collaborate and select clinical topics and outcomes of interest. Moores, Breslin, and Burns (2002) describe the process of talking through problems with peers as a means of bringing the issue into focus as an answerable question.

Another type of resource specific to practices is the type of economic resources available for patient care. If a practice has a largely indigent population, the type of measures readily available may differ from one with a more affluent patient population, unless the practice has additional sources of funding to support patient care needs.

Patient-specific variables must be considered when planning outcome measurement. For instance, patients who tend to seek episodic care are not easily followed over time and short-term outcomes will be important rather than outcomes that are measured over time. For episodic visits, sometimes a performance measure may be helpful, such as the percentage of patients with a given diagnosis who receive or do not receive antibiotics, or the percentage of patients meeting specified criteria who receive appropriate immunization during visits. Of course, efforts to enhance continuity could be implemented and then long-term follow-up included as a measure itself.

In considering relevant outcome measures, ambulatory NPs must also consider what is recommended for select conditions; published clinical recommendations or guidelines provide an excellent source for outcome selection. These often identify a number of measures that could be used to track response to treatment, including specific validated tools. When focusing on a specific condition, it is often favorable to use condition-specific measures that will be more sensitive to change with treatment of that select condition whenever possible. For instance, while asthma affects psychosocial and functional outcomes, these may also be affected by a number of other comorbid conditions, so that these other conditions confound the response to care. By measuring specific asthma variables, outcomes are more easily attributed to treatment of that specific condition. There are scales to assess outcomes of treatment of conditions, such as arthritis, asthma, fibromyalgia, and benign prostatic hyperplasia, in addition to the relevant physiologic markers, such as pulmonary functions, blood glucose, and blood pressure. For varied conditions, generic outcomes could be used. For instance, generic functionality measures, or SF-36 v2 Health Survey, are broadly used. Scales of QOL could be responsive to a number of health changes, as would pain scales.

When the topic of interest has been identified and feasible outcome measures identified based on the characteristics of the practice, patient population, and providers, a plan should be written to guide the continuing effort. While most NPs may be more comfortable with associating the outcome measurement process with continuous quality improvement (CQI) or PI than with more formal "research," outcome measurement is a form of exploratory research (Breslin, Burns, & Moores, 2002) and the methodological issues are important considerations. An important benefit of establishing a written plan early in the planning process is that the plan will help to identify any related costs as well as added resources needed. In addition, even with CQI/PI projects, it is advisable to discuss the plans with a representative from the affiliated institutional review board or research board, to determine whether a formal application and approval are expected.

CASE EXAMPLES

The Shotgun Approach

The first case is an example of the importance of carefully thinking through the outcome measurement approach and how the alternative, using a "shotgun" approach to outcome measurement, can "backfire." A newly hired NP inherited a disease management practice for patients with asthma and/or COPD, finding that her predecessor had created a very broad plan for measuring the outcomes of the practice. At the baseline, initial visit, and again at 3, 6, 12, and 18 months, patients would be assessed with a focused history and physical, as well as by completing the following measures: the Center for Epidemiology Depression Scale, the State-Trait Depression and Anxiety Scale, the SF-36 Medical Outcomes Scale, the Modified Dyspnea Index, a record of peak flow use, history of tobacco use, medication list, a number of VASs (QOL, dyspnea), and a 6-minute walk with pulse oximetry, breath sounds, peak flow, and pulmonary functions before and after. In addition, the system's records were queried at these intervals for any emergency department visits and hospitalizations, as well as the costs and charges for each. Needless to say, even in a 1-hour visit, it was hard to conceive how anyone would accomplish all of the necessary outcome measures, if time were to be spent on patient problem solving, support, and education. The clinic's previous NP provider had recently resigned and, historically, patients rarely returned after the second visit.

The NP manager and interim NP provider reviewed the processes and interviewed some of the practice's patients. Patients shared that they saw little benefit in participating in all of the multi-item scales and found numerous depression, anxiety, medical outcomes, and dyspnea scales difficult to understand and confusing. Moreover, it seemed that collecting outcome measures had become the focus of the clinic, rather than the delivery of care directed toward improving their health.

After reviewing available measures relevant for COPD and asthma, the characteristics of the patient population, and feedback from patients, measurement procedures changed to allow for the emphasis to be on patient-centered care delivery. Necessary outcomes were embedded in the encounter record, with the number of outcomes significantly abbreviated. After testing the new plan, it seemed feasible and beneficial to record responses from dyspnea VAS and other relevant symptom ratings (e.g., shortness of breath, cough, and interrupted sleep), peak flow averages, and tobacco use, as well as to quarterly system queries to document a cost analysis of resource utilization. Subsequently, the continuity of care immediately improved; patients remained in the clinic; and the outcomes improved as time was allotted for shared decision making and education of patients about their conditions. The physiologic measures showed improvement. The population's emergency department visits were cut in half, and the number of hospitalizations was decreased to approximately 15% of the historical data following enrollment to the clinic. On an ongoing basis, the clinic has been able to demonstrate positive outcomes and to serve as a model for other disease-managed clinics.

Triangulation

An earlier chapter describes combining quantitative and qualitative efforts in outcome measurements to provide for triangulation. An NP involved in the pulmonary management described previously monitored tobacco use in her patients. Instituting the "Five-A" approach (ask about patient's habits, advise of consequence of smoking, assess willingness to quit, assist with cessation plan development, and arrange for follow-up) to smoking cessation and providing support based on her patient's level of readiness, she wanted to measure the outcomes of the process.

She asked all newly referred patients whether or not they smoked and, for those who did smoke, the number of cigarettes used per day. Thus, the measures used were tobacco use (Yes/No) and number of cigarettes, collected from each patient at the first visit and again at 3, 6, and 12 months. At baseline and at 3 and 6 months, the percentage of patients who smoked was 45%, 43%, and 49%, respectively, and the number of packs per day for patients who smoked was 0.91, 0.65, and 0.60, respectively. Certainly, the decrease in amount of tobacco used per smoker was positive, but the anticipated outcome had included a decreasing percentage of smokers, not an increase.

The NP instituted a series of interviews with the patients to explore the tobacco use. For instance, she wondered whether prior to the first appointment, a number of patients might have "quit" smoking due to initial concern over their respiratory symptoms, but were unable to maintain abstinence. Instead, she found that the percentage of her patients who smoked was actually stable over time; however, some patients indicated that they had not been forthright in sharing whether they smoked during their initial visit, concerned that their care might be affected or that they would be lectured for the practice. Only after they developed a comfort with the new provider through a couple of visits, were they more likely to be open about their tobacco use.

The series of interviews also identified a number of other issues and challenges related to tobacco use for her patients. When the NP identified that her standard practice was not successful in helping her patients quit smoking, she used the findings to obtain external funding for an individualized tobacco-cessation program. The funded program provided a range of resources for patients during the smoking-cessation process and did result in a decreased percentage of smokers. However, without the qualitative interviews, the necessary information would not have been identified to further improve practice and later outcomes.

APPROACHES TO OVERCOMING POTENTIAL BARRIERS TO OUTCOME MEASUREMENT

There are many potential barriers to outcome measurement. These include lack of confidence, time, and support, as well as limited data analysis resources.

Primary care NPs are likely to struggle with where to start with outcome measurement and to be intimidated by the concept. Primary care is fraught with many competing demands and the need to remain current on the recommended approach to many conditions. This may leave little time for the individual NP to prepare himself or herself for practice in outcome measures and, with the broad range of conditions encountered, to even decide what measures are important. Depending on the practice setting, there may not be a significant level of support for outcome measures or the emphasis may be on the basic performance measures rather than actual outcomes. Finally, given availability of outcome measures, many NPs will lack the initial knowledge of how to analyze the data.

Luckily, there are several resources that will facilitate the outcome measurement process. Resnick (2006) provides a four-step process to implementing outcome research. While her discussion is directed toward implementation of projects that will develop new and generalizable knowledge rather than limited findings to one practice setting, the steps provide examples of how to go about the process as well as encouragement for NPs contemplating the process. The other resources cited earlier also provide guidance.

Key facilitators include the NP's desire to improve practice and to optimize the outcomes of care. In fact, an ideal way to launch outcome measurement may be through practice improvement projects. Practice, or performance, improvement is an area of growing interest by multiple professions. Physicians, in particular, have PI expectations as part of their maintenance of certification requirements. Thus, in multiprofessional ambulatory practices, there is a growing tendency for PI to be implemented and often to involve team efforts—with all providers participating. NPs often are familiar with the PI process, regardless of which particular model they have used in their prior nursing practice. PI encompasses the principles important to overall outcome measurement: the target variables should be important to the practice, based on evidence, designed to measure improvement, and be practical to identify. A benefit of a PI focus is that there are a number of recognized PI models (e.g., plan-do-check-act, model for improvement, or plan-do-study-act [PDSA]) that describe a step-by-step approach for measurement over time.

Another factor facilitating NP efforts in outcome measures is the clinical expertise that NPs bring to their practice. A sound knowledge of a clinical area supports understanding of expected outcomes of care, which should provide direction on how to proceed in measurement activities.

Finally, even when NPs practice in a setting without other providers with similar interests in outcome measurement, it can be very helpful for NPs to establish a collaborative process with providers in other settings who have similar needs. Through collaboration, the providers are able to work together to establish outcome processes and strategies for success. Alternatively, an external mentor can be sought to coach through the process. Finally, there are networks for practice-based research in which providers can participate to become involved in the research process.

SUMMARY

Measuring and documenting outcomes of NP practices in ambulatory and specialty settings is essential in order to identify the impact of the role and to evaluate the care provided. As NPs in primary care settings care for patients with both chronic and acute conditions and manage the range of acute to complex chronic conditions, many opportunities exist for demonstrating the impact of such care. Measures relevant to ambulatory care NP practice span the spectrum from health promotion and disease prevention to management of complex health care conditions and prevention of exacerbations. This chapter has presented an overview of practical considerations for selecting outcomes pertaining to ambulatory NP practice, measurement approaches, examples of how to approach outcome measurement in practice, and resources relevant to primary care outcome measurement.

Answers to Chapter Discussion Questions

1. Physiologic: HbA1C; weight
   Behavioral/knowledge: demonstrated self-injection technique; diabetes knowledge scores

Resource utilization: emergency visits for hyper/hypoglycemia; pharmacotherapy costs

2. NPs in collegial practices can find outcome measurement easier to accomplish when they are able to engage others within the practice, so that the overall requirements are less daunting. Another strategy involves taking advantage of the growing interest in practice improvement methods, selecting one of the recognized models, such as PDSA, to establish a focused project within the practice. Selecting variables that can be abstracted over time and relevant to an identifiable patient population from a well-designed electronic health record is helpful, simplifying the data-collection process.

3. Using the example of asthma guidelines (National Asthma Education Program Report 3: Guidelines for the Diagnosis and Management of Asthma), the following are recommended to monitor asthma periodically in a clinical visit: responses to asthma assessment tools and, taking advantage of the growing interest in practice improvement methods, selecting one of the recognized models to establish a focused project within the practice.

4. Performance measures provide data on the completion of specific activities, depicting the degree to which recommended practices are accomplished. For diabetes, this could relate to documenting the percentage of patients for whom A1c is documented or the percentage of patients with diabetes for whom a retinal examination is documented. Performance measures differ from outcome measures, which would involve documenting the percentage of patients whose A1c was less than a selected level.

WEB LINKS

The following organizations are excellent sources of current and developing measurement resources:

- NCQA: www.ncqa.org
- NQF: www.qualityforum.org
- NQMC: www.qualitymeasures.ahrq.gov
- Office of National Coordinator for Health Information Technology (HITECH): www.healthit.gov
- PQRS: www.cms.gov/medicare/quality-initiatives-patient-assessment-instruments/pqrs

REFERENCES

Breslin, E., Burns, M., & Moores, P. (2002). Challenges of outcomes research for nurse practitioners. *Journal of the American Academy of Nurse Practitioners, 14*, 138–143.

Brown, S., & Grimes, D. (1995). A meta-analysis of nurse practitioners and nurse midwives in primary care. *Nursing Research, 44*, 332–339.

Burl, J., Bonner, A., & Rao, M. (1994). Demonstration of the cost-effectiveness of a nurse practitioner/physician team in primary care teams. *HMO Practice, 8*, 156–157.

Chenowith, D., Martin, N., Penkowski, J., & Raymond, I. (2005). A benefit-cost analysis of a worksite nurse practitioner program: First impressions. *Journal of Occupational and Environmental Medicine, 47*, 1110–1116.

Congressional Budget Office. (1979). *Physician extenders: Their current and future role in medical care delivery.* Washington, DC: U.S. Government Printing Office.

Cunningham, R. (2004). Advanced practice nursing outcomes: A review of selected empirical literature. *Oncology Nursing Forum, 31*, 219–232.

Harvan, J. R., & Cotter, V. (2006). An evaluation of dementia screening in the primary care setting. *Journal of the American Academy of Nurse Practitioners, 18*, 351–360. doi:10.1111/j.1745-7599.2006.00137.x

Horrocks, S., Anderson, E., & Salisbury, C. (2002). Systematic review of whether nurse practitioners working in primary care can provide equivalent care to doctors. *British Medical Journal, 324*, 819–823.

Laurant, M., Reeves, D., Hermens, R., Braspenning, J., Grol, R., & Sibbald, B. (2004). Substitution of doctors by nurses in primary care. *Cochrane Database of Systematic Reviews, 2004*(1). doi:10.1002/14651858.CD001271.pub2

Lenz, E. R., Mundinger, M. O., Kane, R. L., Hopkins, S. C., & Lin, S. X. (2004). Primary care outcomes in patients treated by nurse practitioners or physicians: Two-year follow-up. *Medical Care Research and Review, 61*, 332–351.

Moores, P., Breslin, E., & Burns, M. (2002). Structure and process of outcomes research for nurse practitioners. *Journal of the American Academy of Nurse Practitioners, 14*, 471–474.

Mundinger, M., Kane, R., Lenz, E., Totten, A., Tsai, W., Cleary, P., . . . Shelanski, M. (2000). Primary care outcomes in patients treated by nurse practitioners or physicians: A randomized trial. *Journal of the American Medical Association, 283*, 59–68.

National Organization of Nurse Practitioner Faculties. (2012). Nurse practitioner core competencies, Amended 2012. Retrieved from http://c.ymcdn.com/sites/www.nonpf.org/resource/resmgr/competencies/npcorecompetenciesfinal2012.pdf

Newhouse, R., Stanik-Hutt, J., White, K., Johantgen, M., Bass, E. B., Zangaro, G., . . . Weiner, J. P. (2011). Advanced practice nurse outcomes, 1990–2008: A systematic review. *Nursing Economics, 29*(5), 1–22.

Office of Technology Assessment. (1981). *The cost and effectiveness of nurse practitioners.* Washington, DC: U.S. Government Printing Office.

Office of Technology Assessment. (1986). *Nurse practitioners, physician assistants, and certified nurse midwives: A policy analysis.* Washington, DC: U.S. Government Printing Office.

Paez, K., & Allen, J. (2006). Cost-effectiveness of nurse practitioner management of hypercholesterolemia following coronary revascularization. *Journal of the American Academy of Nurse Practitioners, 18*, 436–444.

Perloff, J., DesRoches, C., & Buerhaus, P. (2016). Comparing the cost of care provided to Medicare beneficiaries assigned to primary care nurse practitioners and physicians. *Health Services Research, 51*(4), 1407–1423.

Resnick, B. (2006). Outcomes research: You do have the time! *Journal of the American Academy of Nurse Practitioners, 18*, 505–509.

Roblin, D., Howard, D., Becker, E., Kathleen Adams, E., & Roberts, M. H. (2004). Use of midlevel practitioners to achieve labor cost savings in the primary care practice of an MCO. *Health Services Research, 39,* 607–626.

Spitzer, W., Sackett, D., Sibley, J., Roberts, R., Gent, M., Kergin, D., . . . Olynich, A. (1974). The Burlington randomized trial of the nurse practitioner. *New England Journal of Medicine, 290,* 252–256.

Virani, S., Maddox, T., Chan, P., Tang, F., Akeroyd, J., Risch, S., . . . Peterson, L. (2015). Provider type and quality of outpatient cardiovascular disease care. *Journal of the American College of Cardiology, 66*(16), 1803–1812.

CHAPTER 8

Assessing Outcomes in Clinical Nurse Specialist Practice

Judy Elisa Davidson, Melissa A. Morse, Cassia Yi, and Mary C. Hellyar

Chapter Objectives

1. List four different categories of outcomes measured as a product of clinical nurse specialist (CNS) work in hierarchical order of importance
2. Describe an example of how to measure time-on activities, process measures, surrogate measures, and actual outcomes of CNS practice
3. Describe how to integrate the CNS spheres of influence and categorical outcomes of a CNS project or activity
4. Describe how outcomes from a project align with organizational goals, objectives, or pillars of performance

Chapter Discussion Questions

1. List four different categories of outcomes discussed in this chapter in hierarchical order of importance.
2. Using your own practice or experience during clinical rotations, how could you personally measure time-on activities, compliance with process measures, a surrogate measure of cost or quality, and an actual impact on patient or staff outcomes? Describe one example.
3. Select one project in which you have been involved or the plan for your capstone project, and make a table to include at least one measure for each of the four categories of outcomes listed in Question 1. Map these outcomes for each sphere of influence, as done in Exhibit 8.9.

4. For the project discussed in question 3, how do the outcomes align to organizational goals or objectives?

5. What are the pros and cons of recording activities and tracking outcomes?

The CNS role was created by the nursing profession to address the increasingly complex needs of patients (National Association of Clinical Nurse Specialists [NACNS], 2004). While the complexity of nursing care continues to increase, there is increasing pressure to contain costs while maintaining quality outcomes. CNSs have an impact on outcomes in three spheres of influence: (a) patients/clients, (b) nurses and nursing practice, and (c) systems and organizations (NACNS, 2004). While the positive impact of CNSs on outcomes is well-documented in the literature (Coen & Curry, 2016; Cunningham, 2004; Dickerson, Wu, & Kennedy, 2006; DiLibero, DeSanto-Madyea, & O'Dongohue, 2016; Duffy, 2002; Fabbruzzo-Cota et al., 2016; Forster et al., 2005; Fulton, 2006; Fulton & Baldwin, 2004; Hamilton & Hawley, 2006; Larsen, Neverett, & Larsen, 2001; Ley, 2001; McCabe, 2005; Prevost, 2002; Willoughby & Burroughs, 2001), the shift in health care to pay-for-performance models requires CNSs to articulate their impact on both clinical and financial outcomes. In this cost-containment environment, the ability to communicate outcomes of CNS practice is paramount to the survival of the CNS role in health care organizations (Davidson, 2010b, 2011; Wojner, 2001). This chapter provides a variety of strategies to select, measure, analyze, and promote outcomes using a hierarchical model familiar to operational leaders. Examples are provided, including a case example crosswalk, to visualize how outcome measures align to the CNS spheres of influence.

FRAMEWORK FOR MEASURING CNS OUTCOMES

In 2010, NACNS revised and published CNS core competencies (National CNS Competency Task Force, 2010). The focus of this document is clearly differentiating CNS practice outcomes from those of other advanced practice registered nurses. While impact on the spheres of influence is important, it may not be meaningful to nonclinical leaders in health care organizations. It is critical to articulate the value of CNSs across health care organizations in an understandable manner. Table 8.1 provides examples of CNS practice outcomes across the three spheres of influence, which are reflective of the CNS competencies. Table 8.2 expands the outline of assessment of CNS practice to include the focus of practice, performance of subroles, and economic impact, in addition to the three spheres of influence. Translating the CNS impact on the three spheres of influence to measurable clinical and fiscal outcomes and communicating this impact across the organization is essential to making a business case for retaining the CNS role during austere economic times (Amber, Carreon, Agan, Johnson, & Cahill, 2012; Davidson, 2010a, 2011).

TABLE 8.1   Categories of Outcomes of CNS Practice and Roles Across Three Spheres of Influence

Patient/Client Sphere	Nursing Personnel Sphere	Organization/Network Sphere
Programs of care are designed for specific populations and new services (e.g., oncology, geriatric, bariatric surgery)	Knowledge and skill development needs of nursing personnel are identified	Issues are trended at the organizational level and action plans are generated to address them
	Nurses maintain evidence-based practice	Systems are created to proactively review practice standards
Nursing therapeutics target specific etiologies	Nurses have access to the evidence supporting their practice	Policies are evidence based and easily accessible by nurses
Nursing therapeutics, in combination with medical therapeutics, where appropriate, result in achievement of goals for prevention, alleviations, or reduction of symptoms, functional problems, or risk behaviors	Nurses articulate how their practice contributes to patient care outcomes	Innovative models of practice are developed, piloted, evaluated, and incorporated as appropriate across the continuum of care
The individualized care plans meet client needs within available resources	Nurses use critical thinking to troubleshoot patient care problems	Innovations in practice contribute to the achievement of quality, cost-effective outcomes for populations of patients
Adverse events and medical errors are prevented	Nurses affect patient outcomes through advocacy behaviors with other providers	Decision makers within the organization are informed of successful innovation or practice changes that result in improved outcomes
Nurse-sensitive outcomes are managed to meet or exceed benchmark	Nurses are provided opportunities for career and professional advancement	Decision makers within the organization are informed regarding practice problems, factors contributing to the problems, and the significance of those problems with respect to outcomes and costs
Patients with unique needs, high-risk or low-volume conditions receive case review	Outdated practice standards are identified and replaced	Nursing care initiatives and programs are aligned with the organization's strategic imperatives, mission, vision, nursing strategic plan, and professional practice model
	Nurses experience job satisfaction	The overall cost of care is reduced through judicious purchase and use of resources while maintaining patient safety
	Nursing personnel are competent	Reports of innovative practice improvements or change are reported through scholarly activities such as presentation and publication
Innovative educational programs for patients, families, and groups are developed, implemented, and evaluated	Nursing personnel are engaged in lifelong learning	
Transitions across the continuum of care are smooth	Educational programs are available for nursing personnel	
Reports of new clinical phenomena and/ or interventions are published	Preceptors are trained in bedside clinical instruction and how to promote critical thinking	

CNS, clinical nurse specialist.
Source: Adapted from the National Association of Clinical Nurse Specialists (2004).

TABLE 8.2 Summary of Assessments of CNS Practice

Focus of Practice	Examples of Types of Assessments/Data	Examples of Sources of Evidence
Performance of subroles	Implementation of job expectation as advanced practice clinician, educator, consultant, and utilizer of research	Time-on activities logs/journals and summaries Peer review CNS end-of-year report Educational materials Summary of educational outcomes (analysis of evaluations) Presentations Publications
Client sphere	Morbidity, mortality data Symptom experience Functional status Mental status Stress level Client satisfaction with care Burden of care Effective self-care behaviors/reduced risk behaviors Avoidance of complications Quality of life Attainment of quality monitoring benchmarks	Case conferencing summaries Ethics review summaries Complaints/Grievances
Nursing personnel sphere	Recruitment and retention Job satisfaction Improvements in nursing personnel competency Decreased cost of products and other resources used in patient care	Recruitment and retention data Job satisfaction data % competency documented % completed orientation records Chart audits for evidence of compliance with practice standards Budget
System sphere	Length of stay, recidivism, use of postdischarge health services Achievement of benchmarks Patient satisfaction Workforce redesign/patient care	Hospital databases Disease registry data Morbidity, mortality, LOS, readmission data Laboratory and x-ray reports Chart audits, risk management information Nurse-sensitive quality indicator reports National quality benchmark data Patient satisfaction data Nursing report cards
Economic impact	Revenue analysis Cost–benefit analysis Cost-effectiveness analysis	Fiscal databases reflecting cost savings, cost avoidance, and revenue generation. Relevant clinical indicators from the three spheres CNS-generated calculations of cost savings or avoidance

CNS, clinical nurse specialist; LOS, length of stay.

▨▨ THE HIERARCHY OF OUTCOME MEASUREMENT

The following hierarchical model (Figure 8.1) is proposed (by these authors) for sorting outcomes by level of value to the organization and is derived from the system widely used to sort levels of evidence (Craig & Smyth, 2007; Melnyk & Fineout-Overholt, 2011; Schmidt & Brown, 2014). The levels are divided from weakest to strongest into (a) time-on

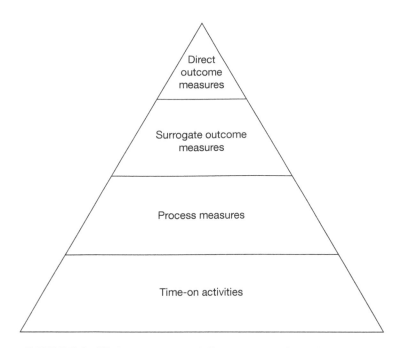

FIGURE 8.1 Clinical nurse specialist outcome hierarchy pyramid.

activities, (b) process measures, (c) surrogate outcome measures, and (d) patient or staff outcomes. The pyramid portrays the fact that the least-valued measure is more easily produced and often used, whereas the strongest measures of patient or staff outcomes are hardest to obtain and least frequently reported. Each level on the pyramid has its place in outcome measurement. For example, it is prudent for every CNS to account for his or her time by keeping track of time spent on projects and outcomes. During the beginning of a practice change, compliance with process measures helps to ensure success during the change process. Patient or nurse outcomes are long-term measures of success. If these end outcomes were the only outcomes measured to determine whether a practice change was successful, it would likely result in failure to course-correct as needed. However, the true success of a practice change depends on measuring the long-term patient or nurse outcomes even though they may take months to measure. In the sections to follow, we will describe examples of each of these forms of outcome measures. An example of measuring educational activities using Kirkpatrick's four-level system will be presented (Kirkpatrick, 2009). In conclusion, a process for developing an end-of-year report will be described.

Time-On Activities

Calendar
One easy strategy to track contributions without spending undue time is for every CNS to keep an electronic calendar populated with actual work done. At the end of the day, just before retiring, go back to the day's calendar and populate the "white space" with projects, rounds, just-in-time education, and so forth. Populate meeting time with major decisions or outcomes. This will take 5 minutes or less if performed while the memory of

the day is fresh. The data can then be used at the end of the month to populate an end-of-month productivity report.

Productivity Report/Organizational Alignment

Productivity reports describing CNS duties are a valuable tool to communicate CNS contributions to health care organizational leadership. To increase visibility of the contributions CNSs make to the organization, record summaries of monthly productivity on a template with subheadings for each of the organization's pillars or key goals (Studer, 2008). Most organizations report a scorecard of metrics to the board of directors according to subheadings such as finance, quality, patient experience, workforce development, and so forth. Instead of hiding activities under the subcategories of the CNS role functions that are known and understood mainly by the CNS community, use the organizational pillars as subheadings, and have each CNS complete the tool at the end of each month. The nursing division likely has a professional practice model and nursing strategic plan. Alignment of project outcomes to these key overarching documents that guide practice should be overtly stated in the report. Proactive thought regarding alignment of project outcomes to organizational and nursing objectives helps CNSs to measure their direct contribution to the organization.

Wherever possible, use cost figures or cost surrogates to estimate impact on finance. A predicted obstacle will be to move the team from qualitative descriptions of their work to quantitative objective outcome reporting. The root of the problem is that most CNSs are not comfortable using estimates of cost reduction or savings, or literature-based cost estimates versus actual values. Because actual savings are difficult to capture, surrogates are acceptable and also save time in hunting for obscure organizational data. This normal business strategy will improve visibility and security. From our experience, moving from paragraph to concrete outcome descriptions took more than a year of practice (Davidson, 2011). In the case where a team is learning how to do this together, it is helpful to have the leader complete one of his or her own, leading by example. The leader's productivity report is distributed to the staff with a timely reminder to complete the end-of-month report. This sets clear expectations for the level of detail. Then the entire team's package can be attached to staff meeting minutes. In this manner, each member of the team can learn from peer examples. The leader of the team may call out especially positive examples and use the documents as a source of staff recognition. Exhibit 8.1 provides an example of how to structure a monthly productivity report. If each CNS submits one, the complete package can be forwarded up the chain of command each month for positive team exposure. The act of sending positive messaging about employees up the chain of command on a regular basis is called "managing up" and is promoted by Studer as a strong business tactic for organizational success (Studer, 2008).

Preformatted Productivity Spreadsheet

This second example is offered for collating monthly performance data. Preformatted electronic spreadsheets provide a quick way to organize CNS activities. The following process was used by a team of CNSs to organize a simple method of tabulating time-on activities. During a retreat, the group brainstormed the categories of activities for which each spent time. The total list was then numbered so that each activity received a unique

EXHIBIT 8.1 **CNS Monthly Productivity Report**

Name _____   Month _____, 2018

	Operational Accountabilities (put activities in this column that never go away, but on which you are making progress)	Time-Limited Projects (put activities in this column that should be time-limited and eventually end)	Quantifiable Data ($ revenue or calculated avoidance, near miss saves related to either time-limited or operational accountabilities)
Financial Performance (any activity that has direct revenue/cost avoidance implications)			
Workforce Development (internal education/ development of practice tools, healthy work environment projects)			
Patient Experience			
Quality			
Meeting Community Needs (community involvement, public speaking, publications)			

CNS, clinical nurse specialist.

identifier. Then, of the total list, individualized lists were made to reflect activities pertinent to each person's scope of practice. The spreadsheets were then autopopulated with time spent on required meetings. At the end of the month, the CNS populated his or her own spreadsheet, which was then forwarded up the chain of command. The process was designed with the goal of spending less than 15 minutes per month tabulating time-on activities. The spreadsheet also provides the ability to capture time within the CNS spheres or within the organizational pillars, which allows the data to be tailored to the target audience (Exhibit 8.2).

Peer Review and CNS Visibility

Another strategy to increase CNS visibility and staff understanding of outcomes generated from activities within the CNS role is the peer evaluation process. One method to obtain peer review is to ensure first that the CNS job description is built according to the published role elements (National CNS Competency Task Force, 2010). The role-specific elements are then abstracted into a peer evaluation along with the standard organizational behaviors required by each employee. The supervisor may send out the peer evaluation electronically to physicians, operational leaders, and staff who work with the CNS on committees, projects, or in their area of practice (Exhibit 8.3). This accomplishes several goals. The recipient can see for what the CNS is accountable, as well as soliciting the input needed for evaluation. When sending out the peer evaluation, a leading message

EXHIBIT 8.2   CNS-Specific Productivity Spreadsheet

Item/Activity	Time (hours)	Units/Items	Pillar	Sphere	Role	Scope
Committee—CNS	120	1				Facility-wide
Committee quality	90	1				Facility-wide
Committee nurse practice council	120	1				Facility-wide
Committee—Restraint	90	1				Facility-wide
Committee—Restraint	120	1				System-wide
Committee—Patient safety	60	1				System-wide
Committee—Delirium		1				Facility-wide
Committee—Delirium		1				System-wide
Security subcommittee	60	1				Facility-wide
Committee—AWS		1				Facility-wide
Committee—AWS		1				System-wide
Care management redesign						System-wide
Patient satisfaction rounding—Assigned unit						Unit specific
Rounding—Restraints						Facility-wide
Rounding—Alcohol withdrawal						Facility-wide
Rounding—Fall reduction						Facility-wide
Rounding—Core measures						Facility-wide
Evidence-based practice review						System-wide
Conduct mortality and morbidities						Facility-wide
Nasal bridle						Facility-wide
Equipment demonstration						Facility-wide
Student precepting						Facility-wide
Occurrence report review						Facility-wide
Auditing						Facility-wide
Community service						Community
Educating staff, managers						System-wide
Rounding—Pain						Facility-wide
Committee						System-wide
Computer screen development						System-wide

Note: This is a CNS-specific productivity report culled from a larger list of possible CNS activities. Standard meeting time is formatted to automatically populate. If viewed electronically, a drop-down list of pillars would appear for selection, as well as the drop-down list of spheres of influence. A drop-down list of CNS role requirements also appears.
AWS, alcohol withdrawal syndrome; CNS, clinical nurse specialist.

EXHIBIT 8.3   Example Script for Peer Evaluation Request

Nancy Nurse, CNS, is due for her yearly evaluation. We are hoping you will e-mail feedback before June 7. Of note, Nancy has chaired the pressure ulcer committee over the past year with a resultant 30% reduction in hospital-acquired pressure ulcers. This reduction is estimated to have saved the organization over $250,000.00 in fines and lost revenue. Nancy has also spearheaded a program to improve compliance with the IHI Bladder Bundle. The Bladder Bundle Team has achieved an overall improvement in protocol compliance from 25% to 96%. There have been no hospital-acquired UTIs reported in the quarter following the launch of the pilot. We congratulate Nancy and the team on this success.

Nancy's evaluation has these subheadings.

Please comment on any of these in the form of a return e-mail:

Influencing Direct Care

Consultation

System Leadership

Collaboration

Coaching

Research

Ethical Decision Making

Problem solving and making improvements

Compliance and organizational alignment

Workplace integrity and accountability

Communicating with others

Working with others

Creating a favorable impression

Serving others

Dependability

Resource utilization

Note: Bold items are subheadings specific to clinical nurse specialist core competencies. Normal text subheadings are specific to required organizational behaviors and will change from facility to facility.
CNS, clinical nurse specialist; IHI, Institute for Healthcare Improvement; UTI, urinary tract infection.

with at least two accomplishments can also be sent to "manage up" the CNS to others (Studer, 2008) and improve visibility of CNS outcomes (Exhibit 8.3). The peer evaluation can easily be sent as an electronic survey with the introductory e-mail to automatically summarize the data according to subheading to cut and paste into the evaluation.

Process Measures

Rounding With a Purpose

It is known that educational offerings do little by themselves to change behavior (Bloom & Bloom, 2005) and, therefore, academic detailing in the form of bedside rounds is imperative to solidify practice change. Table 8.3 summarizes the effectiveness of different methods of education in changing practice (Bloom & Bloom, 2005). There are several forms of rounds that CNSs make during the course of a day. They may round on vulnerable staff, new employees, staff floating outside their normal work environment, or staff working with patients who have unusual diagnoses or complex care. Another form of round is targeted rounds to follow up on new projects, programs, or services. A third form might

TABLE 8.3 Expected Impact of Activity on Change in Practice

Method	High (30%–35%)	Moderate	Low (3%–5%)	None	Total Number of Studies
Didactic (classroom)	0%	15%	35%	50%	20
Information only (e.g., mailings)	0%	15%	23%	61%	13
Clinical practice guidelines	0%	60%	40%	0%	5
Opinion leaders	0%	33%	44%	22%	9
Interactive education	38%	46%	15%	0%	13
Audits with feedback	26%	47%	17%	9%	23
Reminders/prompts	35%	45%	20%	0%	26
Academic detailing (1 to 1)	40%	53%	7%	0%	15

take the form of multidisciplinary rounds or discharge planning rounds. Last, the CNS might be responsible for certain quality metrics, such as restraints, falls, pressure ulcers, or hospital-acquired pneumonia and plans to round on patients with those issues to ensure that standards of care are being met and that the processes designed in meetings actually meet patients' needs without undue burden on staff. In all of these situations, rounds should be performed with a purpose (Studer, 2008) and conducted using tools to gather data and input from staff. The data from these rounds may also be used for monthly productivity reports.

Rounding Tools

The CNS role was originally developed to foster evidence-based practice at the bedside, and this key function remains a critical aspect of the job. Although direct outcomes cannot always be measured, compliance with evidence-based process measures, which have been demonstrated to improve outcomes, can be captured prospectively enabling an opportunity for just-in-time education and practice improvement. CNS-led rounds provide an opportunity to showcase expert assessment and diagnostic skills, while encouraging application of evidence-based nursing interventions in real time.

Johnson et al. (2011) captured the types of evidence-based recommendations made during CNS-led rounds. The rounds were targeted at preventing ventilator-associated pneumonia (VAP), venous thromboembolism, and hospital-acquired infections, as well as use of progressive mobility and improved glycemic management. The number and types of recommendations and the frequency with which the recommendations were carried out could be captured. Johnson et al. found that CNS recommendations were carried out 63% of the time, and over the course of 1 year, CNS-led rounds led to 345 evidence-based interventions. Exhibits 8.4 and 8.5 are examples of tools tailored for data collection from different types of rounds.

Another application of CNS process measurement targets key outcome indicators that change over time. For example, catheter-associated urinary tract infections (CAUTIs) occur infrequently and it may take many months to a year to see if an intervention has been effective. However, the Centers for Disease Control and Prevention has clear guidelines for the prevention of CAUTIs (Gould, Umscheid, Agarwal, Kuntz, & Pegues, 2010), and because CAUTIs are tied to pay for performance, this untoward outcome is ripe for CNS management. Figure 8.2 is an example of process data collected for the reduction of CAUTIs. Bar graphs are especially useful in displaying before and after data for a set of required process elements.

EXHIBIT 8.4   **Outcome Measure: Data-Collection Tool for Outcomes From Rounds**

Follow-Up Items From ICU Multiprofessional Rounds

- Order for occupational therapy/physical therapy for evaluation and treatment
- Order for speech therapy/swallow evaluation and treatment
- Order for intermittent pneumatic compression device
- Order for venous thromboembolism medication
- Complete medication reconciliation form
- Complete vaccination/methicillin-resistant Staphylococcus aureus screening
- Discuss feeding tube placement/nutrition needs
- Discuss weaning from mechanical ventilation or tracheostomy
- Arrange patient/family conference
- Implement the VAP bundle elements
  - Every 4-hour oral care/subglotal suctioning
  - If VAP endotracheal tube present, connect to low continuous suction
  - Venous thromboembolism prophylaxis
  - Head of bed up 30 degrees
  - Daily sedation wake-up/assessment of readiness for weaning and extubation
- Implement appropriate pressure ulcer precautions
  - Placed pressure ulcer order set in chart
  - Order special bed/surface _____
- Review need for central line/Foley catheter
- Consider discontinuation of central line/Foley catheter
- Spiritual care/social work consult
- Consider palliative/pain service consultation
- Recommend medication changes (e.g., PO vs. IV) _____
- Consider transfer out of intensive care unit
- Other _____
- Other _____

ICU, intensive care unit; IV, intravenous; PO, by mouth; VAP, ventilator-associated pneumonia.

EXHIBIT 8.5   Process Measure: Rounding Tool

ICU Multiprofessional Rounds _____   Date: _____

Coordinator _____

Room #	PT/OT/ST	Family conference	Transfer	VAP/Oral care/ HOB/ Sed. hol./ GI proph./Vent wean	VTE proph	Medications: PO vs. IV Duplicate therapy, antibiotics vs. cultures, home medications	Infection control	Diet	Skin	Lines	Foley	Glyc mgt	Other

GI proph., gastrointestinal prophylaxis; Glyc mgt, glycemic management; HOB, head of bed; ICU, intensive care unit; IV, intravenous; OT, occupational therapy; PO, by mouth; PT, physical therapy; Sed. hol., sedation holiday; ST, speech therapy; VAP, ventilator-associated pneumonia; Vent, ventilator; VTE proph, venous thromboembolism prophylaxis.

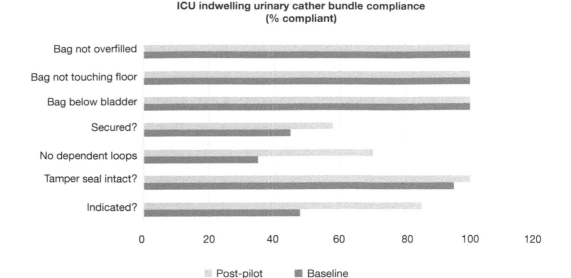

FIGURE 8.2 Process measure: Compliance with urinary catheter bundle.
ICU, intensive care unit.

Reflective Practice and Process Compliance

Another CNS result that can be used as an outcome measure is compliance with a new process standard. At one large academic center, a CNS was responsible for revising the pain assessment and management policy to include the pain assessment hierarchy as outlined by the Society of Critical Care Guidelines (Barr et al., 2013). In the previous version of the pain policy, pain reassessments after analgesia administration were required within 2 hours. The policy was revised to require reassessment dependent on the intervention, thus timing reassessment to the peak effect of the treatment (Pasero, 2010). This seemingly minor revision required a change in nursing culture. Previously, nurses focused on the 2-hour reassessment time frame from the former policy to satisfy regulatory standards. The new policy would require nurses to change practice from a time-based assessment to the critical thinking of a peak-effect-based assessment. Education to the change was rolled out through several different formats and avenues, such as educational symposiums, presentations at shared governance meetings, an online self-learning module, flyers, badge cards, and so on.

To measure the success of the policy change and subsequent education, compliance with pain reassessment was trended. The CNS worked with a pharmacy analyst to use the inpatient medication administration records and the nursing pain assessment documentation to create monthly hospital-wide, unit-specific, and even nurse-specific compliance rates. The compliance rates were distributed monthly to nursing leaders who then distributed them to their respective staff. The compliance rates were generated to the individual staff nurse level. The nursing leaders were also provided with medical record details for each staff nurse listing all as-needed analgesics given in the month along with the documented reassessment times.

Posting the information in a nonpunitive manner, allowing nurses to see the pattern of their own work, is a form of reflective practice. This concept of reflective practice does two things. First, it allows for clinical nurses to use data to evaluate and reflect upon their individual practice. It also allows for nurse leaders to provide data to clinical nursing staff that allows for individual self-reflection, rather than time-intensive auditing and manager to nurse follow-up in a constructive (versus punitive) approach (Lau & Chan, 2005; Lawrence, 2011).

One unexpected result of this reflective practice data was the apparent impact of peer influence. When the data were given to the unit managers it was provided in two different formats. The first format listed the nurses by name; the second format listed them by their employee identification number. The managers were expected to post the unit compliance data in their break room or nursing station. It was up to the managers to decide how the data would be posted, knowing that if posted by employee identification number, the nurses on the unit would be able to identify only their own results.

The CNS kept track of which nursing units were posted by name, and saw an increase in overall compliance compared to those who were posted by employee identification number. Figures 8.3 and 8.4 show the results for two similar units that posted the compliance data starting in February 2016 (see arrows). Figure 8.3 shows that Unit A, which posted by employee identification number only, was unable to increase compliance; the goal was not met. Figure 8.4 shows the results for Unit B, a similar nursing unit, which posted compliance reports by nursing name. This unit saw a 19% increase in compliance.

Surrogate Outcomes

Surrogate Outcome Measures

Cost avoidance and reduction in adverse outcomes can be difficult to capture. Surrogate values are a valuable tool in these circumstances and have been used in medical and allied health literature (Dasta et al., 2010; Fraser, Riker, Prato, & Wilkins, 2001; Stahl et al., 2009).

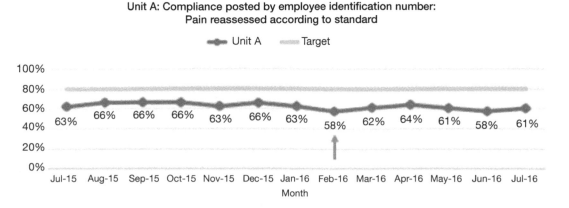

FIGURE 8.3 Compliance posted using employee identification number.

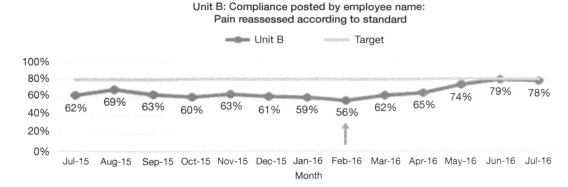

FIGURE 8.4 Compliance posted using employee name.

Costs of a specific test or treatment can be obtained through administrative accounting data providing an actual cost per case figure, which is a better indicator than billing data. When a test or treatment is eliminated from care, the cost of the item plus the cost of staff time spent doing the test or treatment is calculated. Estimates of staff time are described in what follows.

When using a surrogate figure that was published in the literature for an episode of care (e.g., pressure ulcer or VAP), currency of the published figure is evaluated and then adjusted for inflation. If the figure was published in 2010, the inflation factor can be obtained from the department of finance and added to the published cost to bring the cost up to date. The inflation rate methodology is specific to the organization due to geographic variation in inflation. A CNS might find it helpful to proactively keep a list of cost or charge measures for common items such as average salary for each level of employee in the department, average revenue per day of stay, number of admissions per calendar year, average length of stay, and operating room or procedural area charge time in minutes.

Calculating Cost in Staff Time

One of the most desirable outcomes to measure is reduction in wasted time spent on unnecessary activities. For example, streamlined medication passes, decreasing the number of prompts in computerized documentation, or reduced time spent in hunting and gathering supplies could constitute cost savings. If a project has resulted in decreasing wasted process steps in the delivery of care, the hours of saved time can easily be converted into a surrogate figure for dollars saved. To do this, have your supervisor inform the department of finance that you are working on a project that requires this analysis. The data you will be requesting for the calculation is often considered sensitive and will not be granted unless there is verification that you are using it for a business need. If the change in practice will affect only one department, ask for the average nursing salary for that department. If the change will eventually affect all departments, ask for the organizational average salary. Average salary may differ widely based upon seniority. Also ask for the overhead rate that constitutes the percentage over wage that is spent by the organization on provision of benefits. Then, measure the amount of time the wasted process step takes in minutes by conducting a time and motion study. Perform several observations and average the result. Create a spreadsheet using the following variables:

- Minutes of time saved by eliminating this activity
- Average staff hourly wage
- Overhead rate = (express percentage in decimal: e.g., 30% = 0.3)
- Number of times this activity is done in a day
- Number of patients receiving this activity in a day
- Number of times a day the patients receive this activity
- Number of days the activity is expected to occur in a year

Embed formulas within the spreadsheet as shown in Exhibit 8.6 to calculate cost savings. In the example used in Exhibit 8.6, the deleted activity that took 15 minutes to perform and was routinely performed twice a day on 15 patients every day of the year by a nurse whose salary was $55.00 per hour with an organizational overhead rate of 30% resulted in an estimated annual cost savings of $195,731.25.

Because salary figures are sensitive, obtain approval prior to distributing the formula to those outside of the organizational leadership team. For every nonvalue-added activity that is deleted from a nurse's workload, the CNS can promote managing the newly found free time, which is formally referred to as *capacity*, in a way that is desirable to operational leaders. For example, if patients have not been satisfied with discharge education, the report on the project to save time in hunting and gathering could conclude with, "This

EXHIBIT 8.6   **Outcome Measure: Yearly Cost Savings**

	A	C	E
	Variable		Formula Embedded in Column C
4	Average staff hourly wage in dollars	$55.00	
5	Overhead rate (express percentage in decimal: e.g., 30% = .3)	0.3	
6	Total labor/hour	$71.50	(C4*C5) + C4
8	Minutes saved per activity expressed as portion of hour (15 minutes = .25)	25%	
9	Dollars saved/activity	$17.88	C6*C8
11	# Patients receiving activity/day	15	
12	# Times/day patients receive activity	2	
13	Total activity times	30	C11*C12
15	Dollars saved per day	$536.25	C13*C9
17	# Days the activity is expected to occur/year	365	
19	Annual savings	$195,731.25	C17*C15
20	Formula		((C4*C5) + C4)*C8*(C11*C12)*C17

xx minutes of care/day (xx/yr) saved in hunting and gathering could easily correct the problem we currently have with patient education if we manage the transition correctly."

Example of Surrogate Data Use

The following project is explored as an example of the use of surrogates to capture avoidance of cost and adverse outcomes. Gutierrez and Cahill (2011) introduced a nasal gastric tube securement device in their organization and measured reduction in restraints, nursing time, and radiation exposure. Restraint days were measured, pre- and post-implementation, and were reduced from 6.21 to 4.32 days, resulting in 53 restraint days avoided (p <.001). Cost savings from this are calculated to be $12,800, assuming 3 RN hours, 1 charge nurse hour, 1 manager hour, and 0.5 CNS hours per restraint day:

$$([\$41 \times 3] + [\$43 \times 1] + [\$47 \times 1] + [\$55 \times 0.5]) \times 53 = 12,746.50$$

Prior to the new securement device, these patients with nasal gastric tubes had an average of 5.75 abdominal radiographs done, which was reduced to 1.29 after introducing the new product. This resulted in a cost savings of $33,000 as well as a 28,080 millirad reduction in radiation. Because this project was performed over a 3-month period in one hospital, and there was no reason to assume there would be seasonal variation to the number of patients requiring a nasal securement device, the figures could be multiplied by four to obtain and report the estimated yearly savings. The values used in this example were very conservative because the calculation did not account for overhead costs, which are approximately 30% higher than the salary figure.

Calculating Cost of Nursing Time in Education

The time nurses spend in educational programs is costly to the organization. When planning a change in practice, education is often planned as a first step in the change, but the cost of education time is often seen as a burden within any project. As a general principle, the value you anticipate to bring to the change needs to outweigh the burden of the cost of the education. For this reason, limit the didactic education to only what is necessary. Calculate time spent in the classroom using the average wage of the nurse, overhead cost, number of minutes, number of nurses who will be educated, and cost of instructor. Remember to add in replacement figures if the nurse will need to be replaced on the job (back-filled) to attend the class. If the back-fill is anticipated to accrue overtime, account for the overtime by using a replacement factor of 1.5 times the hourly wage.

Because classroom education is so expensive, an alternative that can decrease project burden is to teach 1:1 or in small groups at the bedside while conducting rounds. With careful scheduling and a train-the-trainer approach, many projects can be taught in this manner without adding educational costs while also enhancing valuable CNS exposure to nursing staff at the bedside.

Direct Outcomes

In some instances, direct outcomes of CNS interventions can be measured. This is the highest level of CNS outcome data, but it is also the most difficult to obtain and takes longer to obtain than time-on or process outcomes. Direct outcomes may reflect either patient or staff outcomes.

Staff Outcome

Examples of nurse outcomes are turnover, retention, and satisfaction. The following example describes a project that measured two staff outcomes, engagement and satisfaction, as well as a patient outcome, central-line-associated bloodstream infections (CLABSIs). The beauty of these outcomes is that they were all preexisting normally collected data; engagement from staff meeting minutes, satisfaction from workplace satisfaction surveys, and infections through normal quality monitoring metrics.

Interprofessional Reflective Practice Utilizing Case Studies

This project began as an innovative quality improvement process using case studies and real situations to advance practice through a multiprofessional approach. To promote attendance, the meeting was called "Case Study Investigation" (CSI). It was quickly realized that the implementation of this model of reflective practice as well as a blame-free approach to performance improvement had a powerful effect on participants. Instead of going to a place of blame, it was acknowledged that there might be organizational, power, social, or resource issues that prevent the right thing from happening. By taking time to help the people involved work through the problem to create a better organization, staff expressed feeling cared for and meeting attendance was often standing room only.

Many positive outcomes have resulted from this project. Attendance (staff engagement) has doubled, CAUTI and CLABSI rates dramatically improved, and 100% of meetings have become interprofessionally attended (Figures 8.5–8.7). Employee satisfaction scores were used as preexisting data that directly correlated with the intended outcomes.

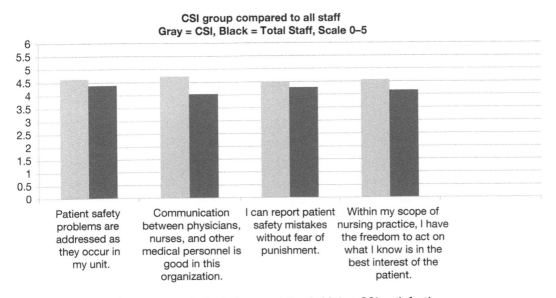

FIGURE 8.5 Bar graph depicting consistently higher CSI satisfaction scores.

CSI, Case Study Investigation.

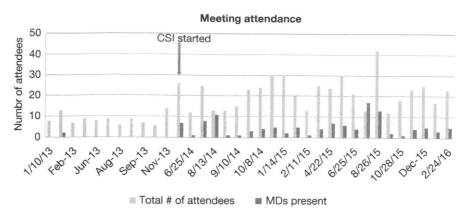

FIGURE 8.6 Staff engagement measured by meeting attendance.
CSI, Case Study Investigation; MDs, medical doctors.

The same questions used in the employee satisfaction surveys were administered to CSI participants making it possible to compare CSI satisfaction with key concepts compared to that of the general staff (Table 8.4).

Patient Outcome
Proactively Meeting Magnet® Standards

For Magnet-designated hospitals it is expected that certain elements of performance are measured with patient or nurse outcomes for at least three data points following a measured baseline of performance within the Magnet-designated timeline. Maintaining and improving several time points following a change demonstrates sustainability of the practice change. For CNSs working in these organizations, it is prudent to set up projects in advance to correctly capture the required displays of outcomes. Recording the exact

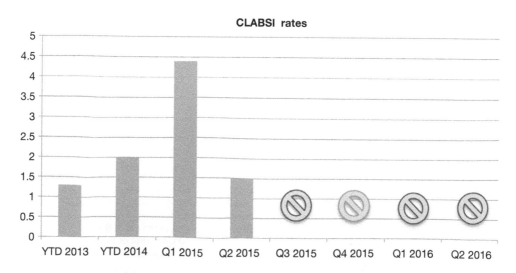

FIGURE 8.7 Patient outcomes measured by CLABSI rates.
CLABSI, central-line-associated bloodstream infection; Q, quarter; YTD, year to date.

TABLE 8.4 Comparison of CSI Satisfaction to Total Staff Satisfaction

Questions	CSI Participants	Total Staff Responses
Patient safety problems are addressed as they occur in my work unit	4.63	4.38
Communication between physicians, nurses, and other medical personnel is good in this organization	4.73	4.04
I can report patient safety mistakes without fear of punishment	4.49	4.27
Patient safety is a priority at this organization	4.59	4.38
Employees in my work unit report adverse events	4.38	4.26
I have the opportunity to influence nursing practice in this organization	4.48	4.23
Within my scope of nursing practice, I have the freedom to act on what I know is in the best interest of the patient	4.56	4.15

CSI, Case Study Investigation.

start date of a project is important because it must fall within the declared window necessary to be reviewed for Magnet designation or redesignation. The baseline and subsequent measurements need to occur at equal intervals. For instance, if the baseline was one quarter before the change, the follow-up measurements need to be quarterly after the change. The table must be prepared with a line or bar chart and a data table underneath (Figure 8.8). Most CNSs would likely be working with many nurses on a variety of projects over time with limited project experience. It is helpful to maintain a template for graphing outcomes that can be repeatedly used to graph outcomes in a Magnet acceptable standard (Exhibit 8.7).

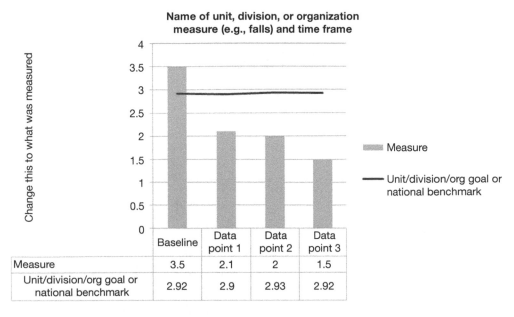

	Baseline	Data point 1	Data point 2	Data point 3
Measure	3.5	2.1	2	1.5
Unit/division/org goal or national benchmark	2.92	2.9	2.93	2.92

FIGURE 8.8 Sample graph according to Magnet standards.

org, organization.

EXHIBIT 8.7 Template for Graphing Magnet Standard Outcome Measures

	A	B	C	D	E	F	G	H
			Instructions	**1.** Delete the word baseline and insert the timeframe to cell D7 (e.g., Q4 2013).	**2.** Change the words 'data point 1' etc. to the timeframe (e.g., Q1 2014 in cells E7, F7, G7).			
			(This table talks to the graph)					
				Baseline	Data Point 1	Data Point 2	Data Point 3	
			Measure	3.5	2.1	2	1.5	
			Unit/Division/Org Goal or National Benchmark	2.92	2.9	2.93	2.92	

3. Change the word "Measure" to what you have measured (e.g., falls/1,000 pt days).

5. Declare where the benchmark came from if you used a national benchmark (e.g., CalNOC).

6. Click on the title to change the words.

4. Change these numbers to your real numbers. Add a row if you have more than one unit or department to report.

7. You can now click on the graph, right click, copy and paste this graph into your paperwork.

CalNOC, Collaborative Alliance for Nursing Outcomes; org, organization; pt, patient; Q, quarter.

Another strategy for demonstrating CNS contributions is measurement of outcomes produced by CNS-led groups. The CNS is often involved in hospital-wide initiatives targeted at nurse-sensitive indicators, such as falls. Whenever available, graphs should be accompanied by a brief text report of achieved outcomes. Do not assume that the audience will correctly interpret the graphs. Provide a concise explanation of whether action or praise is indicated based upon the results.

Linking process measures to outcomes tracked and reported up the chain of command by the department of quality is another strategy to link outcomes with CNS performance. For instance, in the process example described earlier, the CNS conducted rounds focused on compliance with the CAUTI bundle, providing feedback to staff when errors of omission occurred. The department of quality reports urinary tract infections (UTIs) to the infection control committee. Submitting the bundle compliance data highlighting improvement in compliance to the department of quality for inclusion in the report of UTIs to the infection control committee leverages use of existing resources with CNS visibility at a high level within the organization.

MEASURING EDUCATIONAL OUTCOMES

Educational outcomes may also be measured on four levels, similar to the outcome hierarchy. These have been previously described by Kirkpatrick (2009) as reaction, learning, behavior, and results:

Level 1: **Reaction**—How well did the learners like the learning process?

Level 2: **Learning**—What did they learn? (the extent to which the learners gain knowledge and skills)

Level 3: **Behavior**—What changes in job performance resulted from the learning process? (capability to perform the newly learned skills while on the job)

Level 4: **Results**—What are the tangible results of the learning process in terms of reduced cost, improved quality, increased production, efficiency, etc.? (Kirkpatrick, 2009).

For example, a CNS was responsible for executing the organization's preceptor training program. A standard course evaluation was used to measure the reaction to the program: Did participants find it valuable and would they recommend it to others? Knowledge assessment questions were formulated to measure knowledge attainment following the class. Audits were performed of employee files to ensure that preceptors were following the process of completing new nurse orientation paperwork and orientee evaluations. Measuring these types of process/change in behavior outcomes takes time, and requires direct interaction with learners following the program. However, the follow-through increases CNS visibility, which is important to ensure that behaviors change and practice change endures the test of time. If all outcomes are measured through electronic reports, it decreases clinical RN awareness that the outcome is being tracked and is considered important. Direct RN or patient outcomes optimally demonstrate the end result teaching new or expected practice standards in educational programs. However, the change in behavior, which needs to occur to maintain practice standards, also needs to be assessed through in-person onsite activities to optimize results. In this example of preceptor preparation, it was a goal of the organization that nurses have a limit of two preceptors during orientation to improve consistency of education. Adherence to this standard was measured at the third level of evaluation, preceptor and manager behavior, and was collected through new hire audits at 3 months posthire. Turnover data was used as a results (direct) outcome.

PULLING IT ALL TOGETHER

End-of-Year Report

End-of-year reports can be used proactively by the CNS to collate process, surrogate, and outcome data. Usually time-on data are not included in this level of report. Exhibit 8.8 demonstrates an example of how to organize report data. Time the construction of an end-of-year summary so that it can be aggregated to reflect the work of the entire team and be available at the end of each fiscal year. This also becomes a good time to review committee

EXHIBIT 8.8 **End-of-Year Report Template**

DEPARTMENT OF NURSING END-OF-YEAR REPORT

Finance (Put any quantifiable data here including but not limited to reduction in cost of care estimates, cost abatement, avoided fines, avoided reimbursement denials; cite sources for literature-based surrogates at the bottom of the page.):

Quality: Committee reports (List all committees where CNSs serve as chair, cochair, liaison, or have significant impact.)

- Nurse practice council
- Council of scientific inquiry
- Patient satisfaction
- Pain
- Restraint
- Pressure ulcer
- Falls
- Nursing satisfaction
- Pharmacy and therapeutics
- Institutional review board
- Care line committees

Performance improvement/evidence-based practice change projects
Research (List titles, investigators):
Professional projects (Include team leaders' names.):

Workforce Development (List all activities surrounding educating or supporting staff: number of rounds conducted, number of staff affected, courses taught, educational programs developed, and relate to outcomes whenever possible.):

Medical Staff Development (List interdisciplinary projects CNSs conduct in collaboration with physicians in this section. List programs that CNSs develop for medical education.):

Community Benefit

- Lectures to the community (title, speaker)
- Community projects
- Professional presentations (title, speaker, venue)
- Publications (citation)

CNS, clinical nurse specialist.

charters and CNS participation within key committees and projects. In Exhibit 8.8, the organization's pillars are in bold. Change these if your organization's pillars are different. Typical CNS activities are listed under each subheading. At the end of the year, each CNS in the system would submit his or her personal contributions that could be collated and summarized in aggregate. The chief nursing officer could then complete the report with activities not performed by CNSs. The original version provides an overall picture of how the CNSs contribute to organizational goals. The end product will be balanced with contributions by others, but it can be predicted that the bulk of the activity to move the profession forward and enact change to improve important nurse-sensitive outcomes has been affected by the work of a CNS. This template is easily modifiable into an electronic survey that would automatically summarize the data.

PROJECT CASE EXAMPLE AND CROSSWALK

The following project is explored because it was constructed to measure and report a variety of outcomes of a CNS-driven change in practice. Nolan, Burkard, Clark, Davidson, and Agan (2010) developed a new system for conducting mortality and morbidity (M&M) reviews for nurses in an attempt to reduce VAP. Nurses who were directly involved in providing care to each patient with a case of VAP were invited to the review and paid to attend. The primary outcome measure for the project was VAP. However, during the project several other key measures of success were evaluated and reported, such as percentage compliance with elements (process measures) of the Institute for Healthcare Improvement VAP bundle. This investigator also used an unbiased observer to measure nurse accountability by recording how many times the staff used "I" versus "you" statements to reflect accountability for the omissions in care. Satisfaction with the program was measured qualitatively with open-ended comments as well as quantitatively using Likert scale scoring, and included measures of CNS effect within the nursing personnel sphere. Cost of M&M was also measured to reflect an organizational outcome. Last, a surrogate measure for the cost of an episode of VAP was used and multiplied by the number of VAP cases that would have resulted without the M&M intervention. VAP rates were compared in a pretest/ posttest fashion using similar months to account for seasonal variation. Results from the project included overwhelmingly positive nursing satisfaction, improved accountability ($x^2 = 24.041, p < .001$), protocol compliance improvement from 90.1% to 95.2%, and improved VAP rates. The final cost analysis yielded $100,000 prevention in costs associated with VAP per year, even when accounting for the cost of paying nurses to attend M&M reviews. Exhibit 8.9 demonstrates a crosswalk between the outcomes measured in this project and the hierarchical model presented in this chapter plus the spheres of influence.

SUMMARY

CNS outcomes can be measured in a variety of ways. CNS outcome visibility is enhanced when tools and terms understood by operational leaders are used. Time-on activities can be captured from well-kept calendars, committee minutes, and project summaries to be converted into productivity reports and end-of-year reports. Peer evaluations, when constructed and distributed to include examples of CNS outcomes, promote visibility of

EXHIBIT 8.9 Crosswalk of Project Outcomes to Outcome Hierarchy Pyramid and Spheres of Influence

Nursing Morbidity and Mortality Project							
Outcome Measure	Patient/ Client	Nursing Personnel	Organizational/ Network	Time-On	Process	Surrogate Outcome	Outcome
VAP bundle protocol adherence		X			X		
Evidence of nursing accountability in the form of "I" versus "you" statements		X				X	
Qualitative measures of staff satisfaction		X					X
Quantitative measures of staff satisfaction		X					X
VAP	X						X
Cost savings to the organization			X			X	

VAP, ventilator-associated pneumonia.

the individual CNS. All projects can be designed to measure success. Rounds may be performed with the intention to measure and improve protocol adherence following changes in practice. Audits may be performed to measure change in behavior expected following educational activities for new practice standards. Surrogate measures and financial data can be used to create formulas to estimate outcomes affected by streamlining efficiencies or preventing episodes of illness. Finally, direct measurement of improvement in clinical or nurse outcomes can be reported. As highlighted in the NACNS's vision for the future of the CNS, outcome evaluation and measurement is a recommended area of core content specific to CNS practice (Goudreau et al., 2007). Assessing the outcomes of the CNS role to achieve important patient, provider, and health system goals can help to maximize the potential and long-term sustainability of the CNS role (Bryant-Lukosius et al., 2010). Continuing the focus on demonstrating the outcomes of CNS practice will help to ensure recognition of the value and impact of the CNS role.

Answers to Chapter Discussion Questions

1. Time-on activities (least important), process measures, surrogate measures, and outcome measures (most important).
2. Each individual will have a different answer to this question. Time-on activities may include tracking time spent on activities through the use of a calendar or spreadsheet.

Process measures normally include compliance with new changes in practice. Surrogate measures use published costs of care and estimations of events prevented through improved practices to calculate cost reduction. Actual outcome measures may include those focused on patients (e.g., length of stay, mortality, adverse events, readmissions) or staff (e.g., retention, satisfaction, comprehension, change in practice following education).

3. Each individual will create a unique table. If the learner has not yet done a project or planned a capstone, he or she should create a fictitious example based upon the last time he or she was expected to change practice as a nurse in response to a performance improvement project in the area of practice.

4. Answers will be individualized based upon the organization. Organizational objectives and goals normally center around publicly reported metrics and regulatory or accreditation standards, expanded services, and centers of excellence. The general themes of objectives are often clustered under pillars of performance such as finance, quality, workforce development, medical staff engagement, community involvement.

5. Cons include time spent to record and track activities, time and effort to develop tracking tools. Literature-based surrogates are not available for all measures of interest. Extracting actual outcomes from organizational databases can be cumbersome, time-consuming, or restricted. Pros include visibility, promotion/positive imaging of the CNS role, employment security, and justification of additional CNS positions. Tracking outcomes from change may also decrease resistance to change and help to solidify change when positive outcomes are shared with those affected by the change.

ACKNOWLEDGMENTS

We would like to acknowledge the work of Nancy Dayhoff, EdD, RN, CNS, and Brenda Lyon, DNS, CNS, FAAN, who served as the authors for the chapter on assessing outcomes in CNS practice for the 2000 and 2009 editions of this book. We would like to acknowledge Anne W. Alexandrov for her contributions to the 2008 edition of this text.

We would also like to acknowledge the following nurses whose projects have been showcased in this chapter as examples of outcome reporting: Rhonda Amber, MS, RN-BC, CMSRN, CNS; Donna Cahill, MS, RN-BC, CNS, CEN, CHTP; Nancy Carreon, MS, RN; Felipe Gutierrez, MS, RN, FNP; Scot Nolan, DNP, RN, CNS, PhN, CCRN, CNRN.

REFERENCES

Amber, R., Carreon, N., Agan, D., Johnson, M., & Cahill, C. (2012, March). Quantification of clinical nurse specialist outcomes: Clinical nurse specialist rounds. *Clinical Nurse Specialist*, 26(2), E37–E37.

Barr, J., Fraser, G. L., Puntillo, K., Ely, E. W., Gélinas, C., Dasta, J. F., . . . Jaeschke, R. (2013). Clinical practice guidelines for the management of pain, agitation, and delirium in adult patients in the intensive care unit. *Critical Care Medicine*, 41(1), 263–306. doi:10.1097/CCM.0b013e3182783b72

Bloom, B. S., & Bloom, B. S. (2005). Effects of continuing medical education on improving physician clinical care and patient health: A review of systematic reviews. *International Journal of Technology Assessment in Health Care, 21*(3), 380–385.

Bryant-Lukosius, D., Carter, N., Kilpatrick, K., Martin-Misener, R., Donald, F., Kaasalainen, S., . . . DiCenso, A. (2010). The clinical nurse specialist role in Canada. *Nursing Leadership, 23 Spec No 2010*, 140–166.

Coen, J., & Curry, K. (2016). Improving heart failure outcomes: The role of the clinical nurse specialist. *Critical Care Nursing Quarterly, 39*(4), 335–344. doi:10.1097/cnq.0000000000000127

Craig, J. V., & Smyth, R. L. (2007). *The evidence-based practice manual for nurses* (2nd ed.). Edinburgh: Churchill Livingstone Elsevier.

Cunningham, R. S. (2004). Advanced practice nursing outcomes: A review of selected empirical literature. *Oncology Nursing Forum, 31*(2), 219–232. doi:10.1188/04.onf.219-232

Dasta, J. F., Kane-Gill, S. L., Pencina, M., Shehabi, Y., Bokesch, P., Wiesmandle, W., & Riker, R. R. (2010). A cost-minimization analysis of dexmedetomdine compared with midazolam for long-term sedation in the intensive care unit. *Critical Care Medicine, 38*(2), 497–503.

Davidson, J. E. (2010a). *Creation of a role for the DNP prepared nurse in hospital leadership.* Paper presented at the Third National Doctor of Nursing Practice Conference, San Diego, CA.

Davidson, J. E. (2010b). Measuring CNS outcomes. Doctor of Nursing Practice Conference, San Diego, *CA.* Retrieved from http://www.doctorsofnursingpractice.org/third-national-dnp -conference

Davidson, J. E. (2011). *Developing outcomes reporting for the CNS role.* Paper presented at the 2011 Doctor of Nursing Practice Conference, New Orleans, LA. Retrieved from http://www.doctorsof nursingpractice.org/2011-conf-poster-presentations

Dickerson, S. S., Wu, Y. W., & Kennedy, M. C. (2006). A CNS-facilitated ICD support group: A clinical project evaluation. *Clinical Nurse Specialist, 20*(3), 146–153.

DiLibero, J., DeSanto-Madyea, S., & O'Dongohue, S. (2016). Improving accuracy of cardiac electrode placement: Outcomes of clinical nurse specialist practice. *Clinical Nurse Specialist, 30*(1), 45–50. doi:10.1097/nur.0000000000000172

Duffy, J. R. (2002). The clinical leadership role of the CNS in the identification of nursing-sensitive and multidisciplinary quality indicator sets. *Clinical Nurse Specialist, 16*(2), 70–76; quiz 77–78.

Fabbruzzo-Cota, C., Frecea, M., Kozell, K., Pere, K., Thompson, T., Tjan Thomas, J., & Wong, A. (2016). A clinical nurse specialist-led interprofessional quality improvement project to reduce hospital-acquired pressure ulcers. *Clinical Nurse Specialist, 30*(2), 110–116. doi:10.1097/nur.0000000000000191

Forster, A. J., Clark, H. D., Menard, A., Dupuis, N., Chernish, R., Chandok, N., . . . van Walraven, C. (2005). Effect of a nurse team coordinator on outcomes for hospitalized medicine patients. *American Journal of Medicine, 118*(10), 1148–1153. doi:10.1016/j.amjmed.2005.04.019

Fraser, G. L., Riker, R. R., Prato, B. S., & Wilkins, M. L. (2001). The frequency and cost of patient-initiated device removal in the ICU. *Pharmacotherapy, 21*(1), 1–6.

Fulton, J. S. (2006). Disseminating outcome of clinical nurse specialist practice. *Clinical Nurse Specialist, 20*(6), 264–265.

Fulton, J. S., & Baldwin, K. (2004). An annotated bibliography reflecting CNS practice and outcomes. *Clinical Nurse Specialist, 18*(1), 21–39.

Goudreau, K., Baldwin, K., Clark, A., Fulton, J., Lyon, B., Murray, T., . . . Sendelbach, S. (2007). A vision of the future of clinical nurse specialists: Prepared by the National Association of Clinical Nurse Specialists. *Clinical Nurse Specialist, 21*(6), 310–320.

Gould, C. V., Umscheid, C. A., Agarwal, R. K., Kuntz, G., & Pegues, D. A. (2010). Guideline for prevention of catheter-associated urinary tract infections 2009. *Infection Control & Hospital Epidemiology, 31*(4), 319–326. doi:10.1086/651091

Gutierrez, F., & Cahill, D. (2011). *Nasal bridle: Decrease in restraints, nursing time, and X-ray exposure.* Paper presented at the 20th Annual Academy of Medical–Surgical Nurses Conference, Boston, MA.

Hamilton, R., & Hawley, S. (2006). Quality of life outcomes related to anemia management of patients with chronic renal failure. *Clinical Nurse Specialist, 20*(3), 139–143; quiz 144–135.

Johnson, M., Amber, R., Cahill, D., Nolan, S., Azuma, N., & Davidson, J. (2011). Clinical nurse specialist multidisciplinary rounds as a strategy to translate evidence-based practice to the bedside. *Clinical Nurse Specialist, 25*(2), 80.

Kirkpatrick, D. L. (2009). *Implementing the four levels: A practical guide for effective evaluation of training programs: Easyread large Edition.* Oakland, CA: Berrett-Koehler. Retrieved from http://www.readhowyouwant.com

Larsen, L. S., Neverett, S. G., & Larsen, R. F. (2001). Clinical nurse specialist as facilitator of interdisciplinary collaborative program for adult sickle cell population. *Clinical Nurse Specialist, 15*(1), 15–22.

Lau, P. Y., & Chan, C. W. (2005). SARS (severe acute respiratory syndrome): Reflective practice of a nurse manager. *Journal of Clinical Nursing, 14*(1), 28–34. doi:10.1111/j.1365-2702.2004.00995.x

Lawrence, L. A. (2011). Work engagement, moral distress, education level, and critical reflective practice in intensive care nurses. *Nursing Forum, 46*(4), 256–268. doi:10.1111/j.1744-6198.2011.00237.x

Ley, S. J. (2001). Quality care outcomes in cardiac surgery: The role of evidence-based practice. *AACN Clinical Issues, 12*(4), 606–617; quiz 633–605.

McCabe, P. J. (2005). Spheres of clinical nurse specialist practice influence evidence-based care for patients with atrial fibrillation. *Clinical Nurse Specialist, 19*(6), 308–317; quiz 318–309.

Melnyk, B. M., & Fineout-Overholt, E. (2011). *Evidence-based practice in nursing & healthcare: A guide to best practice.* Philadelphia, PA: Lippincott Williams & Wilkins.

National Association of Clinical Nurse Specialists. (2004). *Statement on clinical nurse specialist practice and education.* Harrisburg, PA: Author.

National Clinical Nurse Specialist Competency Task Force. (2010). Clinical nurse specialist core competencies: Executive summary 2006–2008. Retrieved from http://www.nacns.org/docs/CNSCoreCompetenciesBroch.pdf

Nolan, S. W., Burkard, J. F., Clark, M. J., Davidson, J. E., & Agan, D. L. (2010). Effect of morbidity and mortality peer review on nurse accountability and ventilator-associated pneumonia rates. *Journal of Nursing Administration, 40*(9), 374–383. doi:10.1097/NNA.0b013e3181ee427b

Pasero, C. (2010). Safe IV opioid titration in patients with severe acute pain. *Journal of PeriAnesthesia Nursing, 25*(5), 314–318.

Prevost, S. S. (2002). Clinical nurse specialist outcomes: Vision, voice, and value. *Clinical Nurse Specialist, 16*(3), 119–124.

Schmidt, N. A., & Brown, J. M. (2014). *Evidence-based practice for nurses*. Burlington, MA: Jones & Bartlett.

Stahl, K., Palileo, A., Schulman, C. I., Wilson, K., Augenstein, J., Kiffin, C., & McKenney, M. (2009). Enhancing patient safety in the trauma/surgical ICU. *Journal of Trauma Injury, Infection, and Critical Care, 67*(3), 430–435.

Studer, Q. (2008). *Results that last: Hardwiring behaviors that will take your company to the top*. Hoboken, NJ: John Wiley.

Willoughby, D., & Burroughs, D. (2001). A CNS-managed diabetes foot-care clinic: A descriptive survey of characteristics and foot-care behaviors of the patient population. *Clinical Nurse Specialist, 15*(2), 52–57.

Wojner, A. (2001). *Outcomes management: Applications to clinical practice*. Maryland Heights, MO: Mosby.

CHAPTER 9

Outcome Measurement in Nurse-Midwifery Practice

Julie Marfell

Chapter Objectives

1. Present an overview of the historical implementation and importance of outcome measurement in nurse-midwifery practice and discuss the role that outcome measurement has in improving modern health care delivery in the arena of maternal and child health
2. Summarize published examples of nurse-midwifery outcome studies
3. Outline the use of the American College of Nurse-Midwives (ACNM) Benchmarking Project for use in outcome measurement and quality improvement
4. Present the Uniform Data Set as a tool for collection of outcome measures and research

Chapter Discussion Questions

1. Why is outcome measurement an essential practice in nurse-midwifery practice? Briefly describe three reasons.
2. What four areas did the ACNM Benchmarking Project use to evaluate quality nurse-midwifery care?
3. How could the ACNM Benchmarking Project be used for nurse-midwifery quality improvement?
4. What is the Optimality Index?
5. What classifications of outcome measurements are used for nurse-midwifery practice? Name and define at least three.

HISTORICAL PERSPECTIVE

Outcome evaluation of nurse-midwifery practice in the United States is as old as the profession. Mary Breckinridge brought nurse-midwifery to America in 1925 and created the Frontier Nursing Service (FNS). FNS was a demonstration project that provided health care to the rural poor in southeastern Kentucky. Mrs. Breckinridge took the advice of one of her consultants, Dr. McCormack, the health commissioner for the Commonwealth of Kentucky, who said she would be unable to determine the effects of the FNS without a complete assessment of the health status of the community. Her first step in establishing the FNS was to ride over more than 700 square miles to obtain health histories of all the area families so that the impact of the nurse-midwives on horseback could be measured (Breckinridge, 1981).

Meticulous records were kept at the FNS. The Metropolitan Life Insurance Corporation was asked to analyze the data of the first 1,000 births attended by the nurse-midwives at FNS. The results were incredible. Dr. Louis Dublin reported:

> The study shows conclusively that the type of service rendered by the Frontier nurses safeguards the life of mother and babe. If such service were available to the women of the country generally, there would be a saving of 10,000 mothers' lives a year in the United States. There would be 30,000 less stillbirths and 30,000 more children alive at the end of the first month of life. (Breckinridge, 1981)

Measuring nurse-midwifery outcomes started with the first nurse-midwifery service in the United States and has been an integral component of establishing nurse-midwifery as a profession in the United States.

The success of the nurse-midwifery care provided in the home by Frontier nurses from 1925 to 1975 was reported in 1975 on the 50th anniversary of the FNS (Browne & Isaacs, 1976). The study of the first 10,000 births at FNS by the Metropolitan Life Insurance Company found 11 maternal deaths, two of which were not obstetrics related. This was much lower than the national maternal mortality rate of 36.3 per 10,000 live births for the midpoint years 1939 to 1941. There were fewer premature births, stillbirths, and neonatal deaths for FNS than the rest of the country.

Continuing throughout the history of nurse-midwifery in the United States, outcomes have been studied. Initially, they were scrutinized to determine the safety and feasibility of midwifery care. A classic study was conducted in Madera County, California, in the early 1960s to determine if nurse-midwives could be utilized to assist physicians in providing maternity care in a rural underserved area and to measure the outcomes of this new model of care (Montgomery, 1969). At the time, nurse-midwifery was not recognized or licensed in the state of California, so this project utilized nurse-midwives but labeled them nurse obstetric assistants (NOAs). A before-and-after comparison was done that showed the NOAs could provide the needed care, and the birth outcomes improved dramatically. The number of women who received prenatal care in the first trimester doubled. The percentage of women receiving more than six prenatal visits increased almost 10%. Prematurity rates declined by 5% and the neonatal mortality rate went from 23.9 per 1,000 live births to 10.3 per 1,000 live births. This project highlighted the successful utilization of nurse-midwives, and a report of the project was presented to the California

Medical Association (CMA) with the hope that they would endorse legislation to allow NOAs to practice in California. However, the CMA did not endorse NOAs, and nurse-midwives were not recognized in California until 1974 (ACNM, 2012).

It is interesting to note that a follow-up study of the Madera County project compared the birth outcomes before, during, and after the use of NOAs (Levy, Wilkinson, & Marine, 1971). In the 3 years following the termination of the NOAs, 9% more women received no prenatal care. Women who did receive prenatal care received fewer visits. The rate of premature infants rose significantly from 6.6% to 9.8%. Neonatal mortality almost tripled going from 10.3 per 1,000 live births when care was provided by the nurse-midwives to 32.1 per 1,000 live births afterward. The authors concluded that the use of nurse-midwives should be encouraged because the maternity outcomes improved during the interim period when they provided care.

Later, studies demonstrated that midwifery outcomes were excellent and there were added benefits of cost-effectiveness and patient satisfaction. Reid and Morris (1979) evaluated the implementation of nurse-midwifery care for the underserved in Georgia in the 1970s and included analysis of cost-effectiveness. There was a substantial increase in the number of women who received early prenatal care, and a reduction in the number of women giving birth with little or no prenatal care for the 3 years after the implementation of the midwifery services compared with the 2 years before. Birth outcomes showed improvement in neonatal mortality, longer gestations, and higher birth weights. Infant mortality rates dropped significantly in the rural counties studied, while there were no differences in the comparison counties. The authors found the cost of prenatal care and hospital care decreased over the course of the project and they were cautiously optimistic, while recommending that future research should include prospective analysis of health expenditures for midwifery care. Anderson and Anderson (1999) found home births cost 68% less than hospital births.

Outcome measurement was also undertaken to determine whether birth centers, which were specifically designed for the practice of the hallmarks of midwifery, were a safe alternative to hospital birth. The landmark prospective study of birth outcomes for over 11,000 women from 84 birth centers was published in the *New England Journal of Medicine* in 1989 (Rooks et al., 1989). The birth center clients were screened as low risk for maternity complications; hence an out-of-hospital setting was appropriate for their care. There were fewer premature births for women giving birth in the birth center than for all women who gave birth in the United States. The cesarean section rate was 4.4%, which contributed to lower costs for maternity care. The intrapartum transfer rate was 15.8% with 2.3% being emergent transports. The infant outcomes for birth center mothers were comparable to those of women with low-risk pregnancies having hospital births. Patient satisfaction was high with 98.8% of the women who gave birth at the birth centers saying they would recommend a birth center, and 94% would return to the birth center for their next birth. The percentage of satisfaction was slightly lower for the women who were transferred to the hospital during labor with 96.9% recommending it, and 83.3% willing to use it again. The authors concluded that "Few innovations in health services promise lower cost, greater availability, and higher degree of satisfaction with a comparable degree of safety" (p. 1810).

Recent attention has been paid to how the midwifery model of care actually improves pregnancy and birth outcomes, which lowers health care costs for maternity services. The

Cochrane review found that maternity care led by midwives was beneficial for women (Hatem, Sandall, Devane, Soltani, & Gates, 2009). Women randomized to midwifery-led maternity units had fewer antepartum hospitalizations, fetal losses, instrumental deliveries, and episiotomies. They had more spontaneous vaginal births and early breastfeeding initiation. The women were cared for during labor by a midwife they knew, and they felt a sense of control. The authors concluded that for women without significant medical or obstetrical problems, "Midwifery-led care confers benefits and shows no adverse outcomes" (p. 13).

CURRENT EXPANSION OF OUTCOME MEASUREMENT

Benchmarking

ACNM is the professional organization for nurse-midwives with the goal of improving the health and well-being of mothers and infants. The ACNM defines eight standards for the practice of midwifery. One standard specifically addresses the need for evaluation of nurse-midwifery outcomes using a program of quality management that includes data collection, problem identification and resolution, as well as peer review.

To assist midwives to measure the quality of care, ACNM developed a Benchmarking Project in 1997 (Collins-Fulea, Mohr, & Tillett, 2005). This program specifically examined four areas of quality midwifery care. The first area examined functional status that included the physical and emotional well-being of the mother. The second area was cost of care, including both direct and indirect costs. The third area was patient satisfaction, and the fourth area consisted of clinical outcomes. The first benchmarking data were obtained in 2004 from 45 practices attending more than 23,000 births. Results were reported so that each midwifery service could see how it performed compared with the other services for each indicator. Each could contact midwifery services with high performance to learn best practices that could then be modified and incorporated into its own practice for quality improvement. The ACNM Benchmarking Project has continued and expanded. Results from 2011 included data from 203 practices with almost 900 nurse-midwives attending over 69,000 vaginal births (ACNM, 2011).

UNIFORM DATA SET

The American Association of Birth Centers (AABC) developed the Uniform Data Set (UDS; an online data registry) that collects comprehensive data on both the process and the outcomes of the nurse-midwifery model of care. It is intended that the data set be used to simultaneously collect data from all providers in hospital, birth center, and home birth settings. The UDS is stored on a password-protected secured site and is Health Insurance Portability and Accountability Act (HIPAA) compliant. The UDS also provides the provider with comprehensive statistic reports that include required reports for birth center accreditation, benchmarking reports for the ACNM Benchmarking Project, registration logs, delivery logs, incomplete reports, and custom reports (AABC, 2007).

Stapleton (2011) conducted a validation study of the 189-item UDS. Five birth center practices had a random audit of 2% of their records. Data from the health record were compared with data entered into the UDS. There was a high level of consistency between the health records and the UDS with 97.1% of the variables matching. This study shows the reliability of the UDS and encourages its use for research and quality assurance. Using such large data sets will greatly facilitate health policy changes.

Data from the UDS were used in a study by Stapleton, Osborne, and Illuzzi (2013) of 15,574 women planning to give birth in 79 birth centers across the United States. The transfer rate from birth center to hospital was 12% with the majority being nonemergent. Only 6% of the births were by cesarean section with 93% of the women having a vaginal birth. There were no maternal deaths and the fetal and neonatal mortality rate was the same as other studies of births to women with low-risk pregnancies. This study mirrors the results of the National Birth Center Study (NBCS; Rooks et al., 1989) showing the positive and durable results of birth center care.

PURPOSE OF OUTCOME MEASUREMENT IN NURSE-MIDWIFERY PRACTICE

The most compelling rationale for outcome measurement is that it assists in efforts to improve the quality of health care for patients. A recent report by the ACNM (2008) highlights that high-quality care, which includes high levels of client satisfaction and lower cost, is provided by certified nurse-midwives (CNMs) with equal to or better outcomes than those of obstetricians or gynecologists.

Enhanced cost-effectiveness is another reason for evaluating outcomes. In cost-effectiveness studies, alternative methods of obtaining the same goal are compared. Clients with similar conditions may be treated with alternative approaches, often with significantly different costs but with very similar outcomes. Studies that document the cost-effectiveness of nurse-midwifery practice while maintaining clinical outcomes have long been documented (Cherry & Foster, 1982; Lubic, 1981; Oakley et al., 1996; Reid & Morris, 1979; Stewart & Clark, 1982). Jackson et al. (2003) discuss collaborative care with CNM versus traditional physician-based care and the decrease in length of stay and decreased emergency department visits documented for women in collaborative care. The safety outcomes of the neonate in this study were similar across both groups.

Alternatively, clients of CNMs and physicians with similar conditions may be treated with different approaches and one group may experience superior outcomes. An example of this is that physicians more often perform episiotomies, while the CNMs might try different approaches, such as perineal massage, warm packs, or positioning, to reduce the need for episiotomy and reducing overall perineal trauma during childbirth (Hastings-Tolsma, Vincent, Emeis, & Francisco, 2007; Robinson, Noritz, Cohen, & Liberman, 2000). Another example of comparing different approaches to maternity care is the use of the Optimality Index-US (OI-US), which measures optimal maternity care (Cragin & Kennedy, 2006). *Optimal* is defined as obtaining the best outcomes with the least amount of intervention while taking into consideration the woman's physical and emotional status. Cragin and Kennedy (2006) studied 375 women in labor with moderate pregnancy risk status. Midwives provided care for 196 women, and 179 women were cared for by a physician. The mean OI-US was significantly higher for the midwifery care group. The care provided by the midwives included more mobility, oral hydration, nonpharmacologic pain relief, and spontaneous vaginal births than the care provided by the physicians. Yet both groups experienced good perinatal outcomes, thus show-ing that less interventive care during labor for women with moderate-risk factors pro-duces positive outcomes. Finally, outcome measurement gives evidence and support to the practice of midwifery. Examples of how quality outcomes can influence and increase appreciation and accessibility of nurse-midwifery practice in the United States include the 2004 Virginia Governor's Task Force on Health-Care Reform recommendations for the development and funding of pilot birth centers in rural areas. The purpose of these sites is to demonstrate the effectiveness of midwifery care and increase access to high-quality pregnancy-related care. The recommendations call for the pilot sites collecting and annual reporting of data using the American Association of Birth Centers Uniform Data Set (Governor's Health Reform Commission, 2007).

The federal government is also intrigued by the positive outcomes of midwifery care and wants to determine whether the midwifery model of care can be a solution to the problem of a high cost with poor outcome maternity care system. The Center for Medicare and Medicaid Innovation has developed Strong Start for Mothers and Newborns (Center for Medicare and Medicaid Innovation, 2012). This initiative is seeking to fund projects related to group prenatal care, birth centers, and maternity homes, all of which are based on the midwifery model of care.

Research is the basis of all clinical practice, a guiding principle shared by all dis-ciplines. It is this requirement for evidence-based practice that is another rationale for outcome measurement in nurse-midwifery practice. While outcome measurement is not synonymous with research, the two methodologies provide empirical support for evi-dence-based changes in clinical practice.

CLASSIFICATION OF OUTCOME MEASUREMENT FOR NURSE-MIDWIFERY PRACTICE

There are several approaches to the classification of outcomes within nurse-midwifery practice. Each method provides data for evidence-based clinical practice. The following outcome classifications are discussed: physiological, perceptual, psychosocial, cognitive, functional, and fiscal.

Physiological outcomes are those that have to do with the impact of CNM interventions on the process of birth. The division of physiological outcomes is somewhat arbitrary because all nurses utilize a holistic approach to health care, recognizing the interrelated-ness of perceptual and psychosocial outcomes. Physiological outcomes can be further divided into groups of expected birth outcomes as well as adverse outcomes. It may be more helpful in outcome studies to focus on expected birth outcomes and to designate adverse events as variances from the usual and expected outcomes. Both classifications are of interest to CNMs because this information provides direction for clinical care improvement. Examples of physiological outcomes in midwifery practice include blood glucose levels, iron deficiency anemia, fetal heart rate, maternal breathing patterns, and use of relaxation techniques in labor.

Perceptual outcomes are defined in terms of patient satisfaction. This may include satisfaction with CNMs as providers, with the facilities, with the care received, or with the clinical outcomes. It is important to understand that perception refers to the situation as the client views it or understands it. While it may not be entirely congruent with the provider's reality, it does not matter. What does matter is that this is the client's percep-tion of reality. Perceptual outcomes are crucial to the marketing and public acceptance of nurse-midwifery service.

Psychosocial outcomes are those that have to do with such things as the client's affective state, self-image, self-esteem, and interpersonal relationships. Examples of psychosocial outcomes that would be of clinical interest to nurse-midwives include maternal–infant bonding, presence of social support, confidence in the ability to care for the infant, comfort with a pregnant body image, and sense of self-actualization associated with childbirth.

Cognitive outcomes include the knowledge and skills that the client will need to safely and effectively care for herself and/or an infant. These would include the knowledge of prenatal nutrition, the signs and symptoms of postpartum infection, and breastfeeding skills.

Functional outcomes have to do with the maintenance or improvement of physical functioning. While there are standardized measures of functional outcomes, such as various activities of daily living or independent activities of daily living scores, most CNM clients are women involved in a healthy childbearing process. There are standard-ized tools that measure functional outcomes in the postpartum woman; for example, the Childbirth Impact Profile (Tulman, Fawcett, Groblewski, & Silverman, 1990) and the Inventory of Functional Status after Childbirth (Tulman & Fawcett, 1988). Examples of functional outcomes include the ability to care for the infant and readiness to return to a job outside the home.

Fiscal outcomes involve those having to do with the cost of care. Because health care is a business, it is essential that nurse-midwives understand the fiscal aspects of mater-nity care. Fiscal measures include such things as cost per case, hospitalization costs and length of stay, incremental costs of specialized nursing care during labor, reimbursement by payer, and laboratory costs. There are two approaches to the measurement of fiscal outcomes: cost data and charge data.

Charge Data Analysis

Some institutions utilize charges as a proxy measurement for costs. Charges are defined as the charges appearing on the client's bill. Charges are somewhat arbitrary and do include some profit or mark-up amount added to the cost of producing a service or prod-uct. Just as a department store adds a mark-up to the charge for clothing or appliances, so does a health care system add a profit amount to the cost of producing a service. Charges are the same for each client for each procedure and do not reflect policy or group dis-counts. Because contractual payers often receive a provider discount, it is important that charges be studied before the discounts are applied for the purpose of outcome measure-ment. Charges can be collected from both the client billing records and from the provider professional service records.

Cost Analysis

Other institutions have a cost accounting system that will permit the measurement of actual costs of client care, that is, the cost of the service being produced. Cost is a com-plex concept and can be further reduced to a consideration of direct costs (supplies, salaries, and rent) and indirect costs (employee benefits, costs allocated by other departments, e.g., a portion of the building maintenance). Some costs are defined as fixed, that is, they do not change with an increase in client volume. An example of a fixed cost would be heat and light costs. Other costs are variable, meaning that they change with client volume. Laundry and housekeeping costs are examples of variable costs.

What is important in fiscal outcome measurement is that CNMs understand what is included in the costs or charges to make appropriate comparisons. Another consideration is that charges in a clinical practice may be bundled. This means that there is a prospective fee determined by an organization for a particular set of services. For example, hospital charges associated with a normal vaginal delivery may be set at $4,000. This is one all-inclusive fee and there will not be additional charges reflected on the client billing record. This approach does make it difficult to determine variation in fiscal outcomes. If there are no other cost data available when charges are bundled, it is difficult to assess the impact of practice changes on costs.

A decision must be made as to the appropriate interval or timing of charge or cost outcome data collection for nurse-midwifery clients. The purpose of the study will determine the period of measurement. If charges are to represent the entire period of pregnancy, one method to consider is to define the period from the date of determination of pregnancy until 2 months after birth to capture the full scope of the charges for the mother. When collecting fiscal data related to infant outcomes, similar decisions regarding the appropriate measurement interval must be made. Because many infants do not remain within the CNM system but move to pediatrician care, this is an important decision.

DEVELOPING CLIENT OUTCOME MEASURES

Developing client outcome measures is not difficult. It is something that was a part of undergraduate nursing education and included as a step in the nursing process: assessment, analysis, outcome identification, planning, implementation, and outcome evaluation. The CNM builds on that foundation and uses the knowledge and skill base of nurse-midwifery practice to identify and write outcomes supported by evidence-based practice guidelines for clients during the perinatal period. Two basic questions start this process:

1. What results are expected as a result of the implementation of evidence-based guidelines?
2. When will the results likely be achieved by the client and/or family?

When evaluating practice, it is essential to be cognizant of some fundamental principles in outcome analysis. These principles are as follows:

■ Outcomes must be measurable. ACNM outcome that states that "client satisfaction will improve" is not measurable. It is necessary to be explicit about the indicators that will be used to measure satisfaction. The CNM in this case must specify the tool to be used to measure client satisfaction. For example, "Scores on the Picker patient satisfaction tool will increase after CNM care" is a specific measurable outcome.

- The outcome must relate to the care process or intervention. Spontaneous pushing during labor can reasonably be expected to relate to the postpartum perineal condition.
- The outcome should be realistic for both the client and the CNM. While improving client nutrition is a desirable outcome, there will be some clients who have no interest in the outcome and no amount of education and teaching material will impact their knowledge of nutrition and alter intake. It is important, however, to study negative outcomes as well as positive outcomes. There is much to be learned in both directions.
- Outcomes are measured within an accessible time span. If a CNM wishes to study maternal–infant bonding comparing attachment indications at 1 week of age to those at 1 year of age for the same subjects, there will be major difficulties in maintaining the subjects in the study. This is not to negate the value of the study, but to help the CNM to anticipate the inherent challenges in such a design.
- The risk status of the subject population is described. *Risk* is defined as "the presence or absence of selected factors associated with non-optimal outcomes" (Selwyn, 1990). While the typical population of clients of CNMs is described as low-to-moderate risk, there are clinical differences among midwifery practices as to what constitutes low risk. Many studies utilize the risk factors that would preclude admission to the midwifery service as descriptors of the status of the population. This might include such things as: hypertension requiring medication during pregnancy, serious cardiac disease, chronic renal or lung disease, or known multiple gestation. While there is debate in the literature regarding the accuracy of obstetric risk assessment instruments, it is necessary that the risk profile be described in order that appropriate comparisons can be made.
- All data collection has a cost. Often novices at outcome studies ask, "How many subjects are needed?" The only answer is, "It depends." It depends on the size of the population available, the sensitivity of the instrument used to measure outcomes, and the resources available to commit to data collection. More is usually better, but it is necessary to be realistic about the cost of data collection. Some outcomes may be collected for all clients within the midwifery service. At other times, sampling techniques may be used after preliminary analysis of a pilot that would yield sufficient data to conduct a power analysis. Such an analysis is a means of establishing that the study was conducted on a large enough sample to find an effect or relationship among variables if indeed it does exist.

Here are some examples of individual client outcome measures written for a nurse-midwifery practice:

- For a client at the first prenatal visit: client will verbalize an understanding of 2,200 calorie diet, the food pyramid, dietary needs in pregnancy such as iron and calcium, and complete a 3-day intake diary by her next visit
- For a client at the 8-month visit: client will demonstrate knowledge of signs and symptoms of onset of labor and verbalize when to call the CNM
- For a client at her first postpartum visit: breastfeeding at least eight to 12 times per day 1 week after delivery

Note that all of these outcomes are written for an individual client. It is also important to recognize the importance of individual outcomes as well as the aggregate outcomes.

CNMs are concerned with outcome evaluation on both an individual client basis and in aggregate groups. This process helps the CNM to rapidly identify deviations from expected outcomes and to adjust individual client care appropriately.

Outcome measurements on aggregate groups are defined as issues related to a specific, identified population. Outcomes for the aggregate group would be those that are appropriate for all clients within the nurse-midwifery service. These outcomes might include the following:

- Verbalize signs and symptoms of postpartum endometritis before discharge from birthing center
- Demonstrate safety in taking infant temperature, bathing infant, and positioning infant in crib within 24 hours of birth
- Adhere to recommended schedule for follow-up postpartum visits
- Evaluate for the presence and extent of perineal laceration

It is often helpful to utilize a formal approach for identifying clinical outcomes.

It is assumed that the subject of the outcome is the client or an aspect of the client: a blood value, the position of the infant, and blood loss. The client behavior is the observable activity or measurement that the client will demonstrate at some future time. Things such as drink, walk, report, or achievement of specific vital signs or lab values are examples of client behaviors. The criterion of performance sets the parameters for the behavior identified in the outcome (Murray & Atkinson, 2000). In clinical practice, the CNM may want the hemoglobin not to drop below 10.5 g/dL and weight gain not to exceed 35 pounds. The time frame is a realistic estimate of when the client can reasonably be expected to achieve the outcome. Some outcomes are specific to the first trimester (taking supplements that include folic acid, avoiding medications that are possible teratogens), and others begin at the first stage of labor (use of different techniques for relaxation, maintenance of hydration). Finally, a condition may be added if necessary. The CNM might specify the condition under which the behavior specified in the outcome is to occur. Examples of this might include the client will use different types of relaxation techniques with the assistance of the client's mother, the hemoglobin will be stable at 10.5 g/dL after 1 month of iron supplements, or the client will use the food pyramid picture as a strategy to maintain a weight gain not to exceed 35 pounds.

In clinical practice, when thinking of identifying client outcomes, it is important to emphasize that outcomes must be individualized for a particular client. Outcomes that are mutually established with clients are much more likely to be achieved than those that are determined solely by a CNM. There is also a cultural component to outcomes. What is desirable within one culture may be inappropriate in others. For example, in some cultures a grandmother plays a significant role in the care of the infant and the new mother. The CNM needs to incorporate the grandmother as a significant other in the care process, including outcome measurement.

SCHEDULED MEASUREMENTS OF OUTCOMES

Essential to planning any evaluation is determining the measurement of the outcome. This is a major clinical consideration requiring the knowledge of nurse-midwifery practice. One schema used by CNMs is to consider time intervals. The following time periods during pregnancy may be used to evaluate specific objectives related to maternal fetal outcomes: prenatal care (trimesters or weeks), intrapartum care that may be further divided into stages of labor, and postpartum care (first 2 hours, first 12 hours).

Another way to define time intervals might be to consider interim and discharge outcomes. At the completion of the childbirth process, there are some outcomes that signify the completion of the care process for that episode of care. The client may be independent in infant care, may have established a strong maternal–child bond, and may have established new health and wellness patterns reflective of being a family. At this time, usually within 6 to 8 weeks postpartum, the CNM may discharge the client from the care relationship. While some women choose to continue to remain in the practice of CNMs for primary care, the focus shifts from maternity care to well-woman care. Thus, there is the completion of one phase of care. Outcomes may then be classified as interim outcomes, which were those occurring during the care process, and discharge outcomes, those occurring at the completion of the care process. If discharge outcomes are not achieved, it may be an indication that there is a need for additional care. For example, if a mother appears to be experiencing postpartum depression, the CNM may consider a referral to a mental health professional.

VARIANCE FROM EXPECTED OUTCOMES

Variances occur when an expected outcome is not met at all, met later than expected, or even met ahead of the time defined for measurement (Murray & Atkinson, 2000). A rather standard classification system for variances has evolved in recent years. The system attempts to classify variances according to their cause. *System variances* are those that result from variations in the system, perhaps scheduling glitches or computer downtime (Murray & Atkinson, 2000). A patient may not have kept a scheduled appointment because the information was incorrectly entered into the computer and the client did not understand the date of her next appointment, resulting in a missed visit. If the clinical outcome being measured is rate of kept appointments, this will result in a variance.

Another type of variance is *provider* variance. One CNM provider may choose not to do certain lab procedures, feeling that for this particular client it is duplicative or unnecessary. This may result in a variance in lab charges due to provider variance.

The third kind of variance is *client* variance. One client may be physically active, within normal weight range, and accustomed to engage in strenuous cardiovascular exercise three times per week. This client may experience fewer discomforts of pregnancy, less weight gain, a shorter labor, and a faster recovery than defined in clinical outcomes. This is also an example of a positive variance if weight gain and labor length still fall within normal ranges. It is important to understand that not all variances are negative. Variances can mean that the client exceeded the usual outcomes. It is equally important for CNMs to study both positive and negative outcomes to effectively change their clinical practice.

TOOLS FOR OUTCOME DATA COLLECTION

Before selecting and purchasing a data-collection tool or designing a new data-collection tool that might be duplicative or have limited use, it is important to first understand what tools and programs are available and their intended uses and applications. Currently, there are several tools available to assist CNMs in the collection of outcome data, including the UDS developed by the AABC. The UDS is under revision and work is under way to integrate it with electronic medical record.

Additional software programs are available both commercially and through the Centers for Disease Control and Prevention (CDC). These include word processing, epidemiological analysis, and data management programs.

SOURCES OF OUTCOME DATA

Because outcome studies all involve some costs, it is useful to understand some of the existing sources of outcome data available for health care information. These sources may decrease effort and costs when assessing outcome data. These are some sources; not all health care systems will have all of these tools.

- *Routinely collected administrative data.* These typically includes vital statistics (births, deaths), payer source, Medicare/Medicaid, claims data, which include principal diagnosis and procedural codes, complications, comorbidities, and records of adverse events. There may also be a case mix index (CMI), which is a measure of the resources used to treat a clinical population (Adams, 1996). CMI is useful as a tool to make comparisons among populations when there is not another tool to use to adjust for severity of illness. The clients of CNMs could be assumed to typically have a low CMI relative to other hospitalized patients.
- *Birth logs.* Outcome data may also be gathered from birth logs. Hospitals and birth centers routinely keep concise data that usually include information such as place of birth, maternal age, gravity/parity, date of first prenatal visit, number of prenatal visits, total weight gain, significant prenatal events, significant intrapartum events, and infant data. Historically, birth logs have been kept in handwritten logs on birthing units.
- *Data sets.* Data may also be gathered from existing data sets. Data may be collected from data sets, such as the UDS or the ACNM's data set. Many of these sets include comprehensive care and outcome data.
- *Discharge summary.* Upon discharge, hospitals complete a discharge summary that consists of data extracted from the chart. This may include such data elements as Social Security number, medical record number, name, admission and discharge dates, length of stay, disposition (home, nursing home, and subacute facility), total charges, employment status, and race. A cautionary note is that when race is included in this data set, it may be incomplete and unreliable due to diversity within racial categories, the number of people with biracial identities, and differences in self-assignment to potential categories (Alvidrez, Azocar, & Miranda, 1996; Foster & Martinez, 1995).
- *Obstetric discharge summary.* Obstetric units will typically have a department-specific form that will include additional data. This form includes such data elements as intrapartum procedures, postpartum procedures, data related to lacerations, infection, or phlebitis. These data may be entered into a computerized database that permits easy access and retrieval.

- *Program-specific data collection.* Each health care system may collect data related to specific programs. For CNMs this may include newborn screens for hearing loss, medications used during hospitalization, tests ordered, car seats distributed, teen births, and early discharge.
- *Disease registration.* Some institutions participate in registries for various diseases. Programs of interest to CNMs might include sexually transmitted diseases, HIV/AIDS, or birth defects. Some of the registries are required by state law and reporting by providers is mandated.
- *Critical pathways or evidence-based clinical practice guidelines.* These are a form of an interdisciplinary plan of care and are used in many systems. Some perinatal clinical pathways are initiated at the first client visit and outline a plan of care concluding at discharge from the midwifery service. Most pathways contain outcomes that are evaluated at specified times.

One caution when collecting outcome data is the need to protect the confidentiality of the clinical record data. Most institutions maintain rigorous control over who may access data and for what purposes. If a CNM is considering an outcome study that has the potential to be published, the approval of a human subject's protection committee or institutional review board is necessary. This must be done before the initiation of such a study. Typically, the use of data for quality improvement studies does not require such approval but then the CNM must understand that no publication of results is possible. When in doubt, it is recommended to seek consultation with the chairperson of the human subject protection committee at the institution.

REVIEW OF NURSE-MIDWIFERY OUTCOME STUDIES

Discussion of several selected studies will illustrate approaches to outcome measurement within nurse-midwifery clinical practice. While the studies are largely from a research perspective rather than a quality improvement focus, the measurement principles are the same.

The NBCS (Rooks et al., 1989) was a landmark investigation of 18,000 women who enrolled at 84 birth centers across the United States. A full report of the study included descriptions of the birth center clients, birth center care providers, and birth center care. The study measured clinical outcomes of birth centers and compared them with outcomes of low-risk hospital births. Client satisfaction and satisfaction with charges were also measured. Findings from this study led the researchers to conclude that there is no evidence that hospitals are a safer place than birthing centers for low-risk births. While a complete summary is beyond the scope of this chapter, the three articles that provide the complete report are essential reading for CNMs.

A second study (Paine & Tinker Dawkins, 1992) compared two types of bearing-down techniques as they related to fetal and maternal outcomes of arterial umbilical cord blood pH and length of the second stage of labor. In this group, the care process was either using the Valsalva maneuver or spontaneous pushing. Although the subject size was small, the authors concluded that the bearing-down method does not have a negative effect on either the mother or the infant.

In another study, Oakley et al. (1996) compared the outcomes of women cared for by obstetricians and CNMs in a hospital-based setting. The authors reported that fiscal outcomes, specifically hospital charges and professional service fees, were significantly less for women in the nurse-midwife group. The lesser charges are especially interesting because the charge for obstetrician services and CNM services were the same in this institution. There was one bundled charge for all perinatal care, so the differences that existed between providers reflected charges beyond the usual and customary practice. Oakley also reported differences in clinical outcomes of infant–mother separation, extent of perineal laceration, and the number of maternal complications, with CNM providers being significantly lower on each outcome.

A study of macrosomic infant (birth weight greater than 4,000 g) outcomes (Nixon, Avery, & Savik, 1998) asked specific research questions: Is there a difference in Apgar scores, birth morbidity, and shoulder dystocias between infants with birth weights of 2,500 g to 3,999 g, 4,000 g to 4,499 g, and greater than 4,500 g? They also studied route of delivery, maternal position at birth, and antenatal variables that might predict poor infant outcomes. Shoulder dystocia occurred more frequently in large infants but intensive care unit (ICU) admission rates did not. Apgar scores at 1 and 5 minutes were significantly higher for infants weighing greater than 4,500 g. The Apgar differences were not clinically significant. The authors concluded that nurse-midwifery management of the labor of these mothers, in consultation with physicians, produced outcomes similar to those reported in the medical literature.

A study (Sampselle & Hines, 1999) examined the perineal outcomes of 39 women who had spontaneous vaginal births. Chart data were examined for documentation of extent of episiotomy and/or laceration sustained. Findings indicated that women who used spontaneous pushing were more likely to have intact perineum and less likely to have episiotomies and second- or third-degree lacerations. Although the results of this study are consistent with previous findings in the literature, the authors cite the need for conclusive evidence to be gathered in randomized clinical trials.

One comparison study (Jackson et al., 2003) looked at outcomes, safety, and resource utilization differences between traditional physician-based care and a collaborative-(CNM/obstetricians) management birth center. This study included 2,957 low-income pregnant women and their infants who presented for prenatal care at several sites. Data from this study revealed that complications in both groups were similar, while the collaborative care group had a greater number of spontaneous vaginal deliveries and less epidural anesthesia use. The study authors concluded that for low-risk women, both types of care result in safe outcomes for mothers, but there were fewer operative deliveries and less medical resources used in the collaborative-care groups.

A recent comparison study (Cragin & Kennedy, 2006) looked at midwifery and medical care practices and measured optimal perinatal outcomes in 375 moderate-risk women. This pilot study used a new instrument (the OI-US) to compare nurse-midwife and physician care among women who had moderate risk for poor pregnancy outcomes. The instrument consisted of scoring 40 care processes and outcomes across pregnancy, parturition, neonatal condition, and postpartum maternal condition, with higher average OI scores indicating more optimal balance between interventions and outcomes for a given health status. These data were collected from patient records. The authors of this study found that like groups of moderate-risk women cared for by nurse-midwives experienced less use of technology and equal or better health outcomes than women cared for by physicians and had equally positive neonatal outcomes. The researchers acknowledge a limitation of this study was the use of a relatively small convenience sample and recommend additional similar studies using this tool with similar populations of women.

Hastings-Tolsma et al. (2007) examined factors related to perineal trauma in childbirth. This retrospective analysis used recorded birth data from the Nurse Midwifery Clinical Data Set from 510 singleton pregnancies with uncomplicated prenatal courses. Data revealed that for all women, laceration was more likely in lithotomy position for birth. Factors found to be protective of the perineum during birth included perineal massage, warm-compress use, manual support, and birthing in the left lateral position. The authors concluded that side-lying position for birth and perineal support and compress use are important interventions for decreasing perineal trauma during childbirth.

A study published in 2012 by Neal and Lowe presented a partograph to assist with labor assessment in low-risk nulliparous women. The evidence-based tool was designed to correctly identify abnormal labor progression and provide an ongoing evaluation of interventions. The goal is to decrease the cesarean section rate in low-risk nulliparous women.

In 2014 *The Lancet* published a four-part series on the effects of midwifery. For this series the practice of midwifery was defined by the International Confederation of Midwives (2016) in terms of the work of midwives and core competencies and standards for their education and practice:

a midwife is a person who has successfully completed a midwifery education programme that is recognized in the country where it is located and this based on the ICM Essential Competencies for Basic Midwifery Practice and the framework of the ICM Global Standards of Midwifery Education: who has acquired the requisite qualification to be registered and or legally licensed to practice midwifery and use the title midwife and who demonstrates competency in the practice of midwifery.

Nurse-midwifery is included in this definition. A key message from this series regarding midwifery and quality of care from Renfrew et al. (2014) is that there is an improvement in the efficient use of resources and outcomes when midwives are educated in this manner.

Practicing in an environment that promotes effective teamwork, referral methods, and adequate resources increases the effectiveness of midwifery care and supports an integrative health system. A preventive, primary care approach, which focuses on the normal physiologic processes of birth (i.e., support of the mother and the infant including the ability to identify and treat pathology only when needed through interdisciplinary teams and integration across facilities and community settings) has shown to improve outcomes related to maternal and neonatal mortality. These outcomes include fetal loss, maternal morbidity related to preterm birth and reduced use of birth interventions, including cesarean section (Renfrew et al., 2014). Other outcomes that were improved included psychosocial, organizational, and community outcomes.

Homer, Friberg, Dias, Hoope-Bender et al. (2014) looked at the projected effect of scaling up midwifery services. The Lives Saved Tool (LiST) was used to estimate mortality outcomes in 78 countries. The Human Development Index (HDI) was used to classify these counties in terms of life expectancy, education, and income indexes. The countries were grouped into three groups, lowest HDI, low-to-moderate HDI, and moderate-to-high HDI. At all HDI levels about 30% of maternal deaths could be averted by midwifery care over the course of a 15-year period (Homer et al., 2014).

In 2016 Yang, Attanasion, and Kozhimannil (2016) looked at state scope of practice laws and childbirth-related procedures and outcomes. This study found that, in states where contractual agreements or supervision by physicians were not mandated by law, women had a nearly 60% greater chance of having a CNM attend her birth as well 13% lower odds of a cesarean delivery, 13% lower odds of a preterm birth, and 11% lower odds of a low-birth-weight baby. These findings were compared to women giving birth in states where there was a requirement for physician supervision or a contractual agreement. Women who have greater access to nurse-midwifery care have better outcomes.

SUMMARY

In 2009 CNMs attended 8.1% of all births and 11.4% of vaginal births (Declercq, 2012). This was a significant rise from 20 years earlier, when CNM-attended births were noted to represent 0.6% of all births (Martin et al., 2007). As the number of births attended by nurse-midwives increases, it is important to assess outcomes to justify fiscal, quality, and safety goals for the care of women and babies. Nurse-midwives are poised to improve the quality of health care and to act as change agents in the policy arena related to maternal care. This chapter has reviewed outcomes for nurse-midwifery practice. Some suggested outcome classifications in nurse-midwifery practice, including examples of specific client and aggregate data and outcome studies regarding nurse-midwifery practice, were presented. The definition of health care outcomes and the process of evaluating these in relation to nurse-midwifery practice have also been discussed.

Nurse-midwives should use the frameworks presented in this chapter to begin analyzing their practices and evaluating their own practice outcomes based on measurements used in previous studies. Evidence-based practice guidelines and protocols need to be evaluated and updated to reflect current clinical practice. Data demonstrating the safety, quality, and fiscal attributes provided by nurse-midwives need to be widely available for health care providers and consumers to evaluate when making decisions about maternal care. This information will increase the quality and safety of maternity care provided to women and babies and increase the availability of nurse-midwifery services.

Answers to Chapter Discussion Questions

1. Outcome measurement improves the quality of clinical care for patients by defining effective practice protocols. Practices and protocols that are evaluated and found to have best outcomes can be replicated, thus improving care for mothers and babies. Outcome measurement enhances cost-effectiveness. Through the use of

cost-effectiveness studies, alternative methods of obtaining the same goal are com-pared. Practices and protocols with satisfactory outcomes and lower cost can be iden-tified and implemented. Outcome measurement gives evidence and support for the practice of midwifery. Examples of quality outcomes can influence and increase appre-ciation and accessibility of nurse-midwifery practice in the United States.

2. Functional status includes the physical and emotional well-being of the mother; the cost of care, including both direct and indirect costs; patient satisfaction; and clinical outcomes.

3. Data were collected on four specific areas: functional status that includes the physi-cal and emotional well-being of the mother, cost of care including both direct and indirect costs, patient satisfaction, and clinical outcomes. Results of the data collection were compiled and nurse-midwifery services could see how they ranked compared with other practices for each indicator. Individual practices could then contact higher ranking services to learn best practices, which they could incorporate into their own practices.

4. The Optimality Index measures optimal maternity care. Optimal is defined as obtain-ing the best outcomes with the least amount of intervention, while taking into consid-eration the woman's physical and emotional status.

5. Physiological outcomes are those that have to do with the impact of CNM interven-tions on the process of birth. Perceptual outcomes are defined in terms of patient satis-faction. This may include satisfaction with CNMs as providers, with the facilities, with the care received, or with the clinical outcomes. Perception refers to the situation as the client views it or understands it. Psychosocial outcomes are those that have to do with such things as the client's affective state, self-image, self-esteem, and interpersonal relationships. Cognitive outcomes include the knowledge and skills that the client will need to safely and effectively care for herself and/or an infant. Functional outcomes have to do with the maintenance or improvement of physical functioning. Fiscal out-comes involve those having to do with the cost of care (cost per case, hospitalization costs and length of stay, incremental costs of specialized nursing care during labor, reimbursement by payer, and laboratory costs). The two approaches to the measure-ment of fiscal outcomes are cost data and charge data.

WEB LINKS

- AABC homepage: AABC is a multidisciplinary membership organization that com-prises individuals and institutions who support the birth center concept. The UDS registry is located on the organization's site. www.birthcenters.org
- ACNM homepage: The ACNM is the professional organization that represents CNMs and certified midwives (CMs). The site reports on the latest updates on nurse-mid-wifery practice and has links to professional resources, including results of the ACNM Benchmarking Project. www.midwife.org
- Childbirth Connections: This national nonprofit organization evolved from the Maternity Center Association, founded in 1918. It is committed to transforming mater-nity care through evidence-based practice and consumer education. Results from the

Listening to Mothers national survey can be found here. www.childbirthconnection .org/home.asp?Visitor=Professional

Journal of Midwifery & Women's Health. The peer-reviewed journal of the ACNM presents evidence-based practice research in the areas of maternity care, gynecology, primary care for women and newborns, public health, health care policy, and global health. onlinelibrary.wiley.com

REFERENCES

Adams, T. P. (1996). Case mix index: Nursing's new management tool. *Nursing Management, 27*(9), 31–32.

Alvidrez, J., Azocar, F., & Miranda, J. (1996). Demystifying the concept of ethnicity for psychotherapy researchers. *Journal of Consulting and Clinical Psychology, 64*(5), 903–908.

American Association of Birth Centers. (2007). American association of birth centers. Retrieved from http://www.birthcenters.org

American College of Nurse-Midwives. (2008). Nurse-midwifery in 2008: Evidence-based practice. A summary of research on midwifery practice in the United States. Retrieved from http://www .midwife.org/siteFiles/news/nurse_midwifery_in_2008.pdf

American College of Nurse-Midwives. (2011). CNM/CN attended births. Retrieved from http:// www.midwife.org/CNM/CM-attended-Birth-Statistics

American College of Nurse-Midwives. (2012). California state fact sheet. Retrieved from http:// www.midwife.org/index.asp?bid=&cat=11&button=Search&rec=177

Anderson, R. E., & Anderson, D. A. (1999). The cost effectiveness of home birth. *Journal of Nurse Midwifery, 44,* 30–35.

Breckinridge, M. (1981). *Wide neighborhoods: A story of the frontier nursing service.* Lexington: The University Press of Kentucky.

Browne, H. E., & Isaacs, G. (1976). The frontier nursing service: The primary care nurse in the community hospital. *American Journal of Obstetrics and Gynecology, 124*(1), 14–17.

Center for Medicare and Medicaid Innovation. (2012). Strong start for mothers and newborns. Retrieved from http://innovations.cms.gov/initiatives/strong-start/index.html

Cherry, J., & Foster, J. (1982). Comparison of hospital charges generated by certified nurse-midwives' and physicians' clients. *Journal of Nurse-Midwifery, 77*(1), 7–11.

Collins-Fulea, C., Mohr, J. J., & Tillett, J. (2005). Improving midwifery practice: The American college of nurse-midwives' benchmarking project. *Journal of Midwifery & Women's Heath, 50*(6), 461–471.

Cragin, L., & Kennedy, P. (2006). Linking obstetric and midwifery practice with optimal outcomes. *The Association of Women's Health, Obstetric and Neonatal Nurses, 35*(6), 779–785.

Declercq, E. (2012). Trends in midwife-attended births in the United States, 1982–2009. *Journal of Midwifery & Woman's Health, 57,* 321–326.

Foster, S. L., & Martinez, C. R. (1995). Ethnicity: Conceptual and methodological issues in child clinical research. *Journal of Clinical Child Psychology, 24,* 214–226.

Governor's Health Reform Commission. (2007). *Roadmap for Virginia's health: A report of the governor's health reform commission.* Retrieved from http://www.hhr.virginia.gov/Initiatives/HealthReform/MeetingMats/FullCouncil/Health_ReformComm_Draft_Report.pdf

Hastings-Tolsma, M., Vincent, D., Emesis, C., & Francisco, T. (2007). Getting through birth in one piece: Protecting the perineum. *Maternal Child Nursing, 32*(3), 158–164.

Hatem, M., Sandall, J., Devance, D., Soltani, H., & Gates, S. (2009). Midwife-led versus other models of care for childbearing women. *The Cochrane Library, 2009*(3), 1–109.

Homer, C., Friberg, I., Dias, M., et al. (2014). The projected effect of scaling up midwifery. *The Lancet, 384* (9948), 1129–1145.

International Confederation of Midwives. (2016). ICM Definition of the Midwife. Retrieved from http://www.internationalmidwives.org/who-we-are/policy-and-practice/icm-international-definition-of-the-midwife

Jackson, D. J., Lang, J. M., Swartz, W. H., Ganiants, T. G., Fullerton, J., Ecker, J., & Nguyen, U. (2003). Outcomes, safety, and resource utilization in a collaborative care birth center program compared with traditional physician-based perinatal care. *American Journal of Public Health, 93*(6), 999–1006.

Levy, B. S., Wilkinson, F. S., & Marine, W. M. (1971). Reducing neonatal mortality rate with nurse-midwives. *American Journal of Obstetrics and Gynecology, 109*(1), 50–58.

Lubic, R. (1981). Evaluation of an out-of-hospital maternity center for low-risk maternity patients. In L. Aiken (Ed.), *Health policy and nursing practice.* New York, NY: McGraw-Hill.

Martin, J. A., Hamilton, B. E., Sutton, P. D., Ventura, S. J., Menacker, F., . . . Munson, M. L. (2007). Births: Final data for 2005. *National Vital Statistics Reports, 56*(6), 1–103.

Montgomery, T. W. (1969). A case for nurse-midwives. *American Journal of Obstetrics & Gynecology, 105,* 309–313.

Murray, M. E., & Atkinson, L. D. (2000). *Understanding the nursing process in a changing care environment* (6th ed.). New York, NY: McGraw-Hill.

Neal, J., & Lowe, N. (2012). Physiologic partograph improve birth safety and outcomes among low risk, nulliparous women with spontaneous labor onset. *Medical Hypotheses, 76*(2), 319–326.

Nixon, S. A., Avery, M. D., & Savik, K. (1998). Outcomes of macrosomic infants in a nurse-midwifery service. *Journal of Nurse Midwifery, 43*(4), 280–286.

Oakley, D., Murray, M. E., Murtland, T., Hayashi, R., Anderson, H. F., Mayes, F., & Rooks, J. (1996). Comparisons of outcomes of maternity care by obstetricians and certified nurse midwives. *American Journal of Obstetrics & Gynecology, 88*(5), 823–829.

Paine, L. L., & Tinker Dawkins, D. (1992). The effect of maternal bearing-down efforts on arterial umbilical cord pH and length of the second stage of labor. *Journal of Nurse-Midwifery, 37*(1), 61–63.

Reid, M., & Morris, J. (1979). Prenatal care and cost effectiveness: Changes in health expenditures and birth outcomes following the establishment of a nurse-midwife program. *Medical Care, 17*(5), 491–500.

Renfrew, M., McFadden, A., & Bastos, M. H., Campbell, J., Channon, A. A., Cheung, N. F., . . . Declercq, E. (2014). Midwifery and quality care: Findings from a new evidence-informed framework for maternal and newborn care. *The Lancet, 384* (9948), 1129–1145.

Robinson, J., Norwitz, E., Cohen, A., & Lieberman, E. (2000). Predictors of episiotomy use at first spontaneous vaginal delivery. *American Journal of Obstetrics and Gynecology, 96*(2), 214–218.

Rooks, J. P., Weatherby, N. L., Ernst, E. K. M., Stapleton, S., Rosen, D., & Rosenfield, A. (1989). Outcomes of care in birth centers: The national birth center study. *The New England Journal of Medicine, 321,* 1804–1811.

Sampselle, C., & Hines, S. L. (1999). Spontaneous pushing during birth: Relationship to perineal outcomes. *Journal of Nurse-Midwifery, 44*(1), 36–39.

Selwyn, B. J. (1990). The accuracy of obstetric risk assessment instruments for predicting mortality, low birth weight, and preterm birth. In J. Merkatz & J. Thompson (Eds.), *New perspectives on premature care.* New York, NY: Elsevier.

Stapleton, S. R. (2011). Validation of an online data registry for midwifery practices: A pilot. *Journal of Midwifery & Women's Health, 56*(5), 452–460.

Stapleton, S. R., Osborne, C., & Illuzzi, J. (2013). Outcomes of care in birth centers: Demonstration of a durable model. *Journal of Midwifery & Women's Health, 58*(1), 3–14.

Stewart, R., & Clark, L. (1982). Nurse-midwifery practice in an in-hospital birthing center. *Journal of Nurse-Midwifery, 27,* 21–26.

Tulman, L., & Fawcett, J. (1988). Return of functional ability after childbirth. *Nursing Research, 37,* 77–81.

Tulman, L., Fawcett, J., Groblewski, L., & Silverman, L. (1990). Changes in functional status after childbirth. *Nursing Research, 39,* 70–75.

Yang, Y., Attanasio, L., & Kozhimannil, K. (2016). State scope of practice laws, nurse-midwifery workforce, and childbirth procedures and outcomes. *Women's Health Issues: Official Publication of the Jacobs Institute of Women's Health, 26*(3), 262–267.

CHAPTER 10

Outcome Assessment in Nurse Anesthesia

Michael J. Kremer and Margaret Faut Callahan

Chapter Objectives

1. Describe the historical influences on outcome assessment of nurse anesthesia practice
2. List constraining variables that limit research opportunities in the area of nurse anesthesia outcomes
3. Review the outcomes to date of linking pay to performance for surgical procedures
4. Suggest next steps for cost-effectiveness analyses of nurse anesthesia care
5. Examine the role of human patient simulation in knowledge transfer to the clinical area and risk reduction
6. Discuss the risks for certified registered nurse anesthetists (CRNAs) associated with participation in prospective, multicenter anesthesia outcome studies

Chapter Discussion Questions

1. What was the impetus for the development of closed malpractice claims research in anesthesia?
2. What is the relationship between human patient simulation and outcomes in anesthesia care?
3. Why did investigators posit that Surgical Care Improvement Project (SCIP) compliance should not be used to determine Medicare and Medicaid reimbursement rates?

4. Regarding adverse perioperative outcomes, how is the role of anesthesia versus that of surgery in contributing to the adverse outcome determined?

5. What enabling and constraining factors are related to the implementation of evidence-based practice (EBP)?

AN OVERVIEW OF OUTCOME RESEARCH IN NURSE ANESTHESIA

Nurse anesthetists have provided anesthesia care to patients in the United States for more than 150 years. This was the first advanced practice nursing specialty to have a certification exam, implemented in 1956. Successful examinees are known as *certified registered nurse anesthetists* (CRNAs). Some 50,000 CRNAs administer 43 million anesthetics annually in the United States (American Association of Nurse Anesthetists [AANA], 2016a).

Assessing outcomes of nurse anesthesia care is an essential component of CRNA practice. Participating in quality assessment activities is among the *Standards for Accreditation of Nurse Anesthesia Programs, Practice Doctorate* (2016) promulgated by the Council on Accreditation of Nurse Anesthesia Educational Programs (COA, 2016), the *Scope of Nurse Anesthesia Practice* (AANA, 2013a), and the *Standards for Nurse Anesthesia Practice* (AANA, 2013b). Studies have compared outcomes of care provided by various mixes of anesthesia providers (Dulisse & Cromwell, 2010; Hogan, Seifert, Moore, & Simonson, 2010; Lewis, Nicholson, Smith, & Alderson, 2014; Needleman & Minnick, 2009; Negrusa, Hogan, Warner, Schroeder, & Pang, 2016; Simonson, Ahern, & Hendryx, 2007) and have demonstrated satisfactory clinical outcomes with anesthesia provided by CRNAs. However, there are no prospective multicenter studies on anesthesia outcomes.

Methodological challenges in anesthesia outcome research include the various mixes of anesthesia providers and the complexity of health care settings where anesthesia services are delivered. CRNAs provide anesthesia services in hospital operating rooms, labor and delivery suites, and in numerous ancillary areas, including cardiac catheterization laboratories, endoscopy suites, and interventional radiology settings. CRNAs may be the sole anesthesia providers in rural and medically underserved areas as well as in forward-deployed military operations (Liao, Quraishi, & Jordan, 2015). Anesthesia in ambulatory surgery centers and office-based practices may be provided by a CRNA working collaboratively with a surgeon, dentist, or podiatrist. In some clinical settings, an anesthesiologist may work collaboratively with two to four CRNAs administering concurrent anesthetics.

The earliest outcome research in nurse anesthesia was conducted by pioneering nurse anesthetist Alice Magaw. Magaw was a nurse anesthetist at the Mayo Clinic and published a paper in the *Northwestern Lancet* in 1899 detailing over 3,000 ether and chloroform anesthetics she administered without a fatality (Magaw, 1899). These anesthetics were administered to patients undergoing operations ranging from general to orthopedic; ear, nose, and throat; gynecological; and urological surgeries. Note that endotracheal intubation was not common until the mid-20th century, and that Korotkoff did not identify the five sounds associated with blood pressure measurement until 1905. Magaw published a total of five peer-reviewed papers, including "Observations Drawn From

Experiences of Eleven Thousand Anesthesias" (Magaw, 1904) and "A Review of Over Fourteen Thousand Surgical Anaesthesias" (Magaw, 1906).

It is likely that subsequent legal challenges to nurse anesthesia practice were defeated through the documentation of safe, quality care provided by Magaw (Bankert, 1989). Like Nightingale (McDonald, 2001), this nurse anesthesia leader recognized that in addition to clinical excellence, documenting clinical outcomes and disseminating research findings in peer-reviewed literature were requisites of professionalism. Magaw's outcome research also influenced the pivotal 1917 judicial ruling in the *Frank v. South* case where a Kentucky court found that when anesthesia is practiced by a nurse, it is the practice of nursing, and when anesthesia is practiced by a physician, it is the practice of medicine (Blumenreich, 1990).

STUDIES OF ANESTHESIA OUTCOMES

Municipal or state-level study commissions that examined anesthetic morbidity and mortality in the 1930s and 1940s were hampered by the unwillingness of anesthesia providers to share their data (Ruth, 1945). No concerted effort was made to track anesthetic outcomes until the 1950s.

The first large-scale study of anesthesia morbidity and mortality was conducted by Beecher and Todd (1954). Muscle relaxants were found to be significantly associated with anesthetic morbidity and mortality. Almost 60 years later, investigators noted a high incidence of postoperative residual blockade in contemporary anesthesia practices, despite the advances in pharmacology, technology, and provider education (Murphy, 2012).

In the 1970s, a rapid increase in malpractice insurance premiums prompted a new research method for investigating anesthetic outcomes: analysis of closed malpractice claims. Pioneered by the National Association of Insurance Commissioners, this methodology was adopted by the American Society of Anesthesiologists (ASA), which has conducted the largest anesthesia closed claims study to date with nearly 9,000 cases reviewed (Brunner, 1984; Cheney, 2010; Metzner, Posner, Lam, & Domino, 2011). Over 50 publications in peer-reviewed journals have emanated from this study, often with the focus of lessons learned in specific practice-related areas such as equipment, airway management, and specialty practice areas. Recent publications include risk factors associated with ischemic optic neuropathy after spinal fusion surgery (Lee et al., 2012); cervical spinal cord, root and bony spine injuries (Hindman et al., 2011); injury and liability associated with cervical procedures for chronic pain (Ramthell et al., 2011); and malpractice claims associated with medication management for chronic pain (Fitzgibbon et al., 2010).

The American Association of Nurse Anesthetists Foundation (AANAF) has also conducted a closed claims study that is methodologically similar to the ASA study. Peer-reviewed papers related to this study have also focused on lessons learned in specific areas such as preinduction activities and the genesis of perioperative respiratory, peripheral nerve, and other injuries (Jordan & Quraishi, 2015; MacRae, 2007). Distinctions in outcomes among anesthesia providers have not been described in these studies.

Research findings from both the AANAF and ASA studies demonstrate that the process of care, rather than patient acuity or procedure complexity, is most frequently associated with outcomes that are not optimal (MacRae, 2007). Human patient simulation has been used as an instructional tool for clinicians and trainees to foster improved decision making and reinforce principles of care to decrease the incidence of adverse outcomes. Maintenance of certification programs may utilize simulation as well as other instructional methods to assess continued professional competence (AANA, 2016b).

HUMAN PATIENT SIMULATION AND ANESTHESIA PRACTICE

The use of human patient simulation in the context of high-fidelity simulation labs provides trainees and practitioners with opportunities to develop crisis management skills in rarely occurring, potentially fatal scenarios as well as fostering nontechnical skills, such as clinical decision making (Turcato, Roberson, & Covert, 2008; Wunder, 2016). As human patient simulation has been increasingly incorporated in nurse anesthesia education, educators have developed rubrics for evaluation of student performance in simulation scenarios (Overstreet, McCarver, Shields, & Patterson, 2015).

The best features and practices of simulation-based education in health care have been described as:

- Feedback provided to learners
- Deliberate practice that occurs away from the bedside
- Integration of simulation into health sciences curriculum
- Measurement of outcomes that may be influenced by simulation
- Fidelity of simulation
- Acquisition and maintenance of skills, for example, management of difficult airways, placement of central venous catheters
- Mastery learning, for example, the ability to practice skills in the simulation lab before performing the same skills at the bedside
- Transfer of simulation-based learning to clinical practice
- Team training
- High-stakes testing
- Instructor training (McGaghie, Darycott, Dunn, Lopez, & Stefanidis, 2011; McGaghie, Issenberg, Petrusa, & Scaelse, 2010)

The impact and educational utility of simulation-based education in health care are likely to increase in the future. However, simulation labs currently vary significantly in terms of their infrastructure and available resources. The Society for Simulation in Healthcare (SSiH) has developed criteria for the certification of simulation instructors and accreditation standards for simulation labs. At the time of writing, 54 of over 300 simulation labs worldwide have fulfilled the criteria for SSiH accreditation (SSiH, 2015). Recent papers in peer-reviewed journals attest to the growing contributions of human patient simulation in the areas of safety and quality in clinical care (Kim, Park, & Shin, 2016; Stephens, Hunninger, Mills & Freeth, 2016; Wunder, 2016).

There is a developing body of research evidence showing that there is knowledge transfer from the simulation lab to clinical practice with beneficial effects on clinical outcomes. For example, clinicians who participate in simulation-based training on difficult airway management have decreased incidences of failed airway management scenarios.

In addition to decreasing the potential morbidity and mortality associated with airway mishaps, operating room time and professional fees based on time are decreased when less clinical time is required to teach trainees these skills at the bedside. However, there remain critical challenges and gaps in research on the transfer of knowledge, skills, and abilities from the simulation lab to clinical practice (McGaghie et al., 2011).

Another use of human patient simulation that has been described occurs during the interview process for prospective nurse anesthesia students. Applicants are assigned to small groups and provided with a critical scenario in which they must work collaboratively (Penprase et al., 2012). This type of observed interaction and operationalization of critical care nursing skills may provide useful information that is predictive of the potential success of these applicants in a nurse anesthesia program.

CLINICAL OUTCOMES, SAFETY, AND QUALITY

As noted earlier, a methodological and design challenge for outcome research is that anesthetic mortality occurs rarely today, with approximately one death in 200,000 cases (Li, Warner, Lang, Huang, & Sun, 2009). The Centers for Medicare & Medicaid Services (CMS), the American Hospital Association, the ASA, the American College of Surgeons, and the Veterans Administration developed a strategy to reduce surgical morbidity over a 5-year period (Lema, 2003). The result of that collaboration was the SCIP. The goal of SCIP was to reduce surgical complication by 25%. These data are publicly reported on the CMS Hospital Compare website (Medicare, 2016). SCIP measures include the following:

- SCIP Inf-1: prophylactic antibiotics are received within 1 hour before surgical incision
- SCIP Inf-2: prophylactic antibiotic selection for surgical patients
- SCIP Inf-3: prophylactic antibiotics discontinued within 24 hours after surgery end time
- SCIP Inf-4: cardiac surgery patients with controlled 6:00 a.m. postoperative glucose
- SCIP Inf-6: surgery patients with appropriate hair removal
- SCIP Info-10: surgery patients with perioperative temperature management
- SCIP Card-2: surgery patients on beta-blocker therapy before arrival who received a beta-blocker during the perioperative period
- SCIP VTE-1: surgery patients with recommended venous thromboembolism (VTE) prophylaxis ordered
- SCIP VTE-2: surgery patients who received appropriate VTE prophylaxis within 24 hours before surgery to 24 hours after surgery (Thiemann & McFadden, 2010)

SCIP compliance affects Medicare and Medicaid reimbursement rates. Studies have examined compliance with the SCIP surgical site infection (SSI) module, requiring prophylactic antibiotic administration 1 hour prior to surgical incision to determine whether compliance with SCIP correlated with SSI rates reported by the National Surgery Quality Improvement Program (NSQIP) data for the same period. The authors found no statistically significant association in patients whose care failed SCIP Inf-1 guidelines and the rates of SSI. These investigators posited that SCIP compliance should not be used to determine Medicare and Medicaid reimbursement rates because there was no observed correlation between failure of SCIP Inf-1 and SSI (Garcia, Fogel, Baker, Remine, & Jones, 2012). Other studies have demonstrated a modest association with process measures and patient outcomes (Thiemann & McFadden, 2010).

CMS has developed the Ambulatory Surgical Center (ASC) Quality Reporting (ASCQR) Program, which is a pay-for-reporting, quality data program. Under this program, ASCs report quality of care data for standardized measures to "receive the full annual update to their ASC annual payment rate" (CMS, 2016a). These measures include:

- Patient burns
- Patient falls
- Wrong site/wrong side/wrong patient/wrong procedure/wrong implant
- Hospital transfer/admission
- Prophylactic antibiotics within 1 hour of procedure
- Use of patient safety checklist, for example, World Health Organization (WHO) checklist (WHO, 2012). Facility volume data on selected procedures
- Influenza vaccination coverage among health care providers (CMS, 2016a)

As members of multidisciplinary teams providing perioperative care in both inpatient and outpatient settings, CRNAs exert leadership daily, helping to ensure compliance with regulatory guidelines. Measures of compliance with these guidelines reflect the outcomes of direct patient care and leadership provided by CRNAs.

Regarding variables related to anesthesia care, it is difficult to classify anesthesia-specific events versus surgery-specific events. Outcomes such as epidural abscesses following neuraxial anesthesia or patient awareness under general anesthesia are more likely to be associated with anesthesia care. However, there is not a validated algorithm to identify outcomes directly related to anesthesia care (Thiemann & McFadden, 2010).

As noted earlier, there are no ongoing prospective multicenter studies of anesthesia outcomes. Creation of a national health information network (NHIN) will facilitate national quality improvement activities. The NHIN is a set of standards, services, and policies that allow for secure web-supported health information exchange. This network provides a foundation for exchange of health information across diverse entities. NHIN is a simple, secure, scalable standards-based method for participants to send authenticated, encrypted health information directly to known and trusted recipients over the Internet (HealthIT, 2016). Outcomes tracked in this manner can provide data that substantiate the safety and quality of services provided by CRNAs and other advanced practice registered nurses (APRNs).

Performance measures are critical to the national effort to ensure that patients receive appropriate and high-quality care. Pay for performance (P4P), or value-based purchasing, has endeavored to link clinical outcomes with reimbursement. P4P also includes disincentives for negative consequences of care or increased costs for "never" events, for example, wrong-site surgery, operative or postoperative complications, and medication errors (Agency for Healthcare Research and Quality [AHRQ], 2012a).

Investigators used Medicare data to examine 30-day mortality among over 6 million patients who had acute myocardial infarction, congestive heart failure, or pneumonia, or who underwent coronary artery bypass grafting between 2003 and 2009. These researchers found no evidence that the largest hospital-based P4P program led to decreases in

30-day mortality among these patients and suggested that expectations for improved outcomes related to P4P should be modest (Jha, Joynt, Orav, & Epstein, 2012).

Accountable care organizations (ACOs) consist of provider groups that voluntarily collaborate to give high-quality care to Medicare patients. The intent of coordinated care is to limit unnecessary duplication of health care service as well as prevent medical errors. When ACOs deliver high-quality care while containing costs, they share in the savings achieved for Medicare (CMS, 2016b). Given the large number of Medicare beneficiaries who undergo surgery each year, ACOs provide a mechanism to quantify the contributions of CRNAs and other APRNs while contributing to cost containment.

The Physician Quality Reporting System (PQRS) "is a quality reporting program that uses negative payment adjustment to promote reporting of quality information by individual eligible professionals and group practices." Those who do not satisfactorily report data on quality measures for covered Medicare Physician Fee Schedule (MPFS) services furnished to Medicare Part B beneficiaries will be subject to a negative payment adjustment under PQRS (CMS, 2016c). PQRS is applicable to CRNAs, since this provider group has had direct reimbursement under Medicare Part B since 1989.

Guidance on PQRS reporting for CRNAs is reported on the AANA website. Related issues include:

- Verification of correct reporting and whether a payment adjustment will be provided
- Information included in individual PQRS feedback reports
- The process for requesting a review of PRS payment adjustments
- Reasons for receiving a negative payment adjustment

Reimbursement models that reflect clinical outcomes continue to evolve. The Medicare Access and CHIP (Children's Health Insurance Program) Reauthorization Act of 2015 (MACRA) will create two new payment systems for clinicians, affecting more than 600,000 physicians, nurse practitioners, physician assistant and therapists, the majority of the clinicians billing Medicare. In 2019, clinicians will be able to earn higher levels of reimbursement if they adopt new business modes called alternative payment models. That involves a willingness to accept financial risk and reward for performance, reporting quality measures to the government, and using electronic medical records. Most clinical practitioners are expected to follow a track called the merit-based incentive payment system that will feature a more modest financial risk and reward accounting system for quality, efficiency, and use of electronic medical records (Alonso-Zaldivar, 2016).

OUTCOMES IN RURAL SETTINGS

Nurse anesthetists are the primary anesthesia providers in rural America, which enables health care facilities in these medically underserved settings to offer obstetrical, surgical, and trauma stabilization services. In some states, nurse anesthetists are the sole anesthesia providers in nearly 100% of rural hospitals (AANA, 2016a). Little outcome research exists on anesthesia provided in rural America.

Rural CRNAs provide a broad range of anesthesia-related services within and outside of the operating room. One study found significant differences in the employment settings of medically directed and nonmedically directed CRNAs, the availability of certain anesthetic agents and monitoring devices, and the representation of surgical specialists based on the size of the rural community and hospital. However, this study did not examine anesthetic or surgical outcomes (Monti Seibert, Alexander, & Lupien, 2004).

An analysis of cesarean section outcomes showed no difference in complication rates when anesthesia was provided by a CRNA or a CRNA–physician team. Because solo CRNAs often provide anesthesia in rural settings, these findings help to quantify the outcomes of CRNA-provided anesthesia in rural settings (Simonson et al., 2007).

CRNAs provide more anesthesia services to citizens in vulnerable populations, including those with lower incomes, Medicaid-eligible, uninsured, and the unemployed, than do anesthesiologists. This is also reflected in the geographic maldistribution of anesthesia providers, with more CRNAs in rural and medical underserved settings and greater numbers of anesthesiologists in urban areas. The Affordable Care Act seeks to ensure that the population has adequate insurance coverage. Removal of barriers to CRNA scope of practice to maximize the delivery of anesthesia services by CRNAs will facilitate addressing the unmet health care needs of vulnerable populations (Liao et al., 2015).

"Placing unnecessary restrictions via limiting scope of practice for CRNAs may hinder patient access to a readily available workforce where patients may incur a higher indirect cost, i.e., travel expense, time off work, for an anesthesiologist's care when a CRNA is nearby" (Liao et al., 2015). Geographic location as well as socioeconomic factors influence access to anesthesia care.

OUTCOME MEASUREMENT IN NURSE ANESTHESIA

The safety and cost-effectiveness of care provided by CRNAs has been established in research findings (Dulisse & Cromwell, 2010; Hogan et al., 2010; Needleman & Minnick, 2009). The influence of scope of practice laws on outcomes by anesthesia providers has also been studied (Negrusa et al., 2016).

In one large commercial payer database, eight in every 10,000 anesthesia-related procedures have a complication. These complications were four times more likely in inpatient versus outpatient settings. The odds for complication differ with patient characteristics, including comorbidities, as well as the involved procedures. The probability of anesthesia-related complications is higher in procedures related to childbirth. However, the likelihood of anesthesia-related complications occurring is not affected by scope of practice laws or anesthesia delivery models, such as, CRNA only, anesthesiologist only, or mixed anesthesiologist and CRNA team. Patient characteristics, including comorbid conditions and the procedures requiring anesthesia are what affect anesthesia outcomes, independent of the anesthesia provider mix (Negrusa et al., 2016).

A Cochrane review studied the impact of increasing demand for surgery, cost-containment measures, and the anesthesia workforce on anesthesia outcomes. Analysis of six relevant studies with 1.5 million participants from Medicare in the United States and hospital records (Haiti) provided the basis for this review (Lewis et al., 2014).

Research findings demonstrated there was no difference in anesthesia-related mortality based on whether the anesthesia was provided by a nurse anesthetist or an anesthesiologist. The findings of one study indicated that anesthesia-related mortality was lower for solo nurse anesthetists versus nurse anesthetists supervised by anesthesiologists. Variations between studies and complication rates depending on the anesthesia provider were also noted. Since much of the data used for this analysis came from large databases, inaccuracies in reporting may have occurred. Differences that may have accounted for the variability in reported results included patient acuity, analytic methods, and funding sources for the reported research. Since data were not of consistent quality and studies presented inconsistent findings, it was not possible to demonstrate differences in the care provided by anesthesiologists and nurse anesthetists (Lewis et al., 2014).

NURSE ANESTHESIA OUTCOME MEASURES AND PROJECTS

The AANAF began in 1981. The mission of the foundation is "to advance the science of anesthesia through education and research." As the philanthropic arm of the AANA, the foundation raises funds and invests in projects that directly support the nurse anesthesia profession (AANAF, 2016).

The AANA and AANAF support health services research endeavors in these areas:

- Health policy
- Science of anesthesia
- Education
- Practice/clinical
- Leadership (AANA, 2016c)

Continued efforts to fund research in these areas helps to ensure dissemination of findings in peer-reviewed journals. These research findings provide the basis for demonstrating the safety, quality, and cost-effectiveness of nurse anesthesia care to the public, legislators, and regulators.

During the 2016 fiscal year, the foundation supported more than 180 CRNAs and students through awarded scholarships, fellowships, research grants, and poster presentations, conducted workshops that educated 100 CRNAs and students, as well as honoring four exceptional CRNAs (AANAF, 2016). The foundation funds health services research. Research sponsored by the foundation has resulted in findings that substantiate the safety, quality, and cost-effectiveness of anesthesia services provided by CRNAs (Dulisse & Cromwell, 2010; Liao et al.; Needleman & Minnick, 2009; Simonson et al., 2007).

EVIDENCE-BASED PRACTICE

New clinical information is generated more quickly than it can be assimilated by trainees and practicing clinicians. Nurse anesthesia students, faculty, and practitioners need the most current information regarding health care and anesthesia practice. This information need is acute for student registered nurse anesthetists, because they must rapidly learn complex specialty-related content and use this information to justify clinical actions to their faculty (Pellegrini, 2006). Using EBP concepts helps balance the demand for current information with the exponentially increasing supply of specialty-related research information.

EBP has been described as "the integration of individual clinical expertise with the best available external clinical evidence from systematic research" (Sackett, Rosenberg, Gray, Haynes, & Richardson, 2007). Health care professionals may believe that their practices have always reflected evidence-based underpinnings, but performance assessments indicate this is not the case (McGlynn et al., 2003). Current literature advocates increased adoption of EBP, but EBP implementation is inconsistent (Kavey, 2008).

The Institute of Medicine Committee on the Health Professions Education Summit suggested a paradigm shift for health professions education. The principal goal of this process was that "all health professionals will be educated to deliver patient-centric care as members of an interdisciplinary team, emphasizing evidence-based practice, quality improvement approaches, and informatics" (Greiner & Knebel, 2003).

The American Association of Colleges of Nursing (AACN), health educators, and foundations released competencies and action strategies for interprofessional education in 2011. The goal for operationalization of these competencies is transformation of the health care delivery system to provide collaborative, high-quality, and cost-effective care to better serve every patient. The Core Competencies for Interprofessional Collaborative Practice identified four domains of core competencies needed to provide integrated, high-quality care to patients in the current health care delivery system. The panel recommended that future health professionals be able to:

- Assert values and ethics of interprofessional practice by placing the interests, dignity, and respect of patients at the center of health care delivery and embracing the cultural diversity and differences of health care teams
- Leverage the unique roles and responsibilities of interprofessional partners to appropriately assess the health care needs of patients and populations served
- Communicate with patients, families, communities, and other health professionals in support of a team approach to preventing disease and disability, maintaining health, and treating disease
- Perform effectively in various team roles to deliver patient/population-centered care that is safe, timely, efficient, and equitable (AACN, 2011a)

Another report, "Team-Based Competencies, Building a Shared Foundation for Educational and Clinical Practice," was derived from a meeting that was held in 2011 and included 80 leaders from diverse health professions who previewed the Interprofessional Education Collaborative (IPEC) core competencies. These leaders created action strategies to transform health professional education and health care delivery in the United States (AACN, 2011b). Utilization of these competencies in the context of interprofessional education and practice has great potential to positively impact health care, including care delivered by APRNs, including CRNAs.

The paradigm shift that is occurring in health care includes the movement of health care delivery away from the traditional physician-dominated practice toward the concept of the physician as team leader, seeking the best evidence for patient care. Ideally, such physicians and teams will have the ability and expectation to continuously learn and change through utilization of evidence-based clinical support, informatics, and clinical data repositories. The potential scope of this initiative clearly includes all health professionals (Kavey, 2008).

Nurses may have the most experience in using EBP, with a record dating back to the time of Florence Nightingale (McDonald, 2001). Nurses are the largest group of health care providers, numbering 3,100,000 (American Nurses Association [ANA], 2012). The projected job growth in nursing over the time frame of 2008 to 2018 is 581,500, reflecting a 22% growth in nursing employment. The demand for nurse anesthetists is growing at a similar rate.

A survey of 3,000 licensed nurses in the United States demonstrated that almost half of the respondents were unfamiliar with the term "evidence-based medicine." More than half of these survey respondents had not identified a clinical problem that required research, and 43% "sometimes, rarely, or never" read nursing journals or texts (Pravikoff, Tanner, & Pierce, 2005).

Significant information literacy and access to adequate information technology are needed for implementation of EBP with tools such as best-practice databases, clinical practice guidelines, electronic medical records, and computerized physician-order entry. Nurses report that access to evidence-based information can be "extremely difficult." Fewer than 50% of respondents to the Pravikoff et al. (2005) survey reported available workstation access to the Internet. This may be offset by the increasing use of smartphones with functional web browsers. However, attitudes toward EBP are complex, with a majority of nurses identifying a colleague or supervisor as their primary information source, rather than any independent literature source.

One suggested educational direction is to include EBP as a core competency throughout all levels of nursing curricula. Related competencies should include formation of PICOT questions, where P = patient population, I = intervention or area of interest, C = comparison intervention or comparison group, O = outcome, and T = time frame. Students and practitioners need to be able to search for the best evidence, for example, specifically pre-appraised evidence and evidence-based clinical practice guidelines, and integrate the best evidence with their clinical expertise and patient preferences related to clinical decisions. Students also need to be able to assess outcomes based on EBP changes and participate in team EBP projects. Graduate students should be required to demonstrate facility with synthesizing a body of evidence to initiate and evaluate practice changes to improve the health of individuals, lead practice changes based on the best evidence for populations of patients, generate evidence through outcome management, and mentor others in EBP (National League for Nursing [NLN], 2008).

It is difficult for practitioners and trainees to remain current with the relevant advances in their fields of interest. The major bibliographic databases cover less than half of the world's literature and are biased toward English-language publications. Textbooks, editorials, and reviews that have not been systematically prepared may be unreliable. Much evidence is unpublished, and yet unpublished data may have clinical significance. More easily accessible research papers tend to exaggerate the benefits of interventions.

The Cochrane Library consists of a regularly updated collection of EBP databases including The Cochrane Database of Systematic Reviews. This database includes systematic reviews of health care interventions that are produced and disseminated by the Cochrane Collaboration. The Cochrane Library is published quarterly and is available in digital format and online. Abstracts of the reviews are available to browse and search without charge on this website (www.cochrane.org; Cochrane Collaboration, 2012).

Anesthesia-related Cochrane reviews topics include the previously referenced paper comparing anesthesia outcomes by provider types (Lewis et al., 2014).

NURSE ANESTHESIA COMPETENCIES, CURRICULAR MODELS, AND EBP

Organizations seek to identify the core capabilities, or competencies, that have sustainable value and wide applicability to the customers they serve. Professional nursing organizations that serve the interests of patients generally identify role-related competencies that describe their vision of the skills and abilities that the individual must possess (Callahan, 1988). For example, the AANA (2005) *Code of Ethics for the Certified Registered Nurse Anesthetists* describes "competence" as including involvement with lifelong professional educational activities, participating in continuous quality improvement initiatives, and maintaining licensure according to the statutory and regulatory requirements for recertification.

In education, AANA has adopted doctoral-level educational competencies required of the CRNA for entry into practice. These are the acquired knowledge, skills, and competencies in patient safety, perianesthetic management, critical thinking, communication, and the professional role identified by the Council on Accreditation of Nurse Anesthesia Educational Programs (COA, 2016).

The movement of advanced practice nursing education to the practice doctorate level has mandated additional competencies to reflect this educational level. The COA Standards for Accreditation of Nurse Anesthesia Programs, Practice Doctorate (2016) reflect additional doctoral-level competencies. Standard D.14 requires graduates to demonstrate the ability to provide nurse anesthesia services based on evidence-based principles (COA, 2016).

Pellegrini (2006) noted that as nurse anesthesia curricula and clinical practice evolve, instructional methods will need to reflect EBP. The paradigm of using clinical judgment and expertise as the basis for clinical decision making will shift to a structure that incorporates the best available evidence to formulate clinical decisions, as described previously, in the technology and informatics competency, along with clinical experience and expertise. Implementation of EBP principles into nurse anesthesia education will yield a well-informed student along with ensuring that students and faculty remain at the forefront of the latest evidence that is available in the literature (Pellegrini, 2006).

When one is presented with a clinical question, the EBP analysis is as follows:

1. Define the problem or question in terms of the patient or problem, the intervention or comparison interventions used to answer the question, and the findings of the research reviewed.
2. Outline the current steps in one's clinical practice to address the problem.
3. Use a ranking system to determine the quality of evidence available in the literature. This hierarchy, in descending order, consists of findings from systematic review of well-designed clinical studies (meta-analyses); results of one or more appropriately designed studies (randomized trials, cohort studies); results of large case series and case reports; editorial and opinion pieces; animal research; and in vitro research.
4. Identify the resources available to implement any proposed changes to practice to differentiate which evidence is applicable to the current clinical setting.

5. Assess the validity of the research presented with a consistent rubric to review clinical trials that includes these questions:
   a. Did the clinical trials studied include elements such as randomization of subjects, adequate sample size, and appropriate statistical analysis?
   b. Were the results relevant to clinical practice?
   c. Were the therapeutic interventions reported feasible for clinical practice?
   d. Were all research subjects accounted for at the end of the study (Pellegrini, 2006)?

The "pyramid of evidence" is central to EBP. This concept is depicted in Figure 10.1. Utilization of EBP in anesthesia practice is increasing. Longitudinal outcome studies in practices where EBP is employed can determine if associations exist between the implementation of EBP and improved outcomes.

The AANA has recognized the importance of EBP and its importance to health care and society. The AANA realized the need to establish a systematic evidence-based process to analyze and resolve issues of import to the profession and clinical practice as the body of knowledge affecting nurse anesthesia continued to grow. Based on the work of Sackett et al. (2007), the AANA adopted the definition of evidence-based nurse anesthesia practice as "integration and synthesis of the best research evidence with clinical expertise and patient values" in order to optimize the care of patients receiving anesthesia services.

The member side of the AANA website (www.aana.com) lists these components of EBP:

- Patient preferences/values
- Clinical expertise
- Best research evidence

Five steps of the evidence-based process are delineated:

1. Ask a clinical question.
2. Obtain the best research literature.
3. Critically appraise the evidence.
4. Integrate the evidence with clinical expertise and patient preferences.
5. Evaluate the outcomes of the decision.

The AANA notes that as EBP is increasingly adopted, so are the available resources to translate evidence to practice. The AANA Professional Practice website provides information and resources to assist CRNAs and others who seek to learn more about EBP. The available resources include:

- EBP resources
- EBP modules and tutorials
- Guidelines and systematic reviews
- Research terms and definitions
- Types of evidence

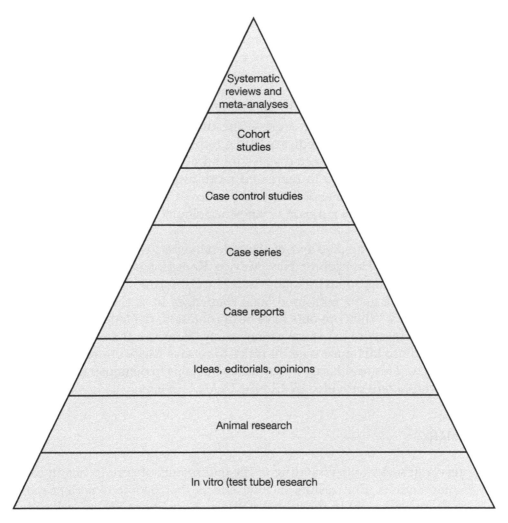

FIGURE 10.1 The evidence pyramid.

This commitment to EBP at the level of the national professional organization is laudable. What is central to this discussion is the impact of promulgating EBP principles on the outcomes of care provided by CRNAs, which requires prospective longitudinal multicenter data collection and analysis.

OUTCOME ECONOMICS AND POLICY DEVELOPMENTS

A cost-effectiveness analysis (CEA) of CRNA practice was conducted in 2010. The investigators found the CRNAs are less costly to train than anesthesiologists and have the potential for providing anesthesia care efficiently. The analysis noted that anesthesiologists and CRNAs can perform the same set of anesthesia services, including relatively rare and difficult procedures such as open-heart surgeries, organ transplantation, and pediatric procedures. In concert with the Institute of Medicine (IOM) report on the future of nursing recommendations to allow nurses to practice at the full scope of their education and training, this CEA has similar recommendations: "As the demand for healthcare continues to grow, increasing the number of CRNAs and permitting them to practice in the most efficient delivery models, will be a key to containing costs while maintaining quality care" (Hogan et al., 2010).

In 2001, the CMS allowed states to opt out of the requirement for reimbursement that a surgeon or anesthesiologist oversee anesthesia care provided by CRNAs. By 2005, 14 states opted out of this Medicare Part A requirement. An analysis of Medicare data from 1999 to 2005 in the affected states found no evidence that opting out of the oversight requirement resulted in increased morbidity or mortality. Based on these findings, the authors recommended that CMS allow CRNAs in every state to work without the supervision of a surgeon or anesthesiologist (Dulisse & Cromwell, 2010; IOM, 2010).

To date, 17 states have opted out of the federal supervision rule: Iowa, Nebraska, Idaho, Minnesota, New Hampshire, New Mexico, Kansas, North Dakota, Washington, Alaska, Oregon, Montana, South Dakota, Wisconsin, California, Colorado, and Kentucky. Some of these opt-outs have withstood legal challenges from the medical societies of their respective states. When opt-outs have been contested, the federal supervision rule was described as a measure to ensure patient safety. However, the supervision rule is a requirement that hospitals must meet in order to receive Medicare reimbursement for anesthesia services. This health care policy initiative helps to demonstrate the safety and quality of anesthesia care provided by CRNAs (AANA, 2016a).

SUMMARY

Outcome research seeks understanding of the end results of certain health care practices and interventions. End results include effects that people experience and care about, such as improvement in functional status and quality of life, as well as morbidity and mortality. Linkage of care provided to the attained outcomes is a function of outcome research, which can lead to improved care. Outcome research has altered the culture of clinical practice and health care research by changing how we assess the end results of health care services. Outcome research is the key to knowing the quality of care that can be achieved, and how providers can move to that level of care (AHRQ, 2012a).

Issues that face advanced practice nursing related to justification of the use of APRNs and the measurement of the effects of APRN services on patients and health care systems are similar but distinct from those faced by individual APRNs evaluating the outcomes of their particular practices. There is clearly a need for well-designed longitudinal assessments of how APRNs, including CRNAs, impact clinical outcomes. Since reimbursement decisions are driven by evidence of provider performance, APRNs who lack valid, reliable data to substantiate their "impactfulness" will struggle for equitable reimbursement (Ingersoll, 2008).

To address the need for addition of APRN-sensitive outcome indicators, development of electronic information systems that identify and track APRN outcome data is required. This process requires national agreement on core outcome indicators germane to APRNs and initiation of standards that support collection of APRN-sensitive data. Health care organizations and third-party payers will be integral to the development of such systems (Ingersoll, 2008).

Outcome measurement is interconnected with every other aspect of the APRN role. Effective outcome measurement and performance reviews related to outcome criteria require APRNs to work collaboratively with others, to plan and organize processes of care and assessment of quality in complex health services environments, and to allow scrutiny of their individual practices by others. In the end, the quality and value of care will improve along with recognition by the community of the impact of the APRN on outcomes of care (Ingersoll, 2008).

Nurses and APRNs, including CRNAs, continue to be interested and involved in the area of outcomes to ensure that patients are represented as more than a composite of physiologic variables or billing data. The use of outcome measures has helped APRNs to articulate their unique value and contributions to the well-being of patients. Many health care outcome measures do not identify or quantify the contributions of nurses. In anesthesia care, the role of CRNAs in patient outcomes has been at times diminished as a result of the economic competition between CRNAs and their physician counterparts.

Given the worsening mismatch between population health care needs and available resources, APRNs and CRNAs must continue to demonstrate their quality and cost-effectiveness. Implementation of the Affordable Care Act will provide an unprecedented opportunity for CRNAs and APRNs to demonstrate the value added to the health care delivery system by this cadre of safe, cost-effective providers.

Historically, quality of care has been described using variables such as morbidity, mortality, length of stay, readmission, and cost. Methods have not been readily available to define quality in terms of the effect of health care delivery on the health of patients. Combined administrative and health-related databases can demonstrate outcome associated with nurse anesthesia practice.

Nurse anesthesia has made outcome research an urgent priority. The benefits of this research in the policy arena are evident in the research findings of Hogan et al. (2010) and Dulisse and Cromwell (2010). Development of methodologically sound outcome research requires the preparation of more scholars within the specialty who have the expertise in research design and measurement. Fortunately, more CRNAs are rising to the challenge of doctoral education, with 3% of AANA members prepared at the doctoral level.

Continuing to strive for the accurate measurement of nurse anesthesia outcomes remains a goal of the nurse anesthesia specialty. Continued research, application of EBP principles, and operationalization of the recommendations of the IOM report *The Future of Nursing* will facilitate attainment of this goal.

Answers to Chapter Discussion Questions

1. The impetus for the development of closed malpractice claims research was a significant rise in anesthesia malpractice premiums in the 1970s.

2. There are gaps in research on the transfer of knowledge, skills, and abilities acquired in human patient simulation. However, there is evidence that simulation-based training in skills such as difficult airway management improves performance as demonstrated by a decreased incidence of failed airway management for those clinicians who have completed simulation-based training in difficult airway management.

3. Investigators believe that SCIP compliance should not be used to determine Medicare and Medicaid reimbursement rates because there was no correlation between SCIP Inf-1 (prophylactic antibiotics are received within 1 hour of surgical incision) and SSI.

4. Determining the contributions of anesthesia and surgery, respectively, to adverse perioperative outcomes is complex. For example, surgical aspects of spine surgery, such as positioning, the duration of surgery, and blood loss associated with the operation, can contribute to the development of postoperative ischemic optic neuropathy. However, factors under the control of the anesthetist, such as temperature regulation, ensuring that pressure points are padded, fluid management, and maintenance of hemodynamic stability, can also impact this problem.

5. The implementation of EBP is limited by the reliance of some clinicians on colleagues for information, rather than seeking information from peer-reviewed sources. Adoption of EBP is more likely with access of clinicians to Internet search engines, through the web browsers in their smartphones, and computer workstations in clinical areas.

WEB LINKS

- CMS Hospital Compare: This consumer-oriented website provides information on how well hospitals provide recommended care to their patients. On this site, the consumer can see the recommended care that an adult should get if being treated for a heart attack, heart failure, pneumonia, or having surgery. The performance rates for this website generally reflect care provided to all U.S. adults with the exception of the 30-day Risk Adjusted Death and Readmission measures and the Hospital Outpatient Medical Imaging measures, which include data from Medicare beneficiaries. www.cms.gov/Medicare/Quality-Initiatives-Patient-Assessment-Instruments/Hospital QualityInits/HospitalCompare.html

- Nationwide Health Information Network: This network is a set of standards, services, and policies that enable secure health information exchange over the Internet. The network will provide a foundation for the exchange of health information across diverse entities, within communities, and across the country. This critical part of the national health IT agenda will enable health information to follow the consumer, be available for clinical decision making, and support appropriate use of health care information beyond direct patient care so as to improve population health. www.healthit.gov/policy-researchers-implementers/ nationwide-health-information-network-nwhin

- ASCQR Program: Developed by CMS, this is a pay-for-reporting, quality data program. Under this program, ASCs report quality of care data for standardized measures to "receive the full annual update to their ASC annual payment rate, beginning with calendar year 2014 payments." www.cms.gov/Medicare/Quality-Initiatives-Patient -Assessment-Instruments/ASC-Quality-Reporting/index.html

REFERENCES

Agency for Healthcare Research and Quality. (2012). Agency for healthcare research and quality: Never events. Retrieved from http://www.psnet.ahrq.gov/primer.aspx?primerID=3

Alonso-Zaldivar, R. (2016). Medicare changing doctors pay rules. *Chicago Tribune*, 8.

American Association of Colleges of Nursing. (2011a). Statement on interprofessional education. Retrieved from http://www.aacn.nche.edu/news/articles/2011/ipec

American Association of Colleges of Nursing. (2011b). Team-based competencies: Building a shared foundation for education and clinical practice. Retrieved from http://www.aacn.nche.edu/news/articles/2011/ipec

American Association of Nurse Anesthetists. (2005). Code of ethics for the CRNA. Retrieved from http://www.aana.com/resources2/professionalpractice/Pages/Code-of-Ethics.aspx

American Association of Nurse Anesthetists. (2013a). Scope of nurse anesthesia practice. Retrieved from http://www.aana.com/resources2/professionalpractice/Pages/Scope-of-Nurse-Anesthesia-Practice.aspx

American Association of Nurse Anesthetists. (2013b). Standards for nurse anesthesia practice. Retrieved from http://www.aana.com/resources2/professionalpractice/Pages/Standards-for-Nurse-Anesthesia-Practice.aspx

American Association of Nurse Anesthetists. (2016a). Certified Registered Nurse Anesthetists fact sheet. Retrieved from http://www.aana.com/ceandeducation/becomeacrna/Pages/Nurse-Anesthetists-at-a-Glance.aspx

American Association of Nurse Anesthetists. (2016b). CPC-facts. Retrieved from http://cpc-facts.aana.com/Pages/index.aspx

American Association of Nurse Anesthetists. (2016c). Research overview. Retrieved from http://www.aana.com/resources2/research/Pages/default.aspx

American Association of Nurse Anesthetists Foundation. (2016). *Annual report.* Retrieved from http://www.aana.com/aanaaffiliates/aanafoundation/Documents/AANA%20Annual%20Report%20all%20pages%20for%20web%20corrected.pdf

American Nurses Association. (2012). Nursing workforce fact sheet. Retrieved from http://nursingworld.org/NursingbytheNumbersFactSheet.aspx

Bankert, M. (1989). *Watchful care: A history of America's nurse anesthetists.* New York, NY: Continuum.

Beecher, H., & Todd, D. (1954). A study of deaths associated with anesthesia and surgery. *Annals of Surgery, 140,* 2–25.

Blumenreich, G. (1990). Is the administration of anesthesia the practice of medicine? *American Association of Nurse Anesthetists Journals, 58,* 185–187.

Brunner, E. (1984). The National Association of Insurance Commissioners closed claims study. *International Anesthesiology Clinics, 22,* 17–30.

Callahan, L. (1988). Competence models: From theory to practical application. *American Association of Nurse Anesthetists, 56,* 5.

Centers for Medicare & Medicaid Services. (2016a). Ambulatory Surgical Center (ASC) Quality Reporting (ASCQR) Program. Retrieved from https://www.cms.gov/Medicare/Quality-Initiatives-Patient-Assessment-Instruments/ASC-Quality-Reporting/index.html

Centers for Medicare & Medicaid Services. (2016b). Accountable care organizations. Retrieved from https://www.cms.gov/Medicare/Medicare-Fee-for-Service-Payment/ACO/index.html ?redirect=/aco

Centers for Medicare & Medicaid Services. (2016c). 2016 Physician Quality Reporting System (PQRS): Implementation Guide. Retrieved from https://www.cms.gov/Medicare/Quality-Initiatives -Patient-Assessment-Instruments/PQRS/Downloads/2016_PQRS_ImplementationGuide.pdf

Cheney, F. (2010). The American Society of Anesthesiologists closed claims project: The beginning. *Anesthesiology, 113*(4), 957–960.

Cochrane Collaboration. (2012). Cochrane reviews. Retrieved from http://www.cochrane.org

Council on Accreditation of Nurse Anesthesia Educational Programs. (2016). *Standards for accreditation of nurse anesthesia educational programs, practice doctorate.* Park Ridge, IL: Author.

Dulisse, B., & Cromwell, J. (2010). No harm found when nurse anesthetists work without supervision by physicians. *Health Affairs, 29*(8), 1469–1475.

Fitzgibbon, D., Ramthell, J., Michna, E., Stephens, L. S., Posner, K. L., & Domino, K. B. (2010). Malpractice claims associated with medication management for chronic pain. *Anesthesiology, 112*(4), 948–956.

Garcia, N., Fogel, S., Baker, C., Remine, S., & Jones, J. (2012). Should compliance with the surgical care improvement project (SCIP) process measures determine Medicare and Medicaid reimbursement rates? *The American Surgeon, 78*(6), 653–656.

Greiner, A., & Knebel, E. (Eds.). (2003). *Health professions education: A bridge to quality.* Washington, DC: The National Academies Press. Retrieved from http://books.google.com/books/about/ Health_Professions_Education.html?id=Ib6pckASxjkC

HealthIT. (2016). Nationwide health information network. Retrieved from https://www.healthit .gov/policy-researchers-implementers/nationwide-health-information-network-nwhin

Hindman, B., Palcek, J., Posner, K., Traynelis, V. C., Lee, L. A., & Sawin, P. D., . . . Domino, K. B. (2011). Cervical spinal cord, root and bony spine injuries: A closed claim analysis. *Anesthesiology, 114*(4), 729–731.

Hogan, P., Seifert, R., Moore, C., & Simonson, B. (2010). Cost effectiveness analysis of anesthesia providers. *Nursing Economics, 28*(3), 159–169.

Ingersoll, G. (2008). Outcomes evaluation and performance improvement: An integrative review of research on advanced practice nursing. In A. Hamric, J. Spross, & C. Hanson (Eds.), *Advanced practice nursing: An integrative approach* (p. 724). St. Louis, MO: Saunders Elsevier.

Institute of Medicine. (2010). *The future of nursing: Leading change, advancing health.* Retrieved from http://www.iom.edu/Reports/2010/The-Future-of-Nursing-Leading-Change-Advancing -Health.aspx

Jha, A., Joynt, K., Orav, E., & Epstein, A. (2012). The long-term effect of premier pay for performance on patient outcomes. *The New England Journal of Medicine, 366*(17), 1606–1615.

Jordan, L., & Quraishi, J. (2015). The AANA Foundation malpractice closed claims study: A descriptive analysis. *American Association of Nurse Anesthetists Journals, 83*, 318–323.

Kavey, R. (2008). IOM roundtable on evidence-based medicine, health professions sector statement. Retrieved from http://www.iom.edu/Object.file/Master/44/388/Health%20Professionsa_ Is%20Sector%20-%20formatted.pdf

Kim, J., Park, J., & Shin, S. (2016). Effectiveness of simulation-based nursing education depending on fidelity: A meta-analysis. *BMC Medical Education, 16*, 152. doi:10.1186/s12909-016-0672-7

Lee, L., Roth, S., Todd, M., Posner, K. L., Polissar, N. L., & Neradilek, M. B. (2012). Risk factors associated with ischemic optic neuropathy after spinal fusion surgery. *Anesthesiology, 116*(1), 15–24.

Lema, M. (2003). Safe anesthetic practice—fact, fantasy, or folly? *American Society of Anesthesiologists Newsletter, 67*(6), 1.

Lewis, S., Nicholson, A., Smith, A., & Alderson P. (2014). Physician anaesthetists versus non-physician providers of anaesthesia for surgical patients. *Cochrane Database of Systematic Reviews,* (7), CD010357. doi:10.1002/14651858.CD010357.pub2

Li, G., Warner, M., Lang, B., Huang, L., & Sun, L. (2009). Epidemiology of anesthesia-related mortality in the United States, 1999–2005. *Anesthesiology, 110*, 759–765.

Liao, C., Quraishi, J., & Jordan, L. (2015). Geographical imbalance of anesthesia providers and its impact on the uninsured and vulnerable populations. *Nursing Economics, 33*, 263–270.

MacRae, M. (2007). Closed claims studies in anesthesia: A literature review and implications for practice. *American Association of Nurse Anesthetists Journal, 75*, 267–275.

Magaw, A. (1899). Observations in anaesthesia. *Northwestern Lancet, 19*, 207–210.

Magaw, A. (1904). Observations drawn from an experience of eleven thousand anesthesias. *Transactions of the Minnesota State Medical Association*, 91–99.

Magaw, A. (1906). A review of over fourteen thousand surgical anaesthesias. *Surgery, Gynecology and Obstetrics, 6*, 795–799.

McDonald, L. (2001). Florence Nightingale and the early origins of evidence-based nursing. *Evidence-Based Nursing, 4*, 68–69.

McGaghie, W., Darycott, T., Dunn, W. Lopez, C., & Stefanidis, D. (2011). Evaluating the impact of simulation on translational patient outcomes. *Simulation in Healthcare, 6*, S42–S47.

McGaghie, W., Issenberg, S. Petrusa, E., & Scaelse, R. (2010). A critical review of simulation-based medical education research: 2003–2009. *Medical Education, 44*(1), 50–63.

McGlynn, E., Asch, S., Adams, J., Keesey, J., Hicks, J., DeCristofaro, A., & Kerr, E. A. (2003). The quality of healthcare delivered to adults in the United States. *New England Journal of Medicine, 348*, 2635–2645.

Medicare. (2016). Surgical care improvement project. Retrieved from www.medicare.gov/hospitalcompare/Data/surgical-care-improvement-project-scores.html

Metzner, J., Posner, K., Lam, M., & Domino, K. (2011). Closed claims' analysis. *Best Practice & Research. Clinical Anaesthesiology, 25*(2), 263–276.

Monti Seibert, E., Alexander, J., & Lupien, A. (2004). Rural nurse anesthesia practice: A pilot study. *American Association of Nurse Anesthetists, 72*, 181–189.

Murphy, G., Szokol, J., Avram, M. et al. (2015). Residual neuromuscular blockade in the elderly: Incidence and clinical implications. Retrieved from http://anesthesiology.pubs.asahq.org/article.aspx?articleid=2463464

National Health Information Network. (2012). National health information network website. Retrieved from https://www.healthit.gov/policy-researchers-implementers/nationwide-health-information-network-nwhin

National League for Nursing. (2008). National League for Nursing: Transforming nursing education: Position statement. Retrieved from http://www.nln.org/aboutnln/positionstatements/transforming052005.pdf

Needleman, J., & Minnick, A. (2009). Anesthesia provider model, hospital resources and maternal outcomes. *Health Services Research, 44*, 464–482.

Negrusa, B., Hogan, P., Warner, J., Schroeder, C., & Pang, B. (2016). Scope of practice laws and anesthesia complications. *Medical Care, 54*, 913–920.

Overstreet, M., McCarver, L., Shields, J., & Patterson, J. (2015). Simulation and rubrics: Technology and grading student performance in nurse anesthesia education. *Nursing Clinics of North America, 50*, 347–365.

Pellegrini, J. (2006). Using evidence-based practice in nurse anesthesia programs. *American Association of Nurse Anesthetists, 74*, 269–273.

Penprase, B., Mileto, L., Bittinger, A., Hranchook, A. M., Atchley, J. A., Bergakker, S. A., . . . Franson, H. E. (2012). The use of high-fidelity simulation in the admissions process: One nurse anesthesia program's experience. *American Association of Nurse Anesthetists Journal, 80*, 43–48.

Pravikoff, D., Tanner, A., & Pierce, S. (2005). Readiness of U.S. nurses for evidence-based practice. *The American Journal of Nursing, 105*, 45–51.

Ramthell, J., Michna, E., Fitzgibbon D., Stephens, L. S., Posner, K. L., Domino, K. B. (2011). Injury and liability associated with cervical procedures for chronic pain. *Anesthesiology, 114*(4), 918–926.

Ruth, H. (1945). Anesthesia study commissions. *Journal of the American Medical Association, 127*, 514–524.

Sackett, D., Rosenberg, W., Gray, J., Haynes, R., & Richardson, W. (2007). Evidence-based medicine: What it is and what it isn't. *Clinical Orthopaedics and Related Research, 455*, 3–5.

Simonson, D., Ahern, N., & Hendryx, M. (2007). Anesthesia staffing and anesthetic complication during cesarean delivery: A retrospective analysis. *Nursing Research, 56*, 9–17.

Society for Simulation in Healthcare. (2015). Fifty-four sim centers have achieved SSH accreditation. Retrieved from http://www.ssih.org/News/ArticleType/ArticleView/ArticleID/1803

Stephens, T., Hunningher, A., Mills, H., & Freeth, D. (2016). An interprofessional training course in crises and human factors for perioperative teams. *Journal of Interprofessional Care, 30*, 685–688.

Thiemann, L., & McFadden, J. (2010). Advancing evidence-based nurse anesthesia practice. *American Association of Nurse Anesthetists Journal, 78*, 279–282.

Turcato, N., Roberson, C., & Covert, K. (2008). Simulation-based education: What's in it for nurse anesthesia educators? *American Association of Nurse Anesthetists Journals, 76*, 257–262.

World Health Organization. (2012). World Health Organization surgical safety checklist. Retrieved from http://www.who.int/patientsafety/safesurgery/ss_checklist/en/index.html

Wunder, L. (2016). Effect of a nontechnical skills intervention on first-year student registered nurse anesthetists' skills during crisis simulation. *American Association of Nurse Anesthetists Journals, 84*, 46–51.

CHAPTER 11

Measuring Outcomes of Doctor of Nursing Practice

Marguerite J. Murphy, Kathy S. Magdic, and Terri L. Allison

Chapter Objectives

1. Examine the current research available related to Doctor of Nursing Practice (DNP) outcomes
2. Explore rationale for the limited numbers of studies of DNP-related outcomes
3. Identify areas for future research related to DNP outcomes

Chapter Discussion Questions

1. Based on the literature supporting the DNP as the entry-level degree for advanced nursing practice and the American Association of Colleges of Nursing (AACN) *The Essentials of Doctoral Education for Advanced Nursing Practice*, what outcomes of DNP-degree-prepared nurses should be evaluated?
2. What factors have influenced the study of DNP outcomes to date?
3. What DNP outcomes should be considered for future study?

Though a practice-doctorate degree in nursing has been offered for more than 20 years, an organized effort to examine and make recommendations for future development of a nursing practice doctorate occurred in 2002 when the AACN convened a task force appointed for this reason (AACN, 2004). In 2004, the AACN proposed the development of practice-doctorate programs for nurses with roles specializing as an advanced practice registered nurse (APRN) or at an aggregate, system, or organizational level (AACN, 2006). Rationale supporting the need for the DNP degree included quality and safety issues in health care addressed in the Institute of Medicine's (IOM's) reports *Crossing the Quality Chasm: A New Health System for the 21st Century* (IOM, 2001) and *To Err Is Human* (IOM, 1999), increasingly complex patient care, rapidly changing health care systems, and the shortage of nursing faculty (AACN, 2004). Advancing the number of doctorally prepared nurses is also supported by the IOM report *The Future of Nursing: Leading Change, Advancing Health* (IOM, 2010). DNP graduates are impacting health and health care outcomes as they implement quality improvement initiatives, apply evidence-based practice (EBP) changes, and explore the impact of system and practice changes. This chapter presents an overview of the DNP degree and reviews the outcome literature related to DNP practice.

AN OVERVIEW OF THE DNP

The DNP curriculum is based on *The Essentials of Doctoral Education for Advanced Nursing Practice* (AACN, 2006), which describes the competencies to be achieved by all DNP graduates and recognizes specialty practice competencies. The DNP *Essentials* comprise eight foundational outcome competencies preparing the graduate to function in complex health care environments (Exhibit 11.1). DNP education is specialty focused; the curriculum incorporates related content developed by national nursing specialty organizations intended to prepare the DNP graduate for specialized advanced nursing practice that is consistent with the DNP *Essentials* (AACN, 2006). Advanced nursing practice may emphasize direct care of patients and families or have a system, aggregate, or organizational focus associated with administration, informatics, or health care policy. The National Organization of Nurse Practitioner Faculties (NONPF) delineated nurse practitioner (NP) core competencies (NONPF, 2011), and in 2015 reaffirmed endorsement of the DNP degree as the entry level for NPs (NONPF, 2015). The American Association

---

EXHIBIT 11.1   AACN *Essentials of Doctoral Education for Advanced Nursing Practice*

I. Scientific underpinnings for practice
II. Organizational and systems leadership for quality improvement and systems thinking
III. Clinical scholarship and analytical methods for evidence-based practice
IV. Information systems/technology and patient care technology for the improvement and transformation of health care
V. Health care policy for advocacy in health care
VI. Interprofessional collaboration for improving patient and population health outcomes
VII. Clinical prevention and population health for improving the nation's health
VIII. Advanced nursing practice

AACN, American Association of Colleges of Nursing.
Source: AACN (2006).

of Nurse Anesthetists (AANA) determines specialty practice competencies for certified registered nurse anesthetists (CRNAs) and adopted the position requiring the doctorate for entry into practice (AANA, 2007; AANA, 2013); The Council on Accreditation of Nurse Anesthesia Educational Programs (COA) requires that nurse anesthetist students graduate with a doctoral degree by 2025 (COA, 2016). In 2015, the National Association of Clinical Nurse Specialists endorsed the DNP degree as a requirement for clinical nurse specialist (CNS) entry to practice, effective 2030 (National Association of Clinical Nurse Specialists, 2015). Other advanced nursing practice organizations have developed competencies for their respective specialties as well, including the American Organization of Nurse Executives (AONE, 2015), American College of Nurse-Midwives (ACNM, 2012), and Healthcare Information and Management Systems Society (HIMSS, 2015).

Early supporters of AACN and the DNP degree cited increasingly diverse and vulnerable populations, rapidly evolving health care systems, and increased complexity of care as needs for better prepared health care providers (Draye, Acker, & Zimmer, 2006; Marion et al., 2003; Mundinger, 2005). The IOM report *The Future of Nursing* (IOM, 2010), the DNP *Essentials* (AACN, 2006), and the AACN *DNP Task Force Report* (AACN, 2015) and various position statements from specialty organizations identify attributes to be achieved through practice-doctorate education preparing nurses in advanced practice to become leaders in the ever-changing future health care environment (Table 11.1). The early rationale and current national acceptance for the DNP degree continues to serve as the impetus for recommending the practice doctorate as the entry into advanced nursing practice.

A survey conducted by O'Dell (2012) of 175 academic institutions with a DNP program and 123 institutions (70.3%) responding, projected a total number of 10,331 DNP graduates in 2012 and 59,872 by 2015 (O'Dell, 2012). By the end of 2013, 251 schools offered

TABLE 11.1   Projected Attributes of DNP-Prepared Advanced Practice Registered Nurses

Attributes	Sources
Leadership in patient care and health care systems	Bellflower and Carter (2006), Drayer et al. (2006), Marion et al. (2003), Marshall and Broome (2017), Montgomery and Porter-O'Grady (2010)
Influence on health care policy	Bellflower and Carter (2006), Nelson, Cook, and Raterink (2013)
Improve quality care and safety issues	Marion et al. (2003), Mundinger (2005), Mundinger et al. (2000), Nelson et al. (2013)
Improve clinical management	Draye et al. (2006), Marion et al. (2003), Mundinger (2005), Mundinger et al. (2000)
Improve interprofessional practice, interprofessional collaboration	Drayer et al. (2006). Nelson et al. (2013), Staffileno, Murphy, and Carlson (2016)
Improve translation of evidence-based practice into health care	Bellflower and Carter (2006), Syler and Levin (2012), Terhaar, Crickman, and Finnell (2016), Waldrop et al. (2014)
Improve health promotion/risk reduction	Draye et al. (2006)
Improve coordination of care	Draye et al. (2006)
Use of technology for data collection and analysis of information	Draye et al. (2006), Montgomery and Porter-O'Grady (2010)
Doctoral-prepared clinical educators	Fang and Bednash (2017), Marion et al. (2003), Staffileno, Murphy, and Carlson (2016)

DNP, Doctor of Nursing Practice.

the DNP degree and 68 additional schools were planning to begin a DNP program (Auerbach et al., 2014; Kirschling, 2014). The actual number of DNP graduates by the end of 2013 was 14,699 (Kirschling, 2014). Based on the AACN 2015 annual survey, 292 DNP programs were available; 62 postbaccalaureate and 66 postmaster's DNP programs were in development; and a total of 4,100 students had graduated from 289 programs during that year (AACN, 2016; D. Fang, personal communication, September 27, 2016).

Although evidence exists in the literature regarding the positive impact advanced nursing practice has on health care outcomes, evidence reflecting the impact of DNP-prepared nurses is limited. Discussion about the need to document DNP outcomes is ongoing (Anderson, 2015; Love, Allison, & McArthur 2014); yet metrics to evaluate the impact of DNP graduates on care delivery are lacking (Berkowitz, 2014). Given the exponential growth in the number of DNP programs and graduates, outcomes associated with doctoral level advanced nursing practice require examination. A literature search using Cumulative Index to Nursing and Allied Health Literature (CINAHL), OVID, PubMed, and commercial search engines, such as Google Scholar and Bing, revealed no research studies specific to the impact of DNP-prepared nurses on health care outcomes. Reasons for this include insufficient number of DNP graduates to effectively study (Cronenwett et al., 2011), and DNP graduates are scattered across varied practice foci decreasing the likelihood of finding a concentrated group of DNP-prepared nurses to include in an outcome study. A landmark study by Aiken, Clarke, Cheung, Slone, and Silber (2003) which was reinforced by a study in 2008 by Aiken, Clark, Sloane, Lake, & Cheney, found that care provided by Bachelor of Science in Nursing (BSN) graduates demonstrated better patient outcomes than care provided by non-BSN graduates. A systematic review conducted by Stanik-Hutt et al. (2013) found that health care quality and patient outcomes associated with care delivered by NPs were comparable to that of physicians. Unlike findings from these two studies, similar aggregate evidence does not yet exist for graduates with a DNP degree. Many singular or anecdotal reports about DNP projects are published in the literature or presented at professional meetings; however, no research studies have been undertaken to evaluate the impact of DNP-prepared nurses on patient and health care system outcomes. Until such studies are conducted to measure the influence of doctoral-level advanced nursing practice, the impact of DNP preparation remains unknown.

DNP OUTCOMES: PERSONAL AND PROFESSIONAL

Anecdotal reports regarding the impact of obtaining a DNP degree on individual graduates' personal outcomes have been reported related to personal satisfaction with degree achievement and professional outcomes related to increased salaries, and movement into more desirable, higher level professional positions (Kung, 2012). A survey of self-selected participants reinforced reports that nurses entered DNP programs for the primary purposes of personal satisfaction, job advancement, or job change (O'Dell, 2012). A small study of 11 DNP graduates reported that all 11 were pleased with their decision to obtain the DNP degree and 10 of the 11 indicated that obtaining the degree had changed their practice (Melnyk, 2013). This study also supported job advancement or change as seven graduates (63.6%) experienced a job shift following graduation, assuming administrative and academic roles (Melnyk, 2013).

TABLE 11.2   Average Annual Nurse Practitioner Salary Based on Education

Nurse Practitioner Degree	2011	2012	2013	2014	2015
Master's	$90,250	$92,867	$98,336	$100, 585	$103,393
Doctorate of Nursing Practice	$98,826	$96,807	$105,021	$113,618	$107,585

Source: Advance Healthcare Network (2015); Advance Healthcare Network (2016); Jones (2013); Pronsanti (2011).

The salary increase reported anecdotally is supported by the findings from the National Salary Survey for Nurse Practitioners and Physician Assistants for years 2011 to 2015, which indicated that the average salary of DNP-prepared NPs is higher than the average annual salary of master's-prepared NPs (Advance Healthcare Network, 2015; Advance Healthcare Network, 2016; Jones, 2013; see Table 11.2). The authors did not explain the reduction of DNP-prepared NP salaries from 2014 to 2015. However, closer evaluation of the survey data indicates that greater than 50% of the respondents in the 2015 survey had 5 years or fewer years of experience (Advance Healthcare Network, 2016). The lower starting salaries of new NPs and growing numbers of DNP-prepared NPs may have impacted the average annual salary toward the lower end.

The DNP degree has been identified as having a positive impact on the empowerment of nurses to influence parity with other health care professionals and to impact health care (Dennison, Payne, & Farrell, 2012; Pritham & White, 2016). The issue of achieving parity with other health care providers is also a rationale provided in the AACN's development of the DNP entry-level proposal (AACN, 2004). Research to determine the degree to which parity and empowerment are being achieved in DNP-prepared nurses is necessary to demonstrate the level to which these goals are being accomplished.

DNP OUTCOMES: DNP COMPETENCIES

The Essentials of Doctoral Education for Advanced Nursing Practice describes the foundational competencies expected of all DNP graduates prepared for specialized advanced nursing practice (AACN, 2006). Competencies in a particular specialty are determined by the national specialty organization for the particular specialty. The hallmark of DNP education is development of skills to search for, evaluate the quality of, and apply evidence to practice to create change and improve patient outcomes. The DNP graduate demonstrates leadership competencies in the translation of evidence for practice, directing quality improvement initiatives, influencing health care policy, leading or participating in interprofessional teams, and utilizing information systems and technology to transform health care (AACN, 2006; Berkowitz, 2014; Pritham & White, 2016; Redman, Pressler, Furspan, & Potempa, 2015).

In 2012, 3 years (2010–2012) of national survey data related to DNP outcomes were collected to answer the question: Are graduates of DNP programs utilizing these core competencies in practice? (O'Dell, 2012). While the number of self-selected respondents was small for each of the 3 years, 294, 359, and 248, respectively, some interesting findings were identified. The DNP degree was established for APRNs with a clinical focus as an

NP, CRNA, nurse-midwife, or CNS, as well as for nurses whose practice specialty focuses on aggregate and systems including nurse executives and nursing informaticists. Data from the O'Dell survey indicated that the majority of students were in programs of clinical concentration, with above 60% of respondents indicating they were APRNs in each year for 2010, 2011, and 2012. The second highest area of DNP program emphasis among participants in the survey, approximately 20%, was advanced nursing practice with a leadership concentration for these same years (O'Dell, 2012). Results from the survey also indicated the number of DNP graduates assuming a nurse faculty role was increasing, a finding supporting one of the initial incentives for the DNP degree—to increase doctoral-prepared clinical faculty (AACN, 2006). Other findings indicated that the majority of DNP graduates feel competent in the DNP policy (Essential V), EBP (Essentials I, III), leadership (Essential II), and practice change (Essential VIII) competencies (O'Dell, 2012).

Professional contributions of DNP graduates include publications in journals and podium and poster presentations (O'Dell, 2012), and is an area that is being recognized and evaluated as a DNP outcome measure (Broome & Riner, 2012; Newland, 2012). A survey by Broome and Riner (2012) identified over 300 articles published in 59 journals from 2007 to 2012, where at least one author displayed DNP credentials. The number of publications increased steadily over the 5-year period with most of the publications being focused on practice. Broome and Riner (2012) also identified interprofessional authorship of medical doctors (MD) and doctors of philosophy (PhD) with doctors of nursing practice (Essential VI). Using a different strategy than Broome and Riner (2012), Redman et al. (2015) conducted a database search for publications between 2005 and 2012 having at least one DNP-prepared author in attempts to determine DNP nurse productivity. The authors used publishing in areas of specialty or relevance to the DNP graduate as an indirect measure of leadership and demonstration of scholarship. Eight focus areas among 690 published articles were noted, including role of the DNP; nursing education; clinical practice; health delivery systems/quality and safety; policy, administration, business, and executive; ethics; and other (Redman et al., 2015). Based on review of the publications, DNPs are engaged in strategic roles in practice and education and have cultivated writing scholarship, consistent with the intended outcomes of the DNP *Essentials*. Redman et al. (2015) validate the need to document outcomes of DNP graduates, particularly measurement of the impact of translation of evidence to practice, ability to lead system and policy changes, and ultimately improvement in health care. The increase in publications and presentations by DNP-prepared nurses indicates the enhanced organizational and system leadership skills and practice impact (Broome & Riner, 2012; O'Dell, 2012; Redman et al., 2015) originally noted in AACN's call for the DNP degree.

While the expected DNP competencies are well-defined, no studies directly link these outcome competencies to the DNP *Essentials*. Case examples and anecdotal reports about the impact of DNP-prepared nurses' scholarly work are found in the literature. Abstracts from podium and poster presentations from professional nursing organizational meetings are abundant. Anderson, Knestrick, and Barroso (2014) and Burson, Moran, and Conrad (2016) describe DNP student projects as exemplars of excellence in clinical practice. Udlis and Mancuso (2015) found that the majority of responders in a study assessing perceptions about the DNP-prepared nurse believed the DNP degree improves the quality of patient care, safety, and outcomes and prepares nurses to be leaders within the health care system, with interprofessional collaboration and in creating change. Pritham and White (2016) describe DNP student outcomes in the context of Essentials I, II, and IV as demonstration of the value of the DNP-prepared graduate and provide recommendations for measuring the impact of the DNP according to all of the DNP *Essentials*. To fully examine the impact of the DNP degree on patient and health care outcomes, methods to assess DNP competencies and outcomes beyond anecdotal reports need to be developed.

DNP OUTCOMES: DNP STUDENT PROJECTS

As previously discussed, there are no published studies comparing the impact on health care outcomes of DNP-prepared graduates to non-DNP-prepared graduates in similar roles. In addition, there are few studies to date documenting the impact of the DNP graduate on the original established goals of improving nursing practice and enhancing leadership skills. The DNP scholarly project is a thread across DNP programs, with components that reflect the DNP competencies and the DNP *Essentials* (AACN, 2015). DNP projects demonstrate impact on patient care at a system or population level, use of EBP to provide innovative care, demonstration of leadership in system and interprofessional teams, influence on patient populations and professional advocacy through policy impact, and demonstration of financial considerations regarding health care decisions. The incorporation of competencies in the DNP project supports the examination of the agglomeration of DNP student projects to answer the question: Do the knowledge and skills gained by this doctoral degree translate into improved patient, system, and educational outcomes?

With the goal to discover areas where DNP graduates are focusing their efforts, an informal web search for DNP projects was performed. In addition, e-mails and phone calls were made to a number of schools with DNP programs requesting a list of DNP project titles and/or abstracts. The search yielded 512 DNP projects from over 51 schools; 243 were accompanied by abstracts. The remainder consisted of simple listings of DNP project titles. Project titles and abstracts were reviewed to identify emerging trends of the foci for DNP projects. If an abstract was not available for review, the project title itself was reviewed. Some titles were detailed enough to clearly identify the focus of the project; however, some titles were either too vague or not explicit enough to clearly appreciate the intent of the project. Broad categories were established in an attempt to categorize elements of the projects with regard to population, setting, and problem. As expected, many of the projects spanned multiple categories. Exhibit 11.2 provides examples of titles of DNP projects from each of the schools sampled.

Summary of DNP Projects

While it was difficult to determine the specific population for each project, the population ages ranged from neonates to the older adult, with the majority of the projects focusing on adult males and females. African Americans were the predominant minority race specifically identified as the population of interest, followed by Latinos, American Indian/Alaskan Natives, and Northwest tribes. International projects included Germany, Nigeria, Central Russia, Costa Rica, and Haitians in Dumay. Interestingly, there was an interest in issues related to veterans. There were a high number of project titles focusing

EXHIBIT 11.2 Examples of DNP Projects

Health Promotion

Empowering Community Health: A Faith-Based Approach

Promoting Nutritional Awareness and Improving Dietary Habits: A Community-Based Approach

Clinical Decision Support System Improves Bone Mineral Density Screening Rates in 65-Year-Old Women

Developing Evidence-Based Evaluation Strategies for a Campus-Workplace Violence Prevention Program

Cardiovascular Disease Awareness: Promoting Healthy Lifestyles in African American Females

Colorectal Cancer Screening in a Free Primary Care Program for the Uninsured

Teenage Pregnancy: An Impact of the Healthy Choices Abstinence Program

An Evidence-Based Toolkit to Prevent Meningococcal Meningitis in College Students

Provider-Focused Process Improvement Project to Enhance Patient Participation in a Tobacco Smoking Cessation Program

Bully Victim Identification and Intervention Program for School Nurses

A Quality Improvement Initiative to Increase HPV Vaccine Uptake and Dose Completion Rates Using an Evidence-Based Educational and Reminder Strategy With Parents of Pre-Teen Girls

Population/Diagnosis Focus

Assessment of Male Partner Needs and Experiences During Labor and Birth

Neonatal Hypoglycemia and Prompted Interventions During the Pre-Transport Phase of Care

Childhood Obesity Prevention in the Context of Family Activity: Development of an Evaluation Tool for the PAK Family Activity Event

Evaluation of a Multidisciplinary Clinical Intervention on Childhood Obesity at Seattle Children's Hospital

Perceptions of Body Image, Body Satisfaction, and Knowledge of Obesity-Related Health Risks Among African American College Students

Improving Diabetes Self-Care Behaviors of Adolescents Through a School-Based Diabetes Care Initiative

Missed Opportunities for the HPV Vaccine in 13-Year-Old Girls Receiving Care at NeighborCare Health

A Transition Checklist for Adolescents with Sickle Cell Disease

Examining the Influence of Structured Diabetes Self-Management Education on Patient Outcomes in an Outpatient Setting

The Predictive Value of Second Trimester Blood Pressures on the Development of Preeclampsia

Improving Patient Satisfaction with Better Pain Management in Hospital Patients

ACES: A Quality Improvement Program to Improve Asthma Outcomes

The Effect of an Evidence-Based Support Intervention to Facilitate Treatment Preference Decision Making by Surrogates of Persons With Incapacitating Dementia

Translation of Autism Screening Research Into Practice

Pressure Ulcer Prevention Protocol of Older Adults in a Nursing Home Setting

Implementing an Evidence-Based Pain Assessment Guideline Within a Pediatric Transitional Hospital Setting

Focus on Veterans

Effectiveness of a Four-Item Screening Tool for Returning Operation Iraqi Freedom/Operation Enduring Freedom Veterans

Gap Analysis: Transition of Health-Care from the Department of Defense to the Department of Veterans Affairs

Cognitive Behavioral Therapy for the Treatment of Sleep Disturbances in Soldiers With Combat-Associated Mild Traumatic Brain Injury

Hospital-Based Care

The Evaluation of the Implementation of an Individualized Educational Program on the 30-Day Readmission Rate for Patients With Heart Failure in a Community Hospital

Application of the Iowa Model of EBP to Promote Quality Care in the Peri-Operative Management of Pacemakers and Implantable Cardioverter-Defibrillators

(continued)

EXHIBIT 11.2   Examples of DNP Projects (*continued*)

Evaluation of Cue vs. Schedule-Based Infant Feeding Protocols in the Neonatal Intensive Care Unit
Implementing an Evidence-Based Risk Assessment Model for Chemotherapy-Induced Neutropenia
Evaluation of an Evidence-Based, Nurse-Driven Checklist Designed to Prevent Hospital-Acquired Catheter-Associated Urinary Tract Infections in Intensive Care Units
Patient Rounding in the LTAC Setting: An Opportunity to Positively Impact Patient Call Light Use, Patient Satisfaction, and Patient Safety
Implementation and Evaluation of an Evidence-Based Oral Care Guideline in a Mechanically Ventilated Patient Population
Improvement of Family-Centered Care Practices in the Neonatal Intensive Care Unit
Evaluation of the Effectiveness of the Ruby Slipper Program in Reducing Falls on a Medical Surgical Unit
Implementation of Early Goal-Directed Therapy in Management of the Septic Patient
Inpatient Fall Prevention Program: Reducing Patient Falls Through Implementation of a Clinical Fall Prevention Team
Quality Improvement Intervention Using Split-Dose Protocol for Bowel Preparation for Colonoscopy
Transition Home for Patients With Heart Failure: A Pilot Program at a Critical Access Hospital
Exploring Coping Mechanisms of Palliative Care Patients in an Acute Care Setting

Psychiatric-Mental Health
Tele-Psychiatry: Pilot Training Program for Washington State Department of Corrections Psychiatric Prescribers
Enhancing Mental Health Services Utilization Among African Immigrants and Refugees in the Northwest
Heightened Mental Health Awareness on a Diverse, Urban Public University Campus Through a Medical Outreach Campaign
Developing a Treatment Guide for PTSD
Evaluation of Alcohol Management Practices in a Community Hospital
Educating Nurses About Postpartum Depression in the Acute Care Setting
Examining the Effectiveness of an Aggression Management Program in an Inpatient Psychiatric Setting
Psychiatric Nurse's Attitudes and Perceived Barriers About Medical Emergency Teams: A Quality Improvement Project
Implementation of a Mental Health Screening Tool by School Nurse Practitioners

Cultural and International Focus
Implementation and Evaluation of a Model of Expanded Nursing Practice in Germany: A Pilot Program
Case Study From the Urban Village in Central Russia: Evaluating Barriers to Vaccine Administration and Vaccine Compliance
Improving Cardiovascular Health for Haitians in Dumay Using a Community Organization Approach
A Multi-Factorial Tailored Intervention to Improve Adherence in Uninsured and Underserved African Americans With Hypertension
Education of Incarcerated African American Males on Sexually Transmitted Diseases
Can an Educational Intervention Lower Blood Sugar Levels in Latinos at Risk for Developing Diabetes Mellitus
Storytelling, a Cognitive Behavior Pain Management Strategy for American Indian and Alaska Natives
Evaluation of the Impact of Information on HPV, Cervical Cancer and PAP Smear Knowledge Among Costa Rican Women Enrolled in HPV Vaccination Trial
Policy Development to Improve Quality of Life Outcomes of Breast Cancer Survivors in a Northwest Tribal Community
Evaluation of Spanish Diabetes Group Visits at a Community Health Center

Technology
Use of the Electronic Health Record in the Measurement of Nurse Practitioner Performance
Tele-Visitation: A Strategy to Reduce Distress Among Isolated Blood and Bone Marrow Transplant Patients Post-Transplantation

(*continued*)

EXHIBIT 11.2   Examples of DNP Projects (*continued*)

Using Computerized Physician Order Entry (CPOE) to Improve Prescribing of Analgesics and Benzodiazepines to Persons 65 and Older

Feasibility of a Webinar for Coaching Patient With COPD on End-of-Life Communication

The Use of Documentation Prompts as an Intervention Strategy for Primary Care Providers Managing Children in Out of Home Placement

Identification and Elimination of Barriers to the Use of a Technology-Based Patient/Family Education System

Crisis Team Training of Perinatal Health-Care Professionals Using Simulation Technology

Treatment Fidelity Evaluation of Tele-Health Stage-Based Motivational Interviewing Interventions

My Papp: An Android App to Educate About Pap Testing

Home But Not Alone: Telephone Support for the First-Time Breastfeeding Mother

Efficacy of an Electronic Integrative Protocol in Managing Alcohol Withdrawal Syndrome: A Quality and Safety Initiative

Development of Smartphone Application to Detect Hypertension in Children and Adolescents

An Evaluation of a Text-Messaging Program to Achieve Smoking Cessation Among Young Adults

---

Health Policy

Policy Development for Prenatal Care Assurance: A Strategic Approach to Improve Maternal and Infant Health Among American Indian and Alaska Native (AIAN) Communities in Washington State

Methicillin-Resistant *Staphylococcus aureus* (MRSA) Infection Control Policy at First Place School: A Policy Development in a Vulnerable Community

Public Policy Involvement and Behavioral Intentions Toward Health Policy Research Among Nurses With Professional Doctorates

---

Professional and Administrative Nursing

Strategies to Improve Patient Flow in an Urgent Care Facility

Nurse Manager Leadership Development Program Evaluation

Transformational Leadership Behaviors of Successful Nurse Managers

Integration of Nurse Practitioner Practice Into a Patient-Centered Medical Home

Roadmap to Improved Trauma Outcomes: The ACNP Practice Model

The Use of Mentoring by a Nurse Executive to Affect Nurse Managers' Use of Transformational Leadership Behaviors

Does the DNP Change Clinical Practice?

Developing a Farm Team: Succession Planning for Nurse Managers

Examining and Reducing Distractions and Interruptions During Medication Administration

Emotional Intelligence and Nurse Managers: Does Coaching and Training Make a Difference?

Education

Acute Pain Management: A Nursing Education Program for Improved Outcomes

Disaster Preparedness and Response: Implication for Nurse Practitioner Education

Predictors of the First-Year Nursing Student at Risk of Early Departure

An Educational Intervention to Implement SBAR for Nurse Provider Telephone Communication

Acute Pain Management: A Nursing Education Program for Improved Outcomes

Evaluation of Nurses' Education Program on End-of-Life Care

Practice Models

MD-NP Collaborative Practice: Models, Barriers and Improvement Strategies

Use of Nurse Case Managers in Diabetic Care

(*continued*)

EXHIBIT 11.2   Examples of DNP Projects (*continued*)
Collaboration in an Outpatient Clinic Setting: Strengthening Care for Patients
Nurse Practitioner–Led Heart Failure Clinic
Development of an Online Learning Module Focusing on the Principles of EBP for Newly Hired Registered Nurses
Integrating Cardiology Acute Care Nurse Practitioners Into a House Staff Model of Care: Development of Performance and Value-Added Outcome Measures
Promoting the Coordination of Care for Patients With a Diagnosis of Chronic Illness and Substance Abuse in a Managed Care Organization
The Development of a National, Multimodal, Multidiscipline Evidence-Based Clinical Practice Guideline for the Prevention and Management of PONV/PDNV in Adult Patients

COPD, chronic obstructive pulmonary disease; DNP, Doctor of Nursing Practice; EBP, evidence-based practice; HPV, human papillomavirus; LTAC, long-term acute care; PAK, physical activity kit; PONV/PDNV, postoperative and post-discharge nausea and vomiting; PTSD, posttraumatic stress disorder; SBAR, situation, background, assessment, recommendation.

on nurses, APRNs, and students. Many of the nurse-focused projects were directed toward education regarding practice change efforts or influence on attitudes. Settings for projects ranged from the community, long-term care, and retail health settings to hospitals and intensive care units.

As might be expected, chronic disease was a major focus, specifically, cardiovascular disease, valvular heart disease, heart failure, stroke, diabetes, hypertension, liver disease, chronic obstructive pulmonary disease (COPD), asthma, and end stage renal disease. Other disease-specific foci included various cancers, HIV, obesity (especially childhood obesity), transplant, dementia, attention deficit disorder, and autism. Pain, end of life, hospice, and palliative care were noted as areas where health care needs were identified. Additional projects addressed women's health, psychiatric mental health, disaster preparedness, and use of technology, informatics, and telemedicine.

Within these populations, settings, and diagnoses, projects were focused on health promotion strategies, development and evaluation of practice guidelines and quality improvement initiatives, practice models, models of care transition, interdisciplinary care, and health policy changes. Projects focusing on academic curriculum development, continuing education, and administrative topics, such as leadership and system changes, were also included. This review supports the practice doctorate's broad scope of impact identified by Burson et al. (2016).

DNP projects have been identified as examples of clinical excellence (Anderson et al., 2014; Burson et al., 2016), demonstrating the impact of the practice doctorate. The use of digital repositories for DNP projects has been recommended by AACN (2015) to "archive and share . . . the work and outcomes [of the DNP projects]" (p. 5). As dissemination of DNP scholarly projects grows through publications, supported by growth of digital repositories, DNP projects will continue to serve as a source to document impact of practice-doctorate outcomes until higher levels of evidence become available.

RECOMMENDATIONS FOR DNP OUTCOME STUDIES

The current focus on health care outcomes, compounded by the ongoing monitoring of educational outcomes, highlights the need for research of DNP-related outcomes to document the impact that DNP-prepared nurses have on quality of care, policy reform, and reduced costs. Research that demonstrates a positive impact in these areas can be used to garner support of key decision makers, such as legislators, health care providers, the community, third-party payers, and administrators (Newland, 2012). Data demonstrating the effectiveness of DNP-prepared nurses is necessary to demonstrate to employers the contributions that DNP-prepared nurses can make to the health care system (Burson et al., 2016; Pritham & White, 2016).

Policy

DNP graduates have impacted policy initiatives primarily at the local and regional levels (O'Dell, 2012); however, nursing has a history of leading policy change at a national level, such as the Magnet® process, which is affiliated with the AACN (American Nurses Credentialing Center, 2008; Leavitt, 2009). The DNP *Essentials* and early supporters of the DNP degree cited leadership in policy reform to improve health care outcomes as a key role. There have been case reports of DNP-prepared nurses being appointed to state and national advisory commissions to shape health care delivery through impacting policy (Pritham & White, 2016). It has been suggested that all nursing researchers should examine policy implications of their research (Leavitt, 2009); however, documentation of widespread transition of research findings into public policy reform led by nurses with practice doctorates is lacking. The analysis, synthesis, application, and evaluation of evidence is a cornerstone of DNP education and practice, placing DNP-prepared nurses in the role to serve as the advocate to champion policy change.

Evidence-Based Practice

As the number of hospitals striving for and maintaining Magnet status increases and the implementation of EBP in health care delivery continues, there will be growing needs for leadership and mentors in this area (Burson et al., 2016; Melnyk, Fineout-Overholt, Gallaher-Ford, & Kaplan, 2012; Syler & Levin, 2012). The DNP-prepared nurse is the logical choice to help fill these roles as one of the main foci of the practice doctorate is the use of EBP to transform health care and policy to improve health care and health care systems (Burson et al., 2016; Melnyk, 2013). The impact of DNP-led EBP changes needs to be documented in the areas of quality care, patient outcomes, cost reduction, and employee satisfaction (Melnyk et al., 2012). Research on the impact of implementation of EBP clinical guidelines on patient care outcomes is warranted in a multitude of settings and a variety of patients. The use of EBP is not limited to the clinical practice setting. Research is needed in academic arenas to determine the most effective teaching modalities, curriculum structure, and the impact that DNP-prepared faculty have on educating nurses of tomorrow.

Quality and Safety Improvement

The Quality and Safety Education for Nurses (QSEN) expanded its recommended knowledge, skills, and attitudes (KSA) to the advanced nursing practice level, with the APRN expected to take the leadership role in combining EBP, information technology, and outcome measures related to quality and safety processes (Cronenwett et al., 2009). These recommendations were supported in word or in spirit by the national organizations representing APRNs. The quality and safety arena is open for research concerning outcomes related to DNP-level nursing practice, to include evaluation of the educational curriculum using the APRN KSA as an outcome measure for DNP students and graduates. The KSA can also be used to select quality and safety outcomes to be monitored and impacted by DNP-prepared nurses.

Academic Education

As the number of DNP programs is expanding across the United States, research to demonstrate the quality and rigor necessary to adequately prepare DNP graduates is vital. DNP graduates require the skillset to be practice change leaders, a skillset that includes "[use of] informatics, secondary data analysis, team science and implementation science" (Broome, 2012, p. 112). What educational methodologies effectively prepare DNP students with this knowledge and these skills? What faculty is necessary to guide the development of leaders at this level? What courses are needed to provide the foundational concepts and encourage application of the concepts to prepare for practice in the future health care setting? These questions need to be answered with research focused on outcomes to guide decisions in the academic arena. Additional research is needed with regard to the impact that DNP-prepared faculty have on the outcomes related to the education of nursing students, the impact of tenure versus non-tenure-track appointments for DNP-prepared faculty, the leadership of DNP-prepared faculty in academic settings, and the impact practice requirements have on DNP APRNs who are full-time faculty.

SUMMARY

Jamesetta Newland reminds her DNP students, "Upon graduation, it can't be business as usual. People have to see a change in how you practice" (Newland, 2016, p. 6). The impact DNP-prepared nurses have on patient, health care, and policy outcomes is becoming more evident as the numbers of DNP graduates increase and studies analyzing these outcomes become more prevalent. The review of the literature demonstrates an increased number of articles about outcomes related to DNP-prepared nurses; however, most of the articles reflect anecdotal comments, include a small sample size, or utilize a case study approach. More robust research related to DNP outcomes has been called for in a number of articles and editorials. Research supports that APRNs educated at the master's level are highly competent, providing care with equal if not better outcomes than physicians (Stanik-Hutt et al., 2013). However, future questions needing answers include: (a) How do outcomes achieved by DNP-prepared nurses compare with outcomes achieved by non-DNP-prepared nurses? and (b) Will the master's-prepared APRN be as well prepared to provide care in the increasingly complex and diverse health care system as the DNP-prepared APRN? Health care policy decisions, such as the Affordable Care Act, and future initiatives proposed by leaders in the field of health care, such as the Josiah Macy Jr. Foundation, the IOM, and the Robert Wood Johnson Foundation, have and will continue to open the door for DNPs to shape the course of health care through projects developed to positively impact outcomes. This, in turn, should drive the need for research as to who is best prepared with the knowledge, skills, and abilities to demonstrate positive outcomes. Will it be the DNP-prepared nurse? The expectation is that it will be; however, research is needed to validate that assumption.

Answers to Chapter Discussion Questions

1. The AACN *Essentials* outline leadership, system change, quality and safety improvement, integration of EBP, informatics, health care policy, interprofessional collaboration, population health, and specialty nursing practice as outcomes that nurses with DNP degrees can positively impact. A review of the literature supports these outcomes as well as outcomes identified by the original supporters of the DNP degree, which included improved health promotion and risk reduction, improved coordination of care, and increased number of doctoral-prepared nursing faculty.

2. Reasons for minimal research available on DNP outcomes to date include an insufficient number of DNP graduates to participate in research studies, and diversity of specialty practice foci among DNP graduates, limiting identification of concentrated groups of DNP graduates to include in outcomes studies. Anecdotal reports about the impact of the DNP degree on individual graduates' practice and scholarship outcomes have been presented related to personal satisfaction with degree achievement, increased salary, and transition to higher levels of professional employment. Survey studies related to the number of DNP programs and graduates and synopses of DNP curricula provide the primary source of data; however, surveys regarding impact of the degree on salary and other professional outcomes are emerging in the literature.

3. Multiple factors will impact the focus of future studies of DNP outcomes. Forthcoming decisions regarding health care policy, reimbursement sources, and increased focus on outcomes in health care and nursing education will require studies of DNP outcomes to support and document the impact of DNP-prepared nurses. The outcome studies should include, but not be limited to, outcomes related to policy reform; clinical practice, specifically care provided by DNP-prepared practitioners compared with MSN-prepared practitioners; development, implementation, and evaluation of EBP guidelines; quality and safety; and the impact of DNP-prepared nurse educators.

WEB LINKS

▪ AACN: This site contains many of the documents related to the organized directive calling for the DNP as the entry-level degree for advanced nursing practice, including: the initial task force report from 2004; *The Essentials of Doctoral Education for Advanced Nursing Practice*, approved in 2006; and *The Doctor of Nursing Practice: Current Issues and Clarifying Recommendations: Report from the Task Force on the Implementation of the DNP* published in 2015, which further outlines the evolution of

DNP education. This site also maintains a list of all academic institutions with DNP programs, as well as fact sheets updated annually to reflect data trends related to DNP enrollment, numbers of graduates, and DNP programs in development. www .aacn.nche.edu/dnp

- Doctors of Nursing Practice, Inc.: This website was developed to serve as a virtual community for DNP-prepared nurses. The site contains abstracts of self-submitted DNP student projects as well as a collection of articles related to the development of the DNP degree. Doctors of Nursing Practice, Inc. is also an organization that hosts an annual conference showcasing presentations by DNP-prepared nurses concerning DNP practice and education. A monthly e-newsletter is published about health care professionals who influence outcomes. www.doctorsofnursingpractice .org
- NONPF, NP Curriculum Material: This site contains a link to DNP scholarly project title exemplars from several universities. NONPF also publishes position statements and competencies related to DNP preparation. www.nonpf.com/displaycommon .cfm?an=1&subarticlenbr=27
- DNP Project Lists and Samples: The following websites provide lists of titles or samples of DNP projects completed by DNP graduates.
  - Doctors of Nursing Practice. www.doctorsofnursingpractice.org/resources/dnp -scholarly-projects
  - Doctor of Nursing Practice Scholarly Projects, Vanderbilt University.
    2016—https://nursing.vanderbilt.edu/dnp/pdf/dnp_scholarlyprojects_2016.pdf
    2015—https://nursing.vanderbilt.edu/dnp/pdf/dnp_scholarlyprojects_2015.pdf
    2014—www.nursing.vanderbilt.edu/dnp/pdf/dnp_scholarlprojects_2014.pdf
    2013—www.nursing.vanderbilt.edu/dnp/pdf/dnp_scholarlprojects_2013.pdf
    2012—www.nursing.vanderbilt.edu/dnp/pdf/dnp_scholarlprojects_2012.pdf

REFERENCES

Advance Healthcare Network. (2015). 2014 NP & PA salary results: NP results by degree. *Advance for NPs & PAs.* Retrieved from http://nurse-practitioners-and-physician-assistants.advanceweb .com/Web-Extras/Online-Extras/2014-NPs-PAs-Salary-Survey-Results.aspx

Advance Healthcare Network. (2016). 2015 NP & PA salary results: NP results by degree and years of experience. *Advance for NPs & PAs.* Retrieved from http://nurse-practitioners-and-physician -assistants.advanceweb.com/Web-Extras/Online-Extras/2015-Salary-Survey-Results.aspx

Aiken, L., Clarke, S. P., Cheung, R. B., Sloane, D. M., & Silber, J. H. (2003). Educational levels of hospital nurses and surgical patient mortality. *Journal of American Medical Association, 290*(12), 1617–1623. doi:10.1001/jama.290.12.1617

Aiken, L., Clark, S. P., Sloane, D. M., Lake, E. T., & Cheney, T. (2008). Effects of hospital care environment on patient mortality and nurse outcomes. *Journal of Nursing Administration, 38*(5), 223–229. doi:10.1097/01.NNA.0000312773.42352.d7

American Association of Colleges of Nursing. (2004). AACN position statement on the practice doctorate in nursing. Retrieved from http://www.aacn.nche.edu/publications/position/ DNPpositionstatement.pdf

American Association of Colleges of Nursing. (2006). The essentials of doctoral education for advanced nursing practice. Retrieved from http://www.aacn.nche.edu/publications/position/DNPEssentials.pdf

American Association of Colleges of Nursing. (2015). *The doctor of nursing practice: Current issues and clarifying recommendations.* Report from the task force on the implementation of the DNP. Retrieved from http://www.aacn.nche.edu/aacn-publications/white-papers/DNP-Implementation-TF-Report-8-15.pdf

American Association of Colleges of Nursing. (2016). Fact sheet: Doctor of nursing practice. Retrieved from http://www.aacn.nche.edu/media-relations/fact-sheets/DNPFactSheet.pdf

American Association of Nurse Anesthetists. (2007). AANA position on doctoral preparation of nurse anesthetists. Retrieved from http://www.aana.com/ceandeducation/educationalresources/Documents/AANA_Position_DTF_June_2007.pdf

American Association of Nurse Anesthetists. (2013). Standards for nurse anesthesia practice. Retrieved from http://www.aana.com/resources2/professionalpractice/Documents/PPM%20Standards%20for%20Nurse%20Anesthesia%20Practice.pdf

American College of Nurse-Midwives. (2012). Core competencies for basic midwifery practice. Retrieved from http://www.midwife.org/ACNM/files/ACNMLibraryData/UPLOADFILENAME/000000000050/Core%20Comptencies%20Dec%202012.pdf

American Nurses Credentialing Center. (2008). ANCC Magnet recognition program. Retrieved from http://www.nursecredentialing.org/Magnet.aspx

American Organization of Nurse Executives. (2015). AONE nurse executive competencies. Retrieved from http://www.aone.org/resources/nurse-leader-competencies.shtml

Anderson, B. A., Knestrick, J. M., & Barroso, R. (Eds.). (2014). *DNP capstone projects: Exemplars of excellence in practice.* New York, NY: Springer Publishing.

Anderson, B. A., Knestrick, J., & Short, G. (2015). *Strategies for NP education: Analyzing completed DNP capstones as exemplars of clinical outcomes.* NONPF 41st Annual Meeting, Baltimore, MD. Retrieved from https://nonpf.confex.com/nonpf/2015md/webprogram/Session4223.html

Auerbach, D. I., Martsolf, G., Pearson, M. L., Taylor, E. A., Zaydman, M., Muchow, A., . . . Dower, C. (2014). *The DNP by 2015: A study of the institutional, political, and professional issues that facilitate or impede establishing a post-baccalaureate doctor of nursing practice program.* Retrieved from http://www.aacn.nche.edu/dnp/DNP-Study.pdf

Bellflower, B., & Carter, M. A. (2006). Primer on the practice doctorate for neonatal nurse practitioners. *Advances in Neonatal Care, 6*(6), 323–332. doi:10.1016/j.adnc.2006.08.001

Berkowitz, B. (2014). The emergence and impact of the DNP degree on clinical practice. In B. A. Anderson, J. M. Knestrick, & R. Barroso (Eds.), *DNP capstone projects: Exemplars of excellence in practice* (pp. 3–16). New York, NY: Springer Publishing.

Broome, M. E. (2012). Doubling the number of doctorally prepared nurses [Editorial]. *Nursing Outlook, 60*(3), 111–113.e1. doi:10.1016/j.outlook.2012.04.001

Broome, M. E., & Riner, M. B. (2012, August). *Contributions of scholarly papers in literature: Dissemination practices of DNP graduates.* Podium presentation at Promoting Quality and Excellence in DNP Education, Chicago, IL.

Burson, R., Moran, K. J., & Conrad, D. (2016). Why hire a doctor of nursing practice-prepared nurse? The value added impact of the practice doctorate. *Journal of Doctoral Nursing Practice, 9*(1), 152–157. doi:10.1891/2380-9418.9.1.152

Council on Accreditation of Nurse Anesthesia Educational Programs. (2016). Accreditation policies and procedures. Retrieved from http://home.coa.us.com/accreditation/Documents/Accreditation%20Policies%20and%20Procedures%20Manual,%20revised%20June%202016.pdf

Cronenwett, L., Dracup, K., Grey, M., McCauley, L., Meleis, A., & Salmon, M. (2011). The doctor of nursing practice: A national workforce perspective. *Nursing Outlook, 59,* 9–17. doi:10.1016/j.outlook.2010.11.003

Cronenwett, L., Sherwood, G., Pohl, J., Barnsteiner, J., Moore, S., Sullivan, D. T.,…Warren, J. (2009). Quality and safety education for advanced nursing practice. *Nursing Outlook, 57,* 338–348. doi:10.1016/j.outlook.2009.07.009

Dennison, R. D., Payne, C., & Farrell, K. (2012). The doctorate in nursing practice: Moving advanced practice nursing even closer to excellence. *Nursing Clinics of North America, 47,* 225–240. doi:10.1016/j.cnur.2012.04.001

Draye, M. A., Acker, M., & Zimmer, P. A. (2006). The practice doctorate in nursing: Approaches to transform nurse practitioner education and practice. *Nursing Outlook, 54*(3), 123–129. doi:10.1016/j.outlook.2006.01.001

Fang, D., & Bednash, G. D. (2017). Identifying barriers and facilitators to future nurse faculty careers for DNP students. *Journal of Professional Nursing, 33*(1), 56–67.

Healthcare Information and Management Systems Society. (2015). TIGER International informatics competency synthesis project. Retrieved from http://www.himss.org/professional-development/tiger-initiative/tiger-international-informatics-competency-synthesis-project

Institute of Medicine. (1999). *To err is human: Building a safer health system.* Retrieved from http://www.nap.edu/catalog.php?record_id=9728#toc

Institute of Medicine. (2001). *Crossing the quality chasm: A new health system for the 21st century.* Retrieved from http://books.nap.edu/openbook.php?record_id=10027

Institute of Medicine. (2010). *Report brief: The future of nursing: Leading change, advancing health.* Retrieved from https://www.nap.edu/download/12956#

Jones, M. (2013). 2012 NP & PA salary results: NP results by degree and years of experience. *Advance for NPs & PAs.* Retrieved from http://nurse-practitioners-and-physician-assistants.advanceweb.com/Web-Extras/Online-Extras/2012-NP-PA-Salary-By-Academic-Degree.aspx

Kirschling, J. M. (2014). *Reflections on the future of doctoral programs in nursing.* Paper presented at the AACN Doctoral Education Conference, Naples, FL. Retrieved from http://www.aacn.nche.edu/dnp/JK-2014-DNP.pdf

Kung, M. (2012, March). How the DNP changed me. *Advance for NPs & PAs.* Retrieved from http://community.advanceweb.com/blogs/np_7/default.aspx

Leavitt, J. K. (2009). Leaders in health policy: A critical role for nursing. *Nursing Outlook, 57*(2), 73–77.

Love, R., Allison, T. L., & McArthur, D. B. (2014). Building a blueprint for evaluation of DNP project outcomes. NONPF 40th Annual Meeting. Retrieved from https://nonpf.confex.com/nonpf/2014co/webprogram/Paper7287.html

Marion, L., Viens, D., O'Sullivan, A. L., Crabtree, K., Fontana, S., & Price, M. M. (2003). The practice doctorate in nursing: Future or fringe? *Topics in Advanced Practice Nursing eJournal, 3*(2), 1–8.

Marshall, E. S., & Broome, M. E. (Eds.). (2017). *Transformational leadership in nursing* (2nd ed.). New York, NY: Springer Publishing.

Melnyk, B. M. (2013). Distinguishing the preparation and roles of doctor of philosophy and doctor of nursing practice graduates: National implications for academic curricula and health care systems. *Journal of Nursing Education, 52*(8), 442–448. doi:10.3928/01484834-20130719-01

Melnyk, B. M., Fineout-Overholt, E., Gallaher-Ford, L., & Kaplan, L. (2012). The state of evidence-based practice in US nurses: Critical implication for nurse leaders and educators. *The Journal of Nursing Administration, 42*(9), 410–417. doi:10.1097/NNA.0b013e3182664e0a

Montgomery, K. L., & Porter-O'Grady, T. (2010). Innovation and learning: Creating the DNP nurse leader. *Nurse Leader, 8*(4), 44–47. doi:10.1016/j.mnl.2010.05.001

Mundinger, M. O. (2005). Who's who in nursing: Bringing clarity to the doctor of nursing practice. *Nursing Outlook, 53*(4), 173–176. doi:10.1016/j.outlook.2005.05.007

Mundinger, M. O., Cook, S. S., Lenz, E. R., Piacentini, K., Auerhahn, C., & Smith, J. (2000). Assuring quality and access in advanced practice nursing: A challenge to nurse educators. *Journal of Professional Nursing, 16*(6), 322–329. doi:10.1053/jpnu.2000.18177

National Association of Clinical Nurse Specialists. (2015). National association of clinical nurse specialists endorses requiring doctor of nursing practice degree for clinical nurse specialists [Press release]. Retrieved from http://www.nacns.org/docs/PR-DNP-Statement1507.pdf

National Organization of Nurse Practitioner Faculties. (2011). Nurse practitioner core competencies. Retrieved from http://www.nonpf.org/associations/10789/files/IntegratedNPCoreCompsFINAL April2011.pdf

National Organization of Nurse Practitioner Faculties. (2015). The doctorate of nursing practice NP preparation: NONPF perspective. Retrieved from http://c.ymcdn.com/sites/www.nonpf.org/ resource/resmgr/DNP/NONPFDNPStatementSept2015.pdf

Nelson, J. M., Cook, P. F., & Raterink, G. (2013). The evolution of a doctor of nursing practice capstone process: Programmatic revisions to improve the quality of student projects. *Journal of Professional Nursing, 29*(6), 370–380.

Newland, J. A. (2012, April). The nurse practitioner salutes the DNP [Editorial]. *The Nurse Practitioner, 37*(4), 5. doi:10.1097/01.npr.0000412897.94383.64

Newland, J. A. (2016, April). The impact of the DNP degree [Editorial]. *The Nurse Practitioner, 41*(4), 6. doi:10.1097/01.NPR.0000481996.54530.26

O'Dell, D. G. (2012, September 22). *The state of DNP degree: Analysis of three years of national survey data*. Presentation at Fifth National DNP Conference, Saint Louis, MO.

Pritham, U. A., & White, P. (2016, April). Assessing DNP impact: Using program evaluations to capture healthcare system change. *The Nurse Practitioner, 41*(4), 41–53. doi:10.1097/01 .NPR.0000481509.24736.c8

Pronsanti, M. P. (2011). National salary report 2011: Advance for NPs and PAs. Retrieved from http://nurse-practitioners-and-physician-assistants.advanceweb.com/Features/Articles/ National-Salary-Report-2011.aspx

Redman, R. W., Pressler, S. J., Furspan, P., & Potempa, K. (2015). Nurses in the United States with a practice doctorate: Implications for leading in the current context of health care. *Nursing Outlook*, *63*(2), 124–129.

Staffileno, B. A., Murphy, M. P., & Carlson, E. (2016). Determinants for effective collaboration among DNP-and PhD-prepared faculty. *Nursing Outlook*, *65*(1), 94–102. doi:http://dx.doi.org/10.1016/j .outlook.2016.08.003

Stanik-Hutt, J., Newhouse, R. P., White, K. M., Johantgen, M., Bass, E. B., Zangaro, G., . . . Weiner, J. P. (2013). The quality and effectiveness of care provided by nurse practitioners. *The Journal for Nurse Practitioners*, *9*(8), 492–500.

Syler, J., & Leving, R. F. (2012). Evidence-based practice: On the doctor of nursing practice (DNP). *Research and Theory for Nursing Practice: An International Journal*, *26*(1) 6–9.

Terhaar, M. F., Crickman, R., & Finnell, D. S. (2016). Project planning and the work of translation. In K. M. White, S. Dudley-Brown, & M. F. Terhaar (Eds.), *Translation of evidence into nursing and health care* (2nd ed., pp. 183–209). New York, NY: Springer Publishing.

Udlis, K. A., & Mancuso, J. M. (2015). Perceptions of the role of the doctor of nursing practice-prepared nurse: Clarity or confusion. *Journal of Professional Nursing*, *31*(4), 274–281. doi:10.1016/j .profnurs.2015.01.004

Waldrop, J., Caruso, D., Fuchs, M. A., & Hypes, K. (2014). EC as PIE: Five criteria for executing a successful DNP final project. *Journal of Professional Nursing*, *30*(4), 300–306.

CHAPTER 12

Resources to Facilitate Advanced Practice Nursing Outcome Research

Denise Bryant-Lukosius, Ruth Martin-Misener, Joan Tranmer, Faith Donald, Linda Brousseau, and Alba DiCenso

Chapter Objectives

1. Describe the impact of dedicated national research programs for building advanced practice nursing (APN) research capacity and expertise
2. Provide an overview of the PEPPA (Participatory, Evidence-Based, Patient-Focused Process for Advanced Practice Nursing Role Development, Implementation, and Evaluation) framework and how it has been enhanced and applied to guide the successful design, implementation, and evaluation of APN roles
3. Describe additional tools and resources developed to support the selection and evaluation of APN-sensitive outcomes relevant to different stages of role development

Chapter Discussion Questions

1. What five features of complex health care interventions are consistent with common characteristics of APN roles?
2. What are common barriers to conducting meaningful APN role evaluations?
3. How can participatory action research (PAR) be used to inform the development and implementation of APN roles? Why is this process important?
4. Provide examples of APN role structures, processes, and outcomes. What are the objectives for evaluating structures, processes, and outcomes at three distinct stages of role development?

Based on UK Medical Research Council guidelines, APN roles meet the criteria of a complex health care intervention (Craig et al., 2008). They involve a number of interacting components, including role competencies and related activities (clinical, educational, research, leadership, consultation, collaboration), which when enacted in combination are greater than the sum of their parts (Canadian Nurses Association [CNA], 2008). These activities are often directed at several target groups (patients and families, nurses and other health care providers, organizations, and health systems) to address difficult health care problems and to achieve a variety of outcomes relevant to each target group. APN roles also need to be highly flexible and responsive to the dynamic needs and contexts of the patient populations they serve and the environments and practice settings in which they work.

Like other complex health care interventions, high-quality and meaningful evaluations of APN roles require a sophisticated research skill set to determine the purpose of the evaluation and to apply the most appropriate methods for examining the role at different stages of development (Bryant-Lukosius, 2009). While numerous reviews document the effective outcomes of APN roles (Morrilla-Herrera et al., 2016; Newhouse et al., 2011; Swan, Ferguson, Change, Larson, & Smaldone, 2015), the quality of the individual APN studies included in the reviews is inconsistent. Advanced practice registered nurses (APRNs) also report that they lack the research knowledge, skills, and experience to evaluate the impact of their roles (DiCenso & Bryant-Lukosius, 2010). A common limitation of APN role evaluations is the failure to use relevant theoretical frameworks and rigorous research methods in designing both the role and the evaluation plan. This limitation contributes to poorly defined roles and evaluation designs that do not improve our understanding about the complexity of the role and the relationships between role activities and outcomes, or how these roles did or did not achieve expected outcomes. Similarly, the lack of clearly defined APN roles and poor agreement among stakeholders about expected outcomes is a barrier to selecting APN-sensitive outcomes and collecting baseline data for future comparative evaluations (Bryant-Lukosius, DiCenso, Browne, & Pinelli, 2004).

This chapter reviews work being done in Canada to further APN outcome research, by providing resources to address these five major barriers (i.e., lack of APN research expertise, guiding frameworks, role clarity, sensitive outcome measures, baseline data) to evaluate these complex health care interventions. These resources include (a) the evolution of a federally funded APN research chair and establishment of a dedicated national research unit designed to build research capacity; (b) mentorship and continuing education to support the development of novice APN researchers at the point of care; (c) guidelines for conducting economic evaluations of APN roles; (d) an enhanced conceptual framework and related toolkit for guiding the APN role design, implementation and evaluation process; and (e) a strategy for identifying sensitive outcome measures, including an APN research data collection toolkit for selecting APN-sensitive outcome measurement tools. An overview of these resources will be provided and their application to promote high-quality outcome assessments of APN roles will be examined.

RESEARCH CHAIR IN APN

From 2001 to 2011, the Canadian government's health research agency funded a chair in APN held by Alba DiCenso, a coauthor of this chapter. The purpose of the chair was to increase Canada's pool of nurse researchers with the ability to lead and conduct applied APN-related research that serves the needs of clinicians, managers, and policy makers in the health sector. Chair activities designed to achieve this goal focused on (a) the education of nurse researchers at the graduate level, (b) linkage and exchange with decision makers to ensure policy relevance and the dissemination and uptake of research results, (c) mentoring junior faculty and postdoctoral fellows to launch an APN-related research program, and (d) conducting research to inform the practice of APRNs across Canada.

Annually, through a competitive process, three Canadian graduate students (master's and PhD level) planning to conduct APN-related health services research were accepted into the Chair Program and awarded a $10,000 bursary. In addition to the university requirements for degree completion, the Chair Program required participating students to (a) enroll in a graduate course, "Research Issues in the Introduction and Evaluation of APN Roles," specifically developed for APN chair students, (b) write an APN-related commentary for the journal *Evidence-Based Nursing*, (c) complete a 90-hour practicum in a policy setting and a 90-hour research internship, (d) identify an interdisciplinary thesis committee to oversee an APN-related health services research study, (e) partner with a decision maker to identify a policy-informing thesis topic, and (f) attend monthly meetings of Chair Program students via remote technology. Chair funding permitted graduate students from across the country to enroll in the APN-related graduate course by covering travel and accommodation costs for face-to-face components.

Impact of the Chair Program on Building APN Research Capacity and Expertise

The Chair Program accepted 24 graduate students from five provinces (6 MSc, 16 PhD, 2 DNP) who were enrolled in nine Canadian and American universities. Those who completed their PhDs were eligible to compete for a junior faculty position funded and supervised by the Chair Program with the goal to secure postdoctoral funding. Three junior faculty were funded through the Chair Program, all of whom were successful in competing for externally funded postdoctoral fellowship awards. These plus two additional postdoctoral fellows supervised by the chair, continued to participate in the Chair Program as McMaster University–based senior faculty or as affiliate faculty from other Canadian universities. In addition to the chair students, 87 APRNs, graduate students, and health care administrators from across Canada completed the graduate course "Research Issues in the Introduction and Evaluation of APN Roles." The final course assignment was the preparation of a research proposal related to the development, implementation, or evaluation of an APN role.

Over the course of 10 years (2001–2011), the APN Chair Program had substantive impact on the capacity to conduct APN research in Canada. The program received over $3.5 million in research funding to complete 48 APN-focused studies. Research trainees and faculty presented their study findings and other scholarly work in 605 oral and 182 poster peer-reviewed presentations at national and international conferences and in 236 peer-reviewed publications and 21 book chapters. Through linkage and exchange activities among graduate students, APRNs, researchers, and health care administrators, the Chair Program fostered the development of other national APN research enterprises, supported national collaboration within research teams conducting APN research, and enabled studies of national importance. For example, one clinical nurse specialist (CNS), who is also a coauthor of this chapter (D.B-L.), transitioned through each research-training opportunity provided by the Chair Program and went on to receive funding to establish a Canadian Centre of Excellence in Oncology APN. This center provides research training, mentorship, and consultative services and promotes the uptake of research findings through knowledge translation focused on APRNs in cancer control. More information about the center can be found online (oapn.mcmaster.ca).

Chair students and faculty from several provinces also collaborated on a landmark national study and interdisciplinary research team, led by two coauthors of this chapter (F.D. and R.M.M.), to examine the role of nurse practitioners (NPs) in long-term care settings (Carter et al., 2016; Donald et al., 2013; Kaasalainen et al., 2013; Martin-Misener, Donald, et al., 2015; Ploeg et al., 2013; Sangster-Gormley et al., 2013). A second national study led by chair faculty and graduate students established the foundation for the next generation of APN research in Canada (DiCenso & Bryant-Lukosius, 2010). The results of this comprehensive study were summarized in a special issue of the *Canadian Journal of Nursing Leadership* that included 10 publications outlining evidence-based recommendations for the individual, organizational, and health system supports required to better integrate CNS and NP roles into the Canadian health care system. A major finding of this study was the need for further research about the outcomes and cost-effectiveness of APN roles. The special issue can be accessed freely online (www.longwoods.com/content/22264?utm_source=Longwoods+Master+Mailing+List&utm_campaign=17b93e9e2d-NL_Vol23SP_Issue_TOC_Alert4_8_2011&utm_medium=email).

CANADIAN CENTRE FOR APN RESEARCH

In July 2011, the 10-year funding for the Chair Program ended but its legacy continues with the establishment of the Canadian Centre for APN Research (CCAPNR) at McMaster University. As evidence of growing research capacity and the importance of succession planning to maintain research productivity and momentum, this center is led by senior and affiliate faculty from three provinces who are graduates of the Chair Program. In contrast to the APN Chair Program, the primary focus of the Center is on conducting research and on knowledge translation, with a continued but less prominent emphasis on the training and mentorship of APN researchers. To further the development of APN research expertise and to strengthen our understanding of these complex roles, CCAPNR has expanded its mandate to support collaborative, interdisciplinary research nationally and internationally. More information on CCAPNR can be found online (fhs.mcmaster.ca/ccapnr).

Five Years of CCAPNR Activities and Influence

Over the past 5 years, CCAPNR's research, evaluation, and knowledge transfer activities and products have made a substantial contribution to APN role introduction, implementation, and sustainability. Topics that have been the focus of CCAPNR research are summarized in Exhibit 12.1. CCAPNR has completed or is currently involved in policy, practice, educational, and research initiatives with organizations at the national level and

EXHIBIT 12.1	Examples of Topic Areas of CCAPNR Research

- Cost-effectiveness of CNS and NP roles
- Optimizing health care system integration of the CNS role
- APN activity and workload
- APN roles and team collaboration
- Navigation roles in primary health care
- Optimizing RN roles in primary health care
- NP competencies and education in primary health care
- Indicators for evaluating the quality of NP services in primary health care
- NP prescribing practices in primary health care
- Impact of NPs in long-term care
- Effectiveness of health coaching in type 2 diabetes
- Effective use of APN roles in cancer control
- Interprofessional models of cancer survivorship care in primary health care

APN, advanced practice nursing; CCAPNR, Canadian Centre for APN Research; CNS, clinical nurse specialist; NP, nurse practitioner.

in more than half of Canadian provinces/territories. Internationally, CCAPNR has provided consultation, education, and leadership to international organizations and in at least eight countries. CCAPNR's knowledge translation tools and research evidence are being used around the world. Some of CCAPNR's accomplishments include:

- Securing over $5.3 million in funded research grants, contracts, and capacity-building initiatives
- Publishing over 100 articles in high-impact international and national peer-reviewed journals
- Giving 100 presentations at international, national, and regional peer-reviewed conferences to researcher, policy-maker, and clinician audiences
- Presenting 70 addresses as invited speakers at a variety of international, national, and regional forums
- Providing leadership to international, national, and regional organizations seeking to establish, expand, or optimize APN and other specialized nursing roles through education, regulation, and policy
- Offering innovative approaches to educate and mentor health care professionals in leading and conducting point-of-care research, quality improvement (QI), or evidence-informed decision-making (EIDM) projects
- Establishing productive, mutually rewarding collaborations with international, national, and regional partners
- Contributing to graduate education about APN beyond expected teaching roles

In summary, CCAPNR has evolved to become known as a leader in: APN research and evaluation; education and policy; and linkage and exchange, both nationally and internationally. Future directions include expanding our membership, and continuing to build our international reach while maintaining the strength of involvement and influence we have in producing and translating evidence related to APN and special-ized nursing in Canada. In the following two sections, specific examples of innovative CCAPNR initiatives are described.

Building APN Capacity to Conduct Point-of-Care Research

The Trillium and Alberta Rose projects involved academic practice partnerships estab-lished between CCAPNR and two health care organizations in different provinces. The aim of these partnerships was to provide an applied research course and mentorship to promote the integration of research into the day-to-day practice of APRNs. The major output from the course was a research proposal or QI/evidence-based project that par-ticipants would implement following completion of the course. Participants were paired with a CCAPNR faculty mentor with similar research interests, to support the develop-ment of their research proposal or project plan and to assist with the development of research competencies over a short period of time (e.g., 4 months). Course topics were led by CCAPNR faculty and included a variety of learning strategies, such as small group seminars, peer review, and videoconferencing. A formative evaluation completed at the end of the course showed that participants were highly satisfied with the course content and the knowledge and expertise of the faculty. A pre- and postcourse evaluation dem-onstrated significant improvement in participants' perceived confidence and competence in conducting research (Harbman et al., 2017).

Advancing Economic Evaluations of APN Roles

Controlling health care costs and improving care quality are important drivers that influence decisions to implement APN roles. To inform these decisions, CCAPNR fac-ulty conducted a systematic review of randomized controlled trials (RCTs) evaluating the economic impact of NP and CNS roles (Donald, Kilpatrick, Reid, Carter, Martin-Misener, et al., 2014). The primary outcomes of interest were health care costs (e.g., professional, family, and hospital costs); resource use (e.g., prescriptions, diagnostic tests and procedures); length of stay; and rehospitalization. Health system utilization was also examined for all patient (e.g., mortality, morbidity, satisfaction with care, qual-ity of life) and provider (e.g., job satisfaction and quality of care) outcomes. Published and unpublished RCTs, in all languages, conducted between January 1980 and July 2012 were eligible for the review. Forty-three RCTs were included in the review and categorized into six groups: NP-outpatient (primary care and long-term care; $n = 11$), NP-transition ($n = 5$), NP-inpatient ($n = 2$), CNS-outpatient ($n = 11$), CNS-transition ($n = 13$), and CNS-inpatient ($n = 1$). Transition roles involved services to safely trans-fer patients from one level of care to another or between settings in a timely manner (Naylor, Aiken, Kurtzman, Olds, & Hirschman, 2011). The review results are published in several papers according to the six groupings (Bryant-Lukosius, Carter, et al., 2015; Donald, Kilpatrick, Reid, Carter, Bryant-Lukosius, et al., 2014; Kilpatrick et al., 2014, 2015; Martin-Misener, Harbman, et al., 2017).

An important aspect of the systematic review was assessment of the quality of eco-nomic evaluations using the Quality of Health Economic Studies (QHES) tool (Marshall et al., 2015). The QHES assesses the quality of health economics studies involving cost-minimization, cost-effectiveness, or cost–utility analyses (Chiou et al., 2003). Based on the QHES tool, most of the 43 RCTs (77%) were found to have poor study quality and only three studies (7%) were of high quality (Marshall et al., 2015). The multifaceted domains and versatility of NP and CNS practice created challenges in applying general economic analysis guidelines to studies evaluating these roles (Marshall et al., 2015). Consequently, the research team determined that the general guidelines required adaptations to adequately address economic analyses of APN roles. Four processes were used to adapt the economic evaluation guidelines: (a) a literature review of theoretical and discussion papers about economic evaluations of CNS and NP roles; (b) a detailed analysis of quality of the 43 RCTs in this study; (c) assessment of current economic evaluation guidelines; and (d) recommendations from a panel of 15 experts from Canada and the United States (Lopatina et al., 2017).

General criteria were identified from a review of economic evaluation tools (e.g., Canadian Agency for Drugs and Technologies in Health, 2006; Drummond, Schulpher, Claxton, Stoddart, & Torrance, 2015). Four criteria were found to be applicable to APN roles without modification:

1. *Specifying the time horizon* or duration of the study that is sufficient to capture important outcomes and costs of the intervention
2. *Applying modeling* techniques using the results from a short-term study to evaluate and project the long-term effect
3. *Using discounting rates* at 5% per year for costs and outcomes that occur beyond 12 months, especially for studies involving patients with chronic conditions
4. *Managing variability and uncertainty* by conducting sensitivity analyses to determine how variations in inputs affect study results and conclusions.

Seven general economic evaluation criteria required adaptation to improve their application to APN studies. A brief overview of these criteria is provided in Table 12.1. A more fulsome summary of the criteria is presented in a manuscript for publication (Lopatina et al., 2017).

ADDITIONAL RESOURCES TO SUPPORT APN ROLE EVALUATION

Two additional resources arising from the Chair Program are the PEPPA framework and the APN Research Data Collection Toolkit. The PEPPA framework was developed by a coauthor of this chapter (D.B-L.) as a doctoral student in the APN Chair Program (Bryant-Lukosius & DiCenso, 2004). As Chair Program students conducted their research, they used existing data collection tools and developed a variety of instruments. The APN Chair Program was often approached by researchers and decision makers for information about APN-related research data collection tools. As a result, the Chair Program, with funding from a provincial decision-maker partner, created the APN Research Data Collection Toolkit. Researchers conducting APN outcome research may find both these resources, the PEPPA framework and the APN Research Data Collection Toolkit, useful. The remainder of this chapter describes these two resources.

TABLE 12.1   Criteria Requiring Adaptation for Economic Evaluations of APN Roles

Criterion	Description
Develop the study question	Include the target population, intervention, comparators, and study perspective. Consider the model of APN care, role domains, and if the role is alternative or complementary to usual care.
Select a suitable method of economic evaluation	*Cost-effectiveness* is applicable for a single unit of outcome, but may not be applicable for multiple outcomes. *Cost–utility analysis* combines several outcomes into a single composite, such as a QALY, but cannot include complex measures of quality of life, nonhealth outcomes, and opportunity costs. *Cost–benefit analysis* values all costs and benefits in the same monetary units to determine the value that people attach to health care services. It can be challenging to place costs on participants' values. *Cost-minimization analysis* can be used when data analysis reveals no differences in outcomes between comparison groups. Only costs are considered. Multiple outcomes may preclude this type of analysis. *Cost–consequence analysis* is recommended for APN role evaluations with multiple outcomes. It provides separate reporting of all costs and outcomes.
Choose a comparator	For alternative APN roles, determine what constitutes "usual care." In complementary models, the APN role may be added to a team to augment care. Evaluations of these roles compare outcomes of teams with and without APRNs.
Decide the study perspective	The perspective (public payer, patient, employer, or society) determines which costs, resources, and consequences are included in the analysis. The public payer perspective is commonly used but fails to capture the benefits or costs from other sectors, cost shifts to the patient and family, productivity costs, or long-term consequences, such as health promotion/prevention costs.
Measure effectiveness	Including at least 10 APRNs in an RCT may minimize bias related to variability in roles and the contexts of care (Donald, Kilpatrick, Reid, Carter, Martin-Misener, et al., 2014).
Value APN outcomes	Some APN outcomes (e.g., access to care, patient satisfaction, quality of care, impact of nonclinical role dimensions) can be challenging to measure from an economic perspective.
Determine resource use and costs	Items typically included in studies of APN roles include prescriptions, diagnostic tests, length or number of visits, length of stay, and so on. The source of the data on these items should be stated (e.g., administrative databases, current literature). A broad and inclusive approach is required for chronic conditions. This may include costs related to lost productivity for patients to attend appointments or for family members to care for sick relatives.

APN, advanced practice nursing; APRNs, advanced practice registered nurses; QALY, quality-adjusted life year; RCT, randomized controlled trial.

The PEPPA Framework

The PEPPA framework was developed to provide APN researchers, health care providers, administrators, and policy makers with a guide to promote the optimal development and deployment of APN roles. A critical feature of this framework is that strategies to support meaningful outcome evaluations of APN roles are incorporated throughout role planning and implementation. The underlying premise of the PEPPA framework is that *the mandate of all APN roles is to maximize, maintain, or restore patient health through innovation in nursing practice and in the delivery of health services* (CNA, 2008; Davies &

EXHIBIT 12.2 **Common Problems Associated With APN Role Implementation**

> ▨ Stakeholder confusion about APN terminology
>
> ▨ Lack of clearly defined roles and role goals or outcomes
>
> ▨ Role emphasis on physician replacement or support
>
> ▨ Underutilization of APN scope of practice and expertise in all role dimensions
>
> ▨ Failure to address role implementation barriers
>
> ▨ Limited use of evidence-based approaches to guide role development, implementation, and evaluation

APN, advanced practice nursing.
Source: Bryant-Lukosius, DiCenso, et al. (2004).

Hughes, 2002). This mandate is consistent with international views of advanced nursing practice. There is a heightened demand worldwide for APRNs, as clinical experts, leaders, and change agents, to assist organizations in developing sustainable models of health care (Bryant-Lukosius, DiCenso, et al., 2004).

An initial review of the international literature identified six frequently reported barriers that were common to the effective implementation of various types of APN roles (Bryant-Lukosius, DiCenso, et al., 2004). A subsequent study involving a review of the international literature and examination of APN role implementation in Canada reconfirmed these challenges (DiCenso & Bryant-Lukosius, 2010). Many of these barriers could be avoided through improved planning and better stakeholder understanding of the roles (Exhibit 12.2). Initial and follow-up reviews of the literature (Bryant-Lukosius, DiCenso, et al., 2004; DiCenso et al., 2010) also indicated that the costs associated with poor APN role implementation planning are high and justify the need for more thoughtful, systematic approaches to role introduction (Exhibit 12.3).

The PEPPA framework builds on earlier models recommending steps for introducing new health providers (Spitzer, 1978) and specifically APN roles (Dunn & Nicklin, 1995; Mitchell-DiCenso, Pinelli, & Southwell, 1996), by incorporating additional steps and strategies to address known barriers to successful APN role implementation. The aims of the framework are to:

- ▨ Use relevant data to support the need and identified goals for a clearly defined role
- ▨ Support advanced nursing practice characterized by patient-centered, health-focused, and holistic care
- ▨ Promote the integration of APN knowledge, skills, and expertise from all role dimensions related to clinical practice, education, research, organizational leadership, and scholarly/professional practice (Canadian Association of Nurses in Oncology [CANO], 2001)
- ▨ Create practice environments that support APN role development by engaging stakeholders from the health care team, practice setting, and health care system in role planning
- ▨ Promote ongoing role development and model of care enhancement through continuous and rigorous evaluation of progress in achieving predetermined outcome-based goals

EXHIBIT 12.3   The Costs of Poor APN Role Implementation Planning

- Poor stakeholder role acceptance
- Role conflict
- Role overload
- Poor APRN job satisfaction
- Difficulty recruiting and retaining highly qualified APRNs
- Negative impact on the quality of patient care and patient safety
- Unrealized opportunity for innovation and benefits from APN expertise for patients, health providers, and the health care system
- Ineffective use of limited health care resources
- Negative impact on long-term role sustainability

APN, advanced practice nursing; APRN, advanced practice registered nurse.
Source: Bryant-Lukosius et al. (2004).

Conceptual Foundations of the PEPPA Framework

The principles of PAR informed the development of the framework. PAR is a democratic, systematic approach that involves individuals from organizations, educational systems, and communities in promoting health and social change (Deshler & Ewert, 1995; Foote Whyte, 1991; Smith, Pyrch, & Lizardi, 1993). Key principles of PAR include: active participation in cycles of reflection and action; valuing what people know and believe by building on their current understanding; collective investigation, analysis, learning, and the conscious production of new knowledge; collective decision making and action in using new knowledge to address problems; and evaluating the impact of these actions (Bowling, 1997; Deshler & Ewert, 1995; Smith, 1997).

The principles of PAR are relevant to APN role development in several ways. First, PAR promotes the use of objective data in health care planning and decisions to develop, implement, and modify an APN role. Early pioneers in the development of APN roles have also emphasized the importance of good data to support the need for new health provider roles, in the same way that research evidence is used to support the introduction of new therapeutic interventions such as medications (Spitzer, 1978). Second, APN practitioners work collaboratively within interprofessional teams and in established relationships with other stakeholders in the health system. Stakeholder roles and relationships are influenced by their values, beliefs, experiences, and expectations. These relationships create the conditions that impact the effective delivery of health care services and can facilitate or obstruct the implementation of APN roles. Therefore, collective learning and consensus decision making in the health planning process, on the part of key stakeholders, are necessary for the effective implementation of APN roles.

The principles of PAR are consistent with research-based approaches recommended for the planning of nursing and health and human resources (Advisory Committee on Health Delivery and Human Resources, 2007; O'Brien-Pallas, Tomblin Murphy, Baumann, & Birch, 2001). These include the principles of collaborative decision making through involvement of appropriate stakeholders, ensuring that target population health care needs are foundational to any process, consideration of environmental trends and drivers (context), and a system approach to ensure comprehensiveness in planning and in the assessment of outcomes.

The PEPPA framework also draws on Donabedian's theory for evaluating the quality of health care by proposing a structure–process–outcome evaluation of the APN role (Donabedian, 1966, 1992). This approach is consistent with other structure–process–outcome models developed to evaluate APN roles (Byers & Brunell, 1998; Grimes & Garcia, 1997; Sidani & Irvine, 1999). "Structures" are factors that affect processes or determine how the APN role is implemented. Role structures may include characteristics of the APN and patient populations; APN education programs; practical and financial resources; nursing and health care policies; regulatory and credentialing mechanisms; the model of care; and the physical, cultural, and organizational environment in which the APN works (Bryant-Lukosius & DiCenso, 2004). "Process" refers to what the APRN does in the role. This includes the types of APN services and how these services are provided. To ensure maximal use of APN expertise and scope of practice, the PEPPA framework recommends that processes be considered across all role dimensions related to clinical practice, education, research, organizational leadership, and scholarly/professional development (CANO, 2001).

"Outcomes" are the results of APN role services and care and thus are affected by both structure and process factors. In the framework, outcomes may be evaluated from the perspectives of patients and families, the APRN, health care providers, the organization, and the broader health care system. Outcomes are determined by goals for improving the delivery of nursing and health care services established early in the role-planning process. A package of APN services and specific role activities for each dimension of advanced nursing practice is developed specifically to achieve these preestablished goals. Strategically linking APN role activities with preset goals and outcomes facilitates the selection of outcome measures that will be most sensitive to APN interventions (Burns, 2001; Minnick, 2001).

The ability to conduct meaningful evaluations of the APN role is further strengthened by linking role structures, processes, and outcomes in the early stages of role development. For example, in the PEPPA framework the APN role is evaluated along with the model of care in which the role is situated. This strategy aids in determining how structures within the model of care, such as other health provider roles, role relationships, and resources, affect APN role processes and outcomes.

Steps of the PEPPA Framework

The PEPPA framework involves a nine-step process (Figure 12.1). These steps reflect the complexity of the roles and are consistent with guidelines for developing and evaluating complex health care interventions that stress the importance of: (a) using the best evidence to design the intervention, (b) developing a theory or clear picture for how the different components of the intervention are expected to lead to desired outcomes, and (c) incorporating process evaluations to test and refine the intervention prior to a full-scale outcome evaluation (Craig et al., 2008). Steps 1 to 6 focus on establishing role structures and processes and developing an evaluation plan. This includes health care planning and decision making about the need for an APN role and to design multicomponents of the role to address identified gaps and to achieve expected outcomes. Step 7 focuses on role processes and initiating the implementation plan and introducing the APN role. Steps 8 and 9 include the short- and long-term evaluations of the APN role and the new model of

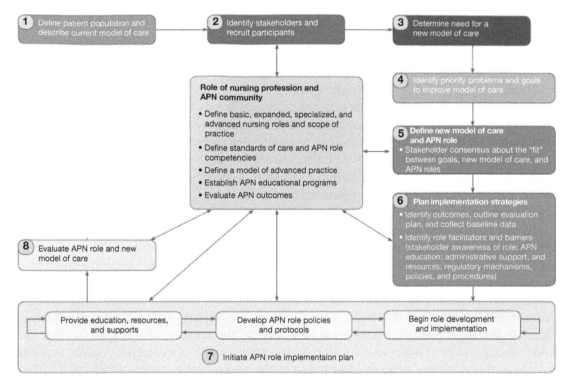

FIGURE 12.1 The PEPPA framework: A Participatory, Evidence-Based, Patient-focused Process for Advanced practice nursing role development, implementation, and evaluation. See color version at http://www.springerpub.com/kleinpell

APN, advanced practice nursing.

Source: Bryant-Lukosius and DiCenso (2004).

care in which it takes place in order to assess progress, refine the role, and promote role sustainability in achieving predetermined goals and outcomes.

Current Applications of the PEPPA Framework

A recent citation analysis examining the spread and use of the PEPPA framework found that it has been used in over 16 countries related to APN research, education, policies, and role development and evaluation (Boyko, Carter, & Bryant-Lukosius, 2016). Researchers and graduate students from non-Canadian universities were the predominant framework users. In several Canadian provinces, PEPPA is incorporated into the curricula of APN educational programs for NPs in primary, acute, and anesthesia care (Boyko et al., 2016; Donald, "The Ontario Primary Health Care Nurse Practitioner Program," 2008; University of Toronto, Lawrence S. Bloomberg Faculty of Nursing, 2008). The APN Chair Program also used the framework as the basis for the graduate nursing course "Research Issues in the Introduction and Evaluation of APN Roles" (McMaster University School of Nursing, Health Sciences Library, 2008). The framework has been used to inform the design of studies and systematic programs of research for APN roles in oncology (Bryant-Lukosius et al., 2007; Martelli-Reid et al., 2007; Slater, Rosenzweig, & Steele, 2009), primary health care (Martin-Misener, Reilly, & Vollman, 2010), and in long-term care (Donald, 2007; Donald et al., 2012; Kaasalainen, DiCenso, Donald, & Staples, 2007). Graduate students have used the PEPPA framework to guide their thesis research about APN roles and services for patients with inflammatory bowel disease (Westin, 2009) and those requiring psychiatric mental health care (Brady, 2010).

In Canada and in other countries, the framework has been recommended by nursing associations and ministries of health as a best practice for implementing APN roles (Boyko et al., 2016; CNA, 2008) as well as nursing roles and models of care involving interprofessional teams (Virani, 2012). The framework is being used by health authorities to introduce NP roles (Sawchenko, Fulton, Gamroth, & Bludeon, 2011) and to develop policies to support the successful implementation of NP and CNS roles (Advanced Practice Nursing Steering Committee, Winnipeg Regional Health Authority, 2012, 2016).

Several published studies and reports document the benefits and illustrate the applicability of the PEPPA framework for the successful implementation of APN roles in varied specialties and for other health provider roles such as: advanced physiotherapist roles for patients undergoing hip and knee replacement surgery (Robarts, Kennedy, MacLeod, Findlay, & Gollish, 2008); advanced radiation therapists in cancer care (Cancer Care Ontario, 2011); and physician assistants in emergency departments (Ducharme, Buckley, Alder, & Pelletier, 2009). In a long-term care setting, the framework's emphasis on stakeholder engagement in order to identify role priorities, establish a common vision, and participate in the planning process contributed to the successful implementation of a unique NP model of care (McAiney et al., 2008). The NPs were found to improve staff confidence and reduce hospital admission rates by 39% to 43% (McAiney et al., 2008). Application of the framework's steps was found to provide the structure for guiding the process and anticipating activities for introducing a new specialized NP in cardiac surgery (McNamara, Giguere, St. Louis, & Boileau, 2009). The PEPPA framework was also an effective change management tool for introducing NPs and physician assistants into the emergency department (Ducharme et al., 2009). Key framework strengths were team-building strategies to motivate and support change and the importance of conducting a needs assessment and environmental scan to identify and address barriers to role implementation. In a project to introduce advanced physiotherapist roles, the flexibility of the framework as a planning guide enabled the redesign process to be completed over a short period of time, fostered quick wins and early buy-in to the role, and led to a new model of care that matched patients' needs with providers with the most appropriate skill set (Robarts et al., 2008).

In a PAR study, we examined the impact of the PEPPA framework, a team facilitator, and a toolkit of resources specific to each step of the framework on the introduction of oncology APN roles for underserved patient populations (Bakker et al., 2009). Similar to other reports (Ducharme et al., 2009; McAiney et al., 2008; Robarts et al., 2008), the high level of team and stakeholder engagement at each step of the framework was important for promoting their support and acceptance of the new APN role. Team function and positive group dynamics also improved over time for implementation teams involved in the role-planning process. The implementation teams also noted that the framework enabled them to identify gaps in care delivery and to develop an APN role job description that was relevant to patient needs. The teams reported that a facilitator with experience in the introduction of APRNs was beneficial for moving the role-planning process along and for implementing the steps in a way that was relevant to their practice setting and patient population.

In this same study, a draft toolkit utilized and evaluated by the implementation teams was found to provide an "essential road map" for guiding the process and keeping the team on track. Varied resources, tools, and activities also aided in the collection of data and facilitated group decision making at each step of the framework. Real-time evaluation data and feedback collected from the implementation teams were used to refine and augment the final toolkit that is available free of charge in an electronic format (Bryant-Lukosius, 2009). One example of a toolkit strategy and resource is a logic model developed in Steps 4 to 6 of the framework. As Figure 12.2 shows, a logic model is very helpful for illustrating the complexity of the APN role and the relationship between role activities and outcomes. Another toolkit, based in part on the PEPPA framework, has also been developed by the Canadian NP Initiative (2006) to support health care planners and administrators with the introduction of NP roles, particularly in primary health care settings.

PEPPA-Plus—An Expanded Framework for APN Role Evaluation

While APN role evaluation is an important component of PEPPA, only three of the framework's nine steps offer broad rather than specific recommendations to facilitate evaluation. Recently, an international group of nurse researchers, educators, APRNs, and health care leaders from Switzerland, Germany, Canada, and the United States completed a project to enhance the PEPPA framework to provide more detailed guidance for designing and planning APN role evaluations (Bryant-Lukosius et al., 2016). The enhanced framework also incorporates strategies to overcome methodological limitations identified in previous APN role evaluations (Bryant-Lukosius, Carter, et al., 2015; Bryant-Lukosius, Cosby, Bakker, Earle, & Burkoski, 2015; Donald, Kilpatrick, Reid, Carter, Martin-Misener, et al., 2014). Dubbed "PEPPA-Plus" for short, the enhanced framework can be applied to inform APN role evaluations at national, regional, practice setting, and health care team levels. Specific evaluation objectives are outlined for three discrete stages of APN role development: introduction, implementation, and long-term sustainability. These objectives help framework users to identify information needs and evaluation questions relevant to different stages of APN role development from varied stakeholder perspectives. Several tools accompany the framework including examples of structure–process–outcome variables and evaluation questions for each stage of APN role development, an evaluation plan template, and a case study demonstrating application of the framework across the three stages.

APN RESEARCH DATA COLLECTION RESOURCES

The ability to monitor and evaluate the direct and indirect roles of APRNs is integral to the PEPPA framework. As previously described, evaluation measures typically quantify processes or outcomes during different stages of APN role development and implementation. The selection of evaluation measures is driven by a number of factors, including, but not limited to: (a) the research or evaluation questions, (b) the theoretical underpinnings or hypothesized effect of the intervention, (c) the availability of data or feasibility of collecting primary data, and (d) the intended user (e.g., decision maker or researcher).

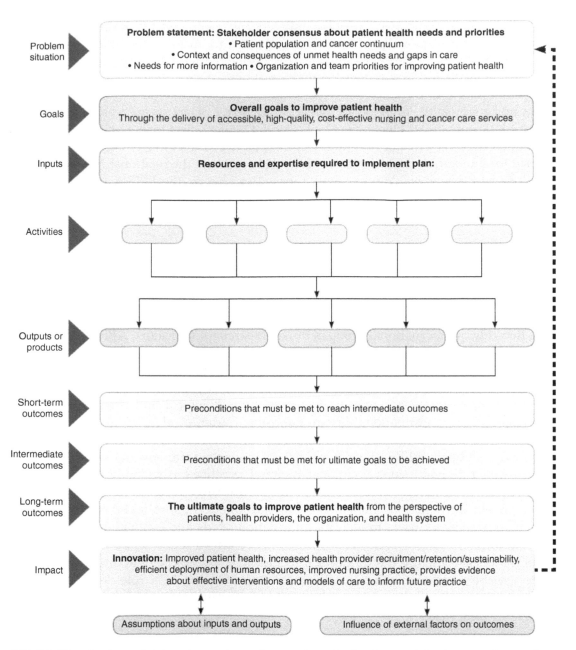

FIGURE 12.2 Logic model for advanced practice nursing role development, implementation, and evaluation. See color version at http://www.springerpub.com/kleinpell
Source: Bryant-Lukosius (2009).

Importantly, within APN-related research and evaluation, measures should be related to APN role activities. Data for objective measures are commonly obtained through the use of secondary data (e.g., administrative or medical record data), clinical assessment, or through patient-reported outcome measures (PROMs). The evaluation plan should be rigorous and strategic.

Many appropriate resources and data collection strategy and tools exist. For example, the Nursing Outcomes Classification (NOC) provides a standardized terminology for nursing-sensitive outcomes for use by nurses across specialties and settings (Moorehead, Johnson, Maas, & Swanson, 2013). These are typically simple Likert scale measures of the area of concern (e.g., mobility) and are relatively easy to collect. Additionally, particularly for research or evaluation at a population level, administrative or medical record data may be used (Tranmer, Edge, Sears, VanDenKerkhof, & Levesque, 2015). Often, the difficulty with secondary data is the ability to link APN role activities to a change in outcomes. The most common evaluation measure used in APN research or evaluation is the use of PROMs. PROMs are psychometric valid measurement instruments completed by the patient or caregiver to obtain information about health status or behaviors. Many PROM instruments are categorized as generic (e.g., 36-Item Short Form [SF-36] health-related quality of life [HRQL]) or condition-specific (assess characteristics particular to a condition). The selection of the most appropriate PROM is difficult; one is encouraged to utilize measures used in previous APN research to facilitate generalizability and comparisons. To facilitate APN-related research, the APN Research Data Collection Toolkit was developed and is accessible via the CCAPNR website (apntoolkit.mcmaster.ca). The objective of the toolkit is to identify instruments that could be used to facilitate data collection for monitoring and measuring a variety of variables relevant to different stages of APN role development. Focused on APN, the toolkit includes instruments that have been used in research related to CNSs as well as to primary and acute care NPs. The toolkit is an ongoing initiative to create a compendium of common instruments used in APN research. It was developed with the following users in mind: APN researchers, graduate students planning APN research, and decision makers who are seeking to evaluate one or more dimensions of APN roles (e.g., structures, processes, outcomes).

The instruments are organized according to the steps of the PEPPA framework, so that users of the website can link the instruments with the distinct steps described in this framework (e.g., needs assessment, describing the model of care, defining the APN role, role implementation, barriers to and facilitators of APN integration, outcome evaluation). The summary developed for each instrument is sent to the instrument developer, who is asked to review it for accuracy. An example of an instrument summary is found in Exhibit 12.4. The APN toolkit is an ever-growing resource that currently houses summaries of over 100 instruments. This toolkit will be an important resource for those introducing and evaluating APN roles by making available existing instruments that have been used, for example, to conduct needs assessments, measure practice patterns, identify barriers and facilitators, and evaluate provider and patient outcomes related to APN.

SUMMARY

The establishment of a nationally funded APN research chair has facilitated the training of the next generation of Canadian nurse researchers who continue to expand knowledge about the effective development and deployment of APN roles to achieve desired patient, provider, and health system outcomes. Initially through the chair in APN and now CCAPNR, APN researchers, educators, health providers, and decision makers have access to critically appraised tools for conducting APN-related research. As a relatively

EXHIBIT 12.4 An Example of an APN-Related Data Collection Tool as Summarized in the APN Data Collection Toolkit

---

Misener Nurse Practitioner Job Satisfaction Scale (MNPJSS)

Original Citation—Misener, T. R., & Cox, D. L. (2001). Development of the Misener nurse practitioner job satisfaction scale. *Journal of Nursing Measurement, 9*(1), 91–108.

Contact Information
De Anna L. Cox
College of Nursing
University of South Carolina
Columbia, SC 29208, USA
Phone: 803-777-4390
dlcox@gwm.sc.edu

Price and Availability—Published in original citation. Contact author for permission to use.

Brief Description of Instrument—Assessment of job satisfaction of primary care NPs.
Scale Format—Forty-four items each measured using a 6-point Likert scale. Response options: "Very Satisfied" 6; "Satisfied" 5; "Minimally Satisfied" 4; "Minimally Dissatisfied" 3; "Dissatisfied" 2; "Very Dissatisfied" 1 point. One item for global satisfaction measured on a 10-point scale, 10 being the highest level of job satisfaction.
Administration Technique—Self-administered questionnaire.
Scoring and Interpretation—Total score is obtained by summing all 44 items. Subscale score is obtained by summing the subscale items.
Factors and Norms—Six factors determined by factor analysis: (a) intrapractice partnership/collegiality, (b) challenge/autonomy, (c) professional, social, and community interaction, (d) professional growth, (e) time, and (f) benefits. Item mean (SD) reported in original citation.
Internal Consistency—Cronbach's alpha on entire scale: 0.96; Cronbach's alphas on subscales range from 0.79 to 0.94.
Content and Face Validity—Instrument development based on literature review, review of existing instruments, and input from numerous NP experts.
Strengths—Easy to administer and score; covers a wide variety of previously published factors associated with job satisfaction.
Limitations—Relies heavily on factor analysis results to justify subscale, lacking theoretical rationale.
Published APN Studies Using Instrument—See original citation.
PEPPA Framework Category—8.

APN, advanced practice nursing; NP, nurse practitioner; PEPPA, Participatory, Evidence-Based, Patient-Focused Process for Advanced Practice Nursing Role Development, Implementation, and Evaluation; SD, standard deviation.
Source: Misener and Cox (2001).

new resource, the PEPPA framework has demonstrated wide applicability for the introduction of advanced nursing and other health provider roles. The enhanced framework (PEPPA-Plus) is suitable for designing and evaluating the complex nature of APN roles and can be employed to inform APN curricula and health care policies in support of APN, establish systematic approaches for role evaluation, and develop APN-focused programs of research.

Answers to Chapter Discussion Questions

1. Like APN roles, complex health care interventions are those that have a number of interacting components, address difficult health care problems or behaviors, target a number of groups or organizations, aim to improve several or variable outcomes, and are flexible or tailored to specific health care contexts (Craig et al., 2008).

2. Common barriers to conducting APN role evaluations that provide meaningful results about role outcomes include: lack of APN research expertise, failure to utilize relevant

theoretical frameworks and rigorous research methods in designing the role and role evaluation plan, lack of clearly defined roles with predetermined outcomes that are linked with APN role activities, lack of baseline data to permit future comparative evaluations, and the use of outcome measures not sensitive to APN role activities (Bryant-Lukosius et al., 2004; DiCenso et al., 2010).

3. Key principles of PAR include: active participation in cycles of reflection and action; valuing what people know and believe by building on their current understanding; collective investigation, analysis, learning, and the conscious production of new knowledge; collective decision making and action in using new knowledge to address problems; and evaluating the impact of these actions (Bowling, 1997; Deshler & Ewert, 1995; Smith, 1997). These principles promote the generation and use of objective data critical for health care planning and introduction of new roles. APN practitioners work collaboratively within interprofessional teams and in established relationships with other stakeholders in the health system. These relationships create the conditions that influence the effective delivery of health care services and can facilitate or obstruct the implementation of APN roles. Therefore, collective learning and consensus decision making in the health planning process are necessary for the effective implementation of APN roles.

4. "Structures" are factors that affect processes or determine how the APN role is implemented (e.g., APN education, patient population, nursing and health care policies). "Process" refers to what the APRN does in the role (e.g., types of APN services and how these services are provided). "Outcomes" are the results of APN role services and care and thus are affected by both structure and process factors (e.g., improved patient quality of life, reduced physician workload, reduction in wait times). The PEPPA framework proposes that the role structures, processes, and outcomes and their relationships within the context of the model of care and organizational environment should be determined during the early stages of role development and evaluated throughout the role implementation journey.

REFERENCES

Advanced Practice Nursing Steering Committee, Winnipeg Regional Health Authority. (2012). A guide for successful integration of a clinical nurse specialist. Retrieved from http://www.wrha .mb.ca/nursing/files/CNS-Toolkit.pdf

Advanced Practice Nursing Steering Committee, Winnipeg Regional Health Authority. (2016). A guide for the successful integration of a nurse practitioner. Retrieved from http://www .wrha.mb.ca/nursing/files/NP-Toolkit.pdf

Advisory Committee on Health Delivery and Human Resources. (2007). *A framework for collaborative pan-Canadian health human resources planning.* Ottawa, ON, Canada: Author.

Bakker, D., Bryant-Lukosius, D., Wiernikowski, J., Conlon, M., Baxter, P., Green, E., . . . DiCenso, A. (2009). *Enhancing knowledge, promoting quality: Evaluating the implementation of oncology APN roles* (Oral presentation). Paper presented at International Conference on Cancer Nursing, Atlanta, Georgia.

Bowling, A. (1997). *Research methods in health: Investigating health and health services.* Philadelphia, PA: Open University Press.

Boyko, J., Carter, N., & Bryant-Lukosius, D. (2016). Assessing the spread and uptake of framework for introducing and evaluating advanced practice nursing roles. *Worldviews on Evidence-Based Nursing, 13*(4), 277–284. doi:10.1111/wvn.12160

Brady, R. L. (2010). *Introducing a new psychiatric mental health nurse practitioner role in a mental health agency* (Master's thesis). Retrieved from ProQuest Dissertations and Theses Database (UMI No. 1475129).

Bryant-Lukosius, D. (2009). *Designing innovative cancer services and advanced practice nursing roles: Toolkit.* Toronto: Cancer Care Ontario. Retrieved from https://www.cancercare.on.ca/cms/one .aspx?pageId=9387

Bryant-Lukosius, D., & DiCenso, A. (2004). A framework for the introduction and evaluation of advanced practice nursing roles. *Journal of Advanced Nursing, 48*, 530–540.

Bryant-Lukosius, D., Carter, N., Reid, K., Donald, F., Martin-Misener, R., Kilpatrick, K., . . . DiCenso, A. (2015). The effectiveness and cost effectiveness of clinical nurse specialist-led hospital to home transitional care: A systematic review. *Journal of Evaluation of Clinical Practice, 21*, 763–781. doi:10.1111/jep.12401

Bryant-Lukosius, D., Cosby, R., Bakker, D., Earle, C., & Burkoski, V. (2015). *Practice guideline on the effective use of advanced practice nurses in the delivery of adult cancer services in Ontario.* Toronto: Cancer Care Ontario. Retrieved from https://www.cancercare.on.ca/common/pages/UserFile .aspx?fileId=340702

Bryant-Lukosius, D., DiCenso, A., Browne, G., & Pinelli, J. (2004). Advanced practice nursing roles: Issues affecting role development, implementation, and evaluation. *Journal of Advanced Nursing, 48*, 519–529.

Bryant-Lukosius, D., Green, E., Fitch, M., Macartney, G., Robb-Blenderman, L., McFarlane, S., . . . Milne, H. (2007). A survey of oncology advanced practice nurses in Ontario: Profile and predictors of job satisfaction. *Canadian Journal of Nursing Leadership, 20*(2), 50–68.

Bryant-Lukosius, D., Spichiger, E., Martin, J., Stoll, H., Degen Kellerhals, S., Fliedner, M., . . . De Geest, S. (2016). Framework for evaluating the impact of advanced practice nursing roles. *Journal of Nursing Scholarship, 48*(2), 201–209.

Burns, S. M. (2001). Selecting advanced practice nurse outcome measures. In R. M. Kleinpell (Ed.), *Outcome assessment in advanced practice nursing* (1st ed., pp. 73–90). New York, NY: Springer Publishing.

Byers, J., & Brunell, M. (1998). Demonstrating the value of the advanced practice nurse: An evaluation model. *AACN Clinical Issues, 9*, 296–305.

Canadian Agency for Drugs and Technologies in Health. (2006). *Guidelines for the economic evaluation of health technologies: Canada* (3rd ed.). Ottawa, ON, Canada: Author. Retrieved from https:// www.cadth.ca/media/pdf/186_EconomicGuidelines_e.pdf

Canadian Association of Nurses in Oncology. (2001). *Standards of care, roles in oncology nursing, role competencies.* Kanata, ON, Canada: Author.

Canadian Nurse Practitioner Initiative. (2006). *Implementation and evaluation toolkit for nurse practitioners in Canada.* Ottawa, ON, Canada: Canadian Nurse Association. Retrieved from https:// nurseone.ca/~/media/nurseone/files/en/toolkit_implementation_evaluation_np_e.pdf?la=en

Canadian Nurses Association. (2008). *Advanced nursing practice: A national framework.* Ottawa, ON, Canada: Author.

Cancer Care Ontario. (2011). *Clinical specialist radiation therapist implementation sustainability project: Toolkit.* Toronto, ON, Canada: Author. Retrieved from https://www.cancercare.on.ca/common/pages/UserFile.aspx?fileId=119464

Carter, N., Sangster-Gormley, E., Ploeg, J., Martin-Misener, R., Donald, F., Wickson-Griffiths, A., . . . Schindel Martin, L. (2016). An assessment of how nurse practitioners create access to primary care in Canadian residential long-term care settings. *Canadian Journal of Nursing Leadership, 29*(2), 45–63.

Chiou, C. F., Hay, J. W., Wallace, J. F., Bloom, B. S., Neumann, P. J., Sullivan, S. D., . . . Ofman, J. J. (2003). Development and validation of a grading system for the quality of cost-effectiveness studies. *Medical Care, 41*(1), 32–44.

Craig, P., Dieppe, P., Macintyre, S., Michie, S., Nazareth, I., & Petticrew, M. (2008). Developing and evaluating complex interventions: The new Medical Research Council guidance. *British Medical Journal, 337*, a1655. doi:10.1136/bmj.a1655

Davies, B., & Hughes, A. M. (2002). Clarification of advanced nursing practice: Characteristics and competencies. *Clinical Nurse Specialist, 16*, 147–152.

Deshler, D., & Ewert, M. (1995). Participatory action research: Traditions and major assumptions. Retrieved from www.oac.uoguelph.ca/~pi/pdrc/articles/article.1

DiCenso, A., & Bryant-Lukosius, D. (2010). *Clinical nurse specialists and nurse practitioners in Canada: A decision support synthesis.* Ottawa, ON: Canadian Health Services Research Foundation. Retrieved from http://www.cfhi-fcass.ca/PublicationsAndResources/ResearchReports/CommissionedResearch/10-06-01/b9cb9576-6140-4954-aa57-2b81c1350936.aspx

DiCenso, A., Bryant-Lukosius, D., Martin-Misener, R., Donald, F., Carter, N., Bourgeault, I., . . . Kioke, S. (2010). Factors enabling advanced practice nursing role integration. *Canadian Journal of Nursing Leadership, 23*, 211–238.

Donabedian, A. (1966). Evaluating the quality of medical care. *Milbank Memorial Quarterly, 44*, 166–203.

Donabedian, A. (1992). Commentary: The role of outcomes in quality assessment and assurance. *Quality Review Bulletin,* 356–360.

Donald, F. (2007). *Collaborative practice by nurse practitioners and physicians in long-term care homes: A mixed method study* (Unpublished doctoral thesis). McMaster University, Hamilton, ON, Canada.

Donald, F., Kilpatrick, K., Reid, K., Carter, N., Bryant-Lukosius, D., Martin-Misener, R., . . . DiCenso A. (2014). Hospital to community transitional care by nurse practitioners: A systematic review of cost-effectiveness. *International Journal of Nursing Studies, 52*, 436–451.

Donald, F., Kilpatrick, K., Reid, K., Carter, N., Martin-Misener, R., Bryant-Lukosius, D., . . . DiCenso, A. (2014). A systematic review of the cost-effectiveness of nurse practitioners and clinical nurse specialists: What is the quality of the evidence? *Nursing Research & Practice, 2014*, 896587. doi:10.1155/2014/896587

Donald, F., Martin-Misener, R., Carter, N., Donald, E. E., Kaasalainen, S., Wickson-Griffiths, A., . . . DiCenso, A. (2013). A systematic review of the effectiveness of advanced practice nurses in long-term care. *Journal of Advanced Nursing, 69*(10), 2148–2161.

Donald, F., Martin-Misener, R., Carter, N., McAiney, C., Kaasalainen, S., Ploeg, J., . . . Dobbins, M. (2012). *The nurse practitioner role in Canadian long-term care settings: A mixed-methods study.* Paper presented at 7th International Council of Nurses International Nurse Practitioner/Advanced Practice Nursing Network (INP/APNN) Conference, London, UK.

Drummond, M. F., Schulpher, M. J., Claxton, K., Stoddart, G. L., & Torrance, G. W. (2015). *Methods for the economic evaluation of health care programmes* (4th ed.). Oxford, UK: Oxford University Press.

Ducharme, J., Buckley, J., Alder, R., & Pelletier, C. (2009). The application of change management principles to facilitate the introduction of nurse practitioners and physician assistants into six Ontario emergency departments. *Healthcare Quarterly, 12*(2), 70–77.

Dunn, K., & Nicklin, W. (1995). The status of advanced nursing roles in Canadian teaching hospitals. *Canadian Journal of Nursing Administration*, 111–135.

Foote Whyte, W. (1991). *Participatory action research*. London, UK: Sage.

Grimes, D. E., & Garcia, M. K. (1997). Advanced practice nursing and work site primary care: Challenges for outcomes evaluation. *Advanced Practice Nurse Quarterly, 3*, 19–28.

Harbman, P., Bryant-Lukosius, D., Martin-Misener, R., Carter, N., Covell, C, Donald, F., . . . Valaitis, R. (2017). Partners in research: Building academic-practice partnerships to education and mentor advanced practice nurses. *Journal of Evaluation in Clinical Practice, 23*, 382–390. doi:10.1111/jep.12630

Kaasalainen, S., DiCenso, A., Donald, F., & Staples, E. (2007). Optimizing the role of the nurse practitioner to improve pain management in long-term care. *Canadian Journal of Nursing Research, 39*(2), 14–31.

Kaasalainen, S., Ploeg, J., McAiney, C., Schindel Martin, L., Donald, L., Martin-Misener, R., . . . Sangster-Gormley, E. (2013). Role of the nurse practitioner in providing palliative care in long term care homes. *International Journal of Palliative Nursing, 19*(10), 477–485.

Kilpatrick, K., Kaasalainen, S., Donald, F., Reid, K., Carter, N., Bryant-Lukosius, D., . . . DiCenso, A. (2014). The effectiveness and cost-effectiveness of clinical nurse specialists in outpatient roles: A systematic review. *Journal of Evaluation in Clinical Practice, 20*(6), 1106–1123. doi:10.1111/jep.12219

Kilpatrick, K., Reid, K., Carter, N., Donald, F., Bryant-Lukosius, D., Martin-Misener, R., . . . DiCenso, A. (2015). A systematic review of the cost effectiveness of clinical nurse specialists and nurse practitioners in inpatient roles. *Canadian Journal of Nursing Leadership, 28*(3), 56–76.

Lopatina, E., Donald, F., DiCenso, A., Martin-Misener, R., Kilpatrick, K., Bryant-Lukosius, D., . . . Marshall, D. A. (2017). Discussion paper: Considerations in the economic evaluation of advanced practice nursing roles. *International Journal of Nursing Studies*. doi.org/10.1016/j.ijnurstu.2017.04.012

Marshall, D. A., Donald, F., Lacny, S., Reid, K., Bryant-Lukosius, D., Carter, N., . . . DiCenso, A. (2015). Assessing the quality of economic evaluations of clinical nurse specialists and nurse practitioners: A systematic review of cost-effectiveness. *NursingPlus Open, 1*, 11–17.

Martelli-Reid, L., Bryant-Lukosius, D., Arnold, A., Ellis, P., Goffin, J., Okawara, G., . . . Hapke, S. (2007). *A model of interprofessional research to support the development of an advanced practice nursing role in cancer care*. Poster presentation at the Canadian Association of Nurses in Oncology Conference, Vancouver, BC, Canada.

Martin-Misener, R., Donald, F., Wickson-Griffiths, A., Akhtar-Danesh, N., Ploeg, J., Brazil, K., . . . Taniguchi, A. (2015). A mixed methods study of the work patterns of full-time nurse practitioners in Canadian nursing homes. *Journal of Clinical Nursing, 24*(9–10), 1327–1337. doi:10.1111/jocn.12741

Martin-Misener, R., Harbman, P., Donald, F., Reid, K., Kilpatrick K., Carter, D., . . . DiCenso, A. (2015). Cost-effectiveness of nurse practitioners in primary and specialized ambulatory care: A systematic review. *BMJ Open, 5*(6), e007167. doi:10.1136/bmjopen-2014-007167

Martin-Misener, R., Reilly, S. M., & Vollman, A. R. (2010). Defining the role of primary health care nurse practitioners in rural Nova Scotia. *Canadian Journal of Nursing Research, 42*(2), 30–47.

McAiney, C. A., Haughton, D., Jennings, J., Farr, D., Hillier, L., & Morden, P. (2008). A unique practice model for nurse practitioners in long-term care homes. *Journal of Advanced Nursing, 62,* 562–571.

McMaster University School of Nursing, Health Sciences Library. (2008). *Finding resources for Nursing 706: Research issues in the introduction and evaluation of advanced practice nursing roles.* Hamilton, ON: McMaster University.

McNamara, S., Giguere, V., St. Louis, L., & Boileau, J. (2009). Development and implementation of the specialized nurse practitioner role: Use of the PEPPA framework to achieve success. *Nursing and Health Sciences, 11,* 318–325.

Minnick, A. (2001). General design and implementation challenges in outcomes assessment. In R. M. Kleinpell (Ed.), *Outcome assessment in advanced practice nursing* (1st ed., pp. 91–102). New York, NY: Springer Publishing.

Misener, T. R., & Cox, D. L. (2001). Development of the Misener nurse practitioner job satisfaction scale. *Journal of Nursing Measurement, 9*(1), 91–108.

Mitchell-DiCenso, A., Pinelli, J., & Southwell, D. (1996). Introduction and evaluation of an advanced nursing practice role in neonatal intensive care. In K. Kelly (Ed.). *Outcomes of effective management practice* (pp. 171–186). Thousand Oaks, CA: Sage.

Moorehead, S., Johnson, M., Maas, M., & Swanson, E. (Eds.). (2013). *Nursing outcomes classification (NOC): Measurement of health outcomes* (5th ed.). St. Louis, MO: Elsevier.

Morrilla-Herrera, J. C., Gracia-Mayor, S., Martın-Santos, F. J., Uttumchandani, S. K., Campos, A. L., Bautista, J. C., & Morales-Ascendio, J. M. (2016). A systematic review of the effectiveness and roles of advanced practice nursing in older people. *International Journal of Nursing Studies, 53,* 290–307.

Naylor, M. D., Aiken, L. H., Kurtzman, E. T., Olds, D. M., & Hirschman, K. B. (2011). The care span: The importance of transitional care in achieving health reform. *Health Affairs, 30*(4), 746–754. doi:10.1377/hlthaff.2011.0041

Newhouse, R. P., Stanik-Hutt, J., White, K. M., Johantgen, M., Bass, E. B., Zangaro, G., . . . Weiner, J. P. (2011). Advanced practice nurse outcomes 1990–2008: A systematic review. *Nursing Economics, 29*(5), 230–250.

O'Brien-Pallas, L., Tomblin Murphy, G., Baumann, A., & Birch, S. (2001). Framework for analyzing health human resources. In *Future development of information to support the management of nursing resources: Recommendations.* Ottawa, ON, Canada: Canadian Institute for Health Information.

Ploeg, J., Kaasalainen, S., McAiney, C., Martin-Misener, R., Donald, F., Wickson-Griffiths, A., . . . Taniguchi, A. (2013). Resident and family perceptions of the nurse practitioner role in long-term care settings: A qualitative descriptive study. *BMC Nursing, 12*(24), 1–11.

Robarts, S., Kennedy, D., MacLeod, A. M., Findlay, H., & Gollish, J. (2008). A framework for the development and implementation of an advanced practice role for physiotherapists that improves access and quality care for patients. *Healthcare Quarterly, 11*(2), 67–75.

Sangster-Gormley, E., Carter, N., Donald, F., Martin-Misener, R., Ploeg, J., Kaasalainen, S., . . . Wickson-Griffiths, A. (2013). A value-added benefit of nurse practitioners in long-term care settings: Increased nursing staff's ability to care for residents. *Canadian Journal of Nursing Leadership, 26*(3), 24–37. doi:10.12927/cjnl.2013.23552

Sawchenko, L., Fulton, T., Gamroth, L., & Bludeon, C. (2011). Awareness and acceptance of the nurse practitioner role in one BC health authority. *Canadian Journal of Nursing Leadership, 24*(4), 101–111.

Sidani, S., & Irvine, D. (1999). A conceptual framework for evaluating the nurse practitioner role in acute care settings. *Journal of Advanced Nursing, 30*(1), 58–66.

Slater, A., Rosenzweig, M., & Steele, C. (2009). Workflow analysis in one community oncology outpatient setting: Advanced practice nurse versus physicians. Online Oncology Nursing Society 34th Annual Congress Podium and Poster Abstracts. *Oncology Nursing Forum, 36*(3), 33.

Smith, S. E. (1997). Deepening participatory action-research. In S. E. Smith & D. G. Willms (Eds.), *Nurtured by knowledge: Learning to do participatory action-research* (pp. 173–264). New York, NY: Apex Press.

Smith, S. E., Pyrch, T., & Lizardi, A. (1993). Participatory action-research for health. *World Health Forum, 14*, 319–324.

Spitzer, W. O. (1978). Evidence that justifies the introduction of new health professionals. In P. Slayton & M. J. Trebilcock (Eds.), *The professions and public policy* (pp. 211–236). Toronto, ON, Canada: University of Toronto Press.

Swan, M., Ferguson, S., Change, A., Larson, E., & Smaldone, E. (2015). Quality of primary care by advanced practice nurses: A systematic review. *International Journal of Quality in Health Care, 27*(5), 396–404.

Tranmer, J., Edge, D., Sears, K., VanDenKerkhof, E., & Levesque, L. (2015). A retrospective cohort study of the prescribing trends of nurse practitioners to older adults in Ontario: 2000–2010. *Canadian Medical Association Journal* (open), *3*(3), E299–E304.

University of Toronto, Lawrence S. Bloomberg Faculty of Nursing. (2008). *Nurse Practitioner in Anesthesia Care Program. Course outlines.* Toronto, ON, Canada: Author.

Virani, T. (2012). *Interprofessional collaborative teams.* A Commissioned Report for the Canadian Nurses Association and published by the Canadian Health Services Research Foundation. Retrieved from http://www.chsrf.ca/Libraries/Commissioned_Research_Reports/Virani-Interprofessional-EN.sflb.ashx

Westin, L. (2009). *Advanced nursing practice in nurse-led inflammatory bowel disease support service* (Master's thesis). Retrieved from https://dspace.library.uvic.ca:8443//handle/1828/4120

Index

AABC. *See* American Association of Birth Centers

AACN. *See* American Association of Colleges of Nursing

AANA. *See* American Association of Nurse Anesthetists

AANAF. *See* American Association of Nurse Anesthetists Foundation

academic education, 241

accountable care organizations (ACOs), 213

ACNP. *See* acute care nurse practitioner

ACOs. *See* accountable care organizations

acute care nurse practitioner (ACNP), 47, 53

acute coronary syndrome, 97

acute or critical care clinical nurse specialist, 47–49

advanced practice nursing (APN)
  cardiovascular, 88–134. *See also* outcome measures
  economic evaluation, 20–33
  locating instruments and measures, 69–80
  outcome measures, 45–56
  research outcomes, 250–265

advanced practice registered nurse (APRN)
  capturing impact, 2–4
  Choosing Wisely initiative, 13–14
  outcome metrics, 3–4
  overview of, 1–2
  quality metrics, 4–14

Agency for Healthcare Research and Quality (AHRQ), 78

aggregate data, 55–56

AHRQ. *See* Agency for Healthcare Research and Quality

ambulatory nurse practitioner outcomes
  behavioral activities and knowledge, 147
  case examples
    shotgun approach, 150–151
    triangulation, 151–152
  functional status, 147
  overview of, 144
  patient perception, 148
  physiologic status, 147
  psychosocial status, 147
  resource utilization, 148
  symptom control, 148

American Association of Birth Centers (AABC), 190

American Association of Colleges of Nursing (AACN), 216

American Association of Nurse Anesthetists (AANA), 208, 213, 215, 219

American Association of Nurse Anesthetists Foundation (AANAF), 209, 215

American Board of Internal Medicine Foundation, 13–14

American Nurses Association, 77

American Society of Anesthesiologists (ASA), 209

analytic issues, outcome assessment (OA) design, 64–65

APN. *See* advanced practice nursing

APRN. *See* advanced practice registered nurse

APRN-directed pain management intervention, 50–51

APRN-role-sensitive outcome measures, 46–47
ASA. *See* American Society of
    Anesthesiologists

benchmarking, 91, 190
bias, 104
bibliographic databases, 73
birth logs, 196
BLS. *See* Bureau of Labor Statistics
Bureau of Labor Statistics (BLS), 31
Buros Institute of Mental Measurement
    Mental Measurements Yearbooks, 71–72
    Tests in Print, 72

Canadian Centre for APN Research
    (CCAPNR)
    conducting point-of-care research, 254
    economic evaluations, 254–256
    five years of activities and influence, 252–254
    research areas, 253
cardiac risk factors, reduction of, 97
cardiovascular advanced practice nursing
    acute coronary syndrome, 97
    after coronary artery bypass graft, 98–99
    after percutaneous transluminal
        angioplasty/stent placement, 98
    heart failure, 97–98
    instruments and approaches, 99–100
    literature review, 116–120
    organizations' websites and quality
        measures, 100
    outcome methods
        advantages and disadvantages, 102–103
        case–control study design, 106
        cohort study design, 106
        correlation, 105
        descriptive research design, 105
        EBP, 109–110
        ex post facto design, 106–107
        mixed design methods, 108–109
        nonexperimental/observational designs,
            104–105
        qualitative research design, 107–108
        quality improvement, 110–113
        quasi-experimental design, 103–104
        randomized controlled trials, 101–103
        research utilization, 109–110

Patient Navigator Program
    outcome measures, description, and data
        source, 131–133
    overview of, 129–130
    risk model and interventions, 130–131
    project framework, goals, and criteria
        interventions for project development and
            implementation, 120–125
        limitations, 128
        outcomes identified, 125
        results before and after project
            implementation, 125–128
    reduction of cardiac risk factors, 97
    role of APRN, 113–116
Carolinas HealthCare System (CHS), 8–10
case–control study design, 106
cause and effect, outcome assessment (OA)
    design, 63–64
CBA. *See* cost–benefit analysis
CCA. *See* cost–consequence analysis
CEA. *See* cost-effectiveness analysis
certified registered nurse anesthetists
    (CRNAs), 208, 212–214
charge data analysis, 193
Children's Health Insurance Program
    (CHIP), 2
CHIP. *See* Children's Health Insurance
    Program
CHS. *See* Carolinas HealthCare System
client variance, 197
clinical nurse specialist (CNS)
    assessments of, 160
    educational outcomes, 178–179
    end-of-year report, 179–180
    framework for, 158
    hierarchical model. *See* hierarchical model
        of clinical nurse specialist
    nursing personnel sphere, 159
    organization/network sphere, 159
    patient/client sphere, 159
    project case example, 180–181
clinical outcome measures, 52–53, 88, 90–91
CMA. *See* cost-minimization analysis
CNS. *See* clinical nurse specialist
Cochrane databases, 74–75
Cochrane Library, 217
cognitive outcomes, 193
cohort study design, 106
comparative-effectiveness research, 20

confounding variable, 104
Consolidated Health Economic Evaluation
    Reporting Standards (CHEERS)
    checklist, 35–37
consumer price index (CPI), 31
corporate websites, 78
correlation method, 105
cost analysis, 193–194
cost–benefit analysis (CBA), 24–25
cost–consequence analysis (CCA), 22
cost-effectiveness analysis (CEA)
    checklist for Journal Report, 34–35
    decision tree, 23–24
    definition of, 23
cost-minimization analysis (CMA), 21–22
cost–utility analysis (CUA), 24
CPI. See consumer price index
CRNAs. See certified registered nurse
    anesthetists
CUA. See cost–utility analysis
Cumulative Index to Nursing and Allied
    Health (CINAHL) database, 70, 73

data sets, 198
descriptive correlation, 105
descriptive research design, 105
direct costs, 28
discharge summary, 198
discounting, 32
disease registration, 199
Dissertation Abstracts, 76
DNP. See Doctor of Nursing Practice
Doctor of Nursing Practice (DNP)
    competencies, 233–235
    individual, personal, and professional
        outcomes, 232–233
    overview of, 230–232
    recommendations for studies
        academic education, 241
        evidence-based practice, 240
        policy, 240
        quality and safety improvement, 240–241
    student projects, 235–239
Donabedian's model of quality health care, 112

EBP. See evidence-based practice
economic evaluation

CEA checklist, 34–35
CHEERS checklist, 35–37
cost–benefit analysis, 24–25
cost–consequence analysis, 22
cost-effectiveness analysis, 23–24
cost-minimization analysis, 21–22
cost–utility analysis, 24
steps in, 26
terminology in, 27
economic evaluation issues
    costs of resources, 28–32
    discounting, 32
    framing analysis, 25–28
    selecting type of, 25
    sensitivity analysis, 32–33
educational outcomes, 178–179
Education Resources Information Center
    (ERIC), 75
efficiency outcomes, 53–54
ERIC. See Education Resources Information
    Center
ethnography, 107
evidence-based clinical practice guidelines,
    199
evidence-based practice (EBP)
    components, 110
    Doctor of Nursing Practice, 240
    frameworks, 111
    nurse anesthesia, 215–218
    research utilization vs., 109–110
evidence pyramid, 220
ex post facto designs, 106–107

failure modes and effects analysis (FMEA),
    112
financial outcomes, 54
fiscal outcomes, 89, 193
FMEA. See failure modes and effects analysis
FNS. See Frontier Nursing Service
framing analysis, 25–28
friction costs, 28
Frontier Nursing Service (FNS), 188
functional outcomes, 89, 193
functional status, 147

Google, 76
Google Scholar, 76

government sites, locating instruments, 78–79
grounded theory, 107–108

HDI. *See* Human Development Index
Health and Psychosocial Instruments (HaPI), 73–74
Health Resources and Services Administration (HRSA), 78
heart failure, 97–98
Heart Failure Handbook, 120–121
Heart Failure Medication Management Patient Information, 122, 124
hierarchical model of clinical nurse specialist
  direct outcome measures
    interprofessional reflective practice utilizing case studies, 174–175
    overview of, 173–174
    proactively meeting Magnet standards, 175–178
  process measures
    reflective practice and process compliance, 169–170
    rounding tools, 166–168
    rounding with purpose, 165–166
  surrogate outcome measures
    cost in staff time, 171–173
    example of data use, 173
    nursing time cost in education, 173
    overview of, 170–171
  time-on activities
    calendar, 161–162
    peer review and visibility, 163, 165
    preformatted productivity spreadsheet, 162–163
    productivity report/organizational alignment, 162
Hinari, 71, 79
hospital benchmark data, 55–56
hospital of University of Pennsylvania, 7–8
HRSA. *See* Health Resources and Services Administration
Human Development Index (HDI), 202
human patient simulation, 210–211

ICER. *See* incremental cost-effectiveness ratio
incremental cost, 21
incremental cost-effectiveness ratio (ICER), 23
indirect costs, 28

Institute of Medicine (IOM), 1–2
international literature and databases, 71, 79
International Society of Pharmacoeconomics and Outcomes Research (ISPOR), 24
Internet resources, 71, 76
interprofessional reflective practice, 174–175
IOM. *See* Institute of Medicine
ISPOR. *See* International Society of Pharmacoeconomics and Outcomes Research

locating instruments and measures
  bibliographic databases, 73
  Cochrane databases, 74–75
  corporate websites, 78
  Dissertation Abstracts, 76
  ERIC, 75
  government sites, 78–79
  Health and Psychosocial Instruments, 73–74
  international literature and databases, 71, 79
  Internet resources, 71, 76
  levels of evidence, 73
  medical applications (apps), 77
  MEDLINE/PubMed, 74
  mobile/handheld devices, 77
  online library resources, 76
  open access to journals and institutional repositories, 79–80
  professional association sites, 77–78
  Proquest Dialog, 76
  PsycINFO, 75
  standard textbooks
    Mental Measurements Yearbooks, 71–72
    Tests in Print, 72
  University Library Websites, 76

MACRA. *See* Medicare Access and CHIP Reauthorization Act of 2015
medical applications (apps), 77
Medical Literature Analysis and Retrieval System Online (MEDLINE) database, 73–74
Medicare Access and CHIP Reauthorization Act of 2015 (MACRA), 2, 213
medication reconciliation
  definition of, 116–117
  monthly audit tool, 126
Memorial Sloan Kettering Cancer Center (MSKCC), 10–12

Mental Measurements Yearbooks (MMYBs), 71–72
metrics, 91. *See also* quality metrics
mixed design method, 108–109
MMYBs. *See* Mental Measurements Yearbooks
mobile/handheld devices, 77
MSKCC. *See* Memorial Sloan Kettering Cancer Center
multivariate sensitivity analysis, 33

National Guideline Clearinghouse, 78
national health information network (NHIN), 212
National Library of Medicine's databases, 74
National Organization of Nurse Practitioner Faculties, 146
National Patient Safety Goals for Hospitals, 53
National Quality Forum (NQF), 91
National Technical Information Service, 78–79
New England Journal of Medicine, 189
NHIN. *See* national health information network
NOAs. *See* nurse obstetric assistants
nonexperimental design, 104–105
NQF. *See* National Quality Forum
nurse anesthesia
  clinical outcomes, safety, and quality, 211–213
  competencies and curricular models, 218–220
  evidence-based practice, 215–220
  human patient simulation, 210–211
  outcome economics and policy developments, 220–221
  outcome measurement, 214–215
  outcome measures and projects, 215
  overview of, 208–209
  in rural settings, 213–214
  studies of, 209–210
nurse-midwifery practice
  benchmarking, 190
  charge data analysis, 193
  client outcome measures, 194–196
  cognitive outcomes, 193
  cost analysis, 193–194
  data-collection tools, 197–198
  data sources, 198–199
  fiscal outcomes, 193

functional outcomes, 193
  historical perspective, 188–190
  perceptual outcomes, 192–193
  physiological outcomes, 192
  psychosocial outcomes, 193
  purpose of outcome measurement, 191–192
  review of studies, 199–202
  scheduled measurements, 196–197
  Uniform Data Set, 190–191
  variance from expected outcomes, 197
nurse obstetric assistants (NOAs), 188–189
nurse-sensitive outcomes, 92
nursing outcomes, 92–93
nursing personnel sphere, 159

OA. *See* outcome assessment
observational design, 104–105
obstetric discharge summary, 198
Ongoing Professional Practice Evaluation (OPPE) process, 5
online library resources, 76
open access resources, 71, 79–80
opportunity costs, 30
optimal maternity care, 191
organizational competencies, 5
organization/network sphere, 159
outcome assessment (OA)
  clinical nurse specialists, 158–181
  design and implementation
    analytic issues, 64–65
    linking purpose and design, 60–61
    selecting outcomes, 61–63
    tracing cause and effect, 63–64
  nurse anesthesia, 208–221
outcome evaluation, 99
outcome indicators, 91
outcome management, 99
outcome measures
  in advanced practice nursing, 93–99
  aggregate data, 55–56
  clinical, 52–53, 88, 90–91
  Doctor of Nursing Practice, 229–241
  efficiency outcomes, 53–54
  financial outcomes, 54
  hospital benchmark data, 55–56
  nurse-midwifery practice, 188–202
  satisfaction, 49–52, 89
outcome research, 99–100
outcomes classification, 93

PAR. *See* participatory action research
participatory action research (PAR), 258
Participatory, Evidence-Based, Patient-Focused Process for Advanced (PEPPA) framework
    conceptual foundations, 258–259
    current applications, 260–262
    expanded framework, 262
    overview of, 256–258
    steps of, 259–260
Patient-Centered Outcomes Research Institute (PCORI), 20
patient/client sphere, 159
Patient Navigator Program (PNP)
    outcome measures, description, and data source, 131–133
    overview of, 129–130
    risk model and interventions, 130–131
patient outcomes, 90–91
patient perception, 148
Patient Protection and Affordable Care Act, 91
Patient-Reported Outcome and Quality of Life Instruments (ProQolid), 78
PCORI. *See* Patient-Centered Outcomes Research Institute
perceptual outcomes, 192–193
phenomenology, 107
physician quality reporting system (PQRS), 145–146, 213
physiological outcomes, 192
physiologic status, 147
PLAN. *See* plan–do–check–act
plan–do–check–act (PLAN), 112
PNP. *See* Patient Navigator Program
PQRS. *See* physician quality reporting system
practice-specific competencies, 5
practice-specific quality metrics, 13–14
predictive correlation, 105
preformatted productivity spreadsheet, 162–163
primary care outcome measurement
    literature of, 146
    overcoming potential barriers, 152–153
    practical outcomes, 149–150
    purpose/importance of, 144–146
proactively meeting Magnet standards, 175–178
probabilistic sensitivity analysis, 33
productivity costs, 29

productivity report/organizational alignment, 162
professional association sites, 77–78
program-specific data collection, 199
project implementation challenges, 65–67
"Project Re-Engineered Discharge," 118–119
ProQolid. *See* Patient-Reported Outcome and Quality of Life Instruments
Proquest Dialog, 76
provider variance, 197
PsycINFO, 75
psychosocial outcomes, 88–89, 193
psychosocial status, 147
PubMed, 74

QALY. *See* quality-adjusted life year
QI. *See* quality improvement
QSEN. *See* Quality and Safety Education for Nurses
qualitative research designs, 107–108
quality-adjusted life year (QALY), 24
Quality and Safety Education for Nurses (QSEN), 240–241
quality improvement (QI), 110–113
quality metrics
    Carolinas HealthCare System, 8–10
    Memorial Sloan Kettering Cancer Center, 10–12
    practice-specific, 13–14
    University of Pennsylvania hospital, 7–8
    Vanderbilt University Medical Center, 4–6
quality/safety metrics, 13
quasi-experimental designs, 103–104

Rand Corporation, 78
random error, 104–105
randomized controlled trials (RCTs), 101–103
rapid response team (RRT) metric methodology, 10–11
RCTs. *See* randomized controlled trials
REDCap. *See* Research Electronic Data Capture
Research Electronic Data Capture (REDCap), 14
research outcomes
    Canadian Centre
        conducting point-of-care research, 254
        economic evaluations, 254–256

five years of activities and influence, 252–254

Chair Program impact on building APN research capacity and expertise, 251–252

data collection resources, 262–264

PEPPA framework
  conceptual foundations, 258–259
  current applications, 260–262
  expanded framework, 262
  overview of, 256–258
  steps of, 259–260

research utilization method, 109–110

resource utilization, 148

risk, definition of, 195

role-specific competencies, 5

role-specific metrics, 13

root cause analysis, 112

rounding tools, 166–168

routinely collected administrative data, 198

sample patient medication list, 123

satisfaction, outcome measures, 49–52, 89

scholarly communication, 80

SCIP. *See* Surgical Care Improvement Project

sensitivity analysis, 32–33

shotgun approach, 150–151

Six Sigma, 112

Society for Simulation in Healthcare (SSiH), 210

SSiH. *See* Society for Simulation in Healthcare

Surgical Care Improvement Project (SCIP), 210–211

surrogate outcome measures
  cost in staff time, 171–173
  example of data use, 173
  nursing time cost in education, 173
  overview of, 170–171

Survey Monkey, 78

symptom control, 148

system variance, 197

Tests in Print (TIP), 72

time horizon, 28

time-saving outcomes, 53–54

TIP. *See* Tests in Print

total quality management and continuous quality improvement (Deming), 112

Toyota Lean, 112

traditional metrics, 13

transfer costs, 30

triangulation, 151–152

UDS. *See* Uniform Data Set

Uniform Data Set (UDS), 190–191

univariate sensitivity analysis, 33

University Library Websites, 76

Vanderbilt University Medical Center (VUMC), 4–6

variances, 197

VUMC. *See* Vanderbilt University Medical Center

Lightning Source UK Ltd.
Milton Keynes UK
UKHW031829190720
366807UK00004B/18